# Contrast Media in Radiology

## Appraisal and Prospects

First European Workshop – Proceedings – Lyon 1981

---

Edited by M. Amiel
With the Collaboration of J.F. Moreau

With 141 Figures

Springer-Verlag
Berlin Heidelberg New York 1982

Prof. Dr. Michel Amiel
Service de Radiologie
Hôpital Cardio-Vasculaire et
Pneumologique Louis Pradel
B.P. Lyon Montchat
F-69394 Lyon Cédex 3
France

Library of Congress Cataloging in Publication Data
Main entry under title: Contrast media in radiology.
Bibliography: p. Includes index.
1. Diagnosis, Radioscopic--Congresses. 2. Contrast media--Toxicology--Congresses. I. Amiel, M. (Michel), 1934– . II. Moreau, J.F. [DNLM: 1. Contrast media--Adverse effects. WN 160 C7646]
RC78.A1C66 1982 616.07'572 82-5866

ISBN-13: 978-3-540-11534-2 e-ISBN-13: 978-3-642-68584-2
DOI: 10.1007/978-3-642-68584-2



Typesetting: Schreibsatz Service Weihrauch, Würzburg

2127/3321-543210

# Opening Address

Presidents, Ladies and Gentlemen, Dear Colleagues,

I would like to welcome participants of this meeting to Lyon and to greet particularly the famous specialists, some of whom have come from far abroad to bring us their experience and to make their contribution to this workshop.

Why such a meeting in Lyon, 2 1/2 years after the one in Colorado Springs?

First it seemed an opportune time to look at today's progress on the numerous contrast media being used in laboratories, or already commercialized. During this meeting we have chosen to prefer studies of uroangiographic contrast media, or those intended to be used in new imaging systems.

Then it seemed both natural and desirable that Europe, rich in manufacturers of contrast media (Guerbet, Schering, Bracco, Nyegaard) and research teams working on this subject, should provide its contribution to the international scientific community. I hope that this meeting will present the opportunity to start fruitful scientific exchanges between us in Europe and our colleagues from North America, Japan, and Australia.

On the other hand, I wanted to give the officials of the French research councils the opportunity to understand the major contribution that contrast media provide in improving diagnostic imaging.

The present meeting should help to point out the still unknown efforts of some French teams who have oriented their research toward this field.

Finally I would like to thank particularly those who have helped and encouraged me in this undertaking:

Manufacturers of contrast media, mainly Guerbet (France) and Schering (France and West Germany), but also Wintrop (France), Bracco (Italy), Nyegaard (Norway), Lafayette (United States), and Berlex (United States),

Professor Tavernier, President of the French Association of University Radiologists,

Professor Mornex, Vice-President of the Medical Research Faculty in Lyon,

Professor Revillard, Director of the Medical Research Faculty in Lyon,
Professor Louisot, Member of Scientific Council of Inserm.

I proclaim the First European Workshop open and hope that it will be followed by many other meetings.

M. Amiel

# Preface

Journalists, always very direct and in search of sensation, essentially asked me two questions on the occasion of this workshop:
What were the goals of the meeting?
With the improvement of diagnosis through the development of image techniques, didn't the contrast media already have their future behind them?

Many answers were provided during the course of the workshop, and in order to best answer the journalists I proposed the following synopsis.

1. Since the 1979 Colorado Springs workshop organized by E. Lasser, progress has been so rapid and the newly available works so numerous that another meeting on an international level for the purpose of presenting and discussing these advances appeared indispensable. Why not then in Europe and why not in Lyon?

To expand on this progress, by 1981 the new contrast media with less-hyperosmolar molecules, still in the trial stage in 1979, were almost all available commercially for angiography, albeit at prohibitive prices. The advantages of these various media are becoming better known; moreover, in the wake of Lasser's work, our understanding of the pathophysiology of their noxious effects is also advancing rapidly owing to the use of models (for the target organs: heart, vessel wall, nervous system, kidney; and for the more general reactions: blood cells, coagulation, complement system, circulating enzymatic systems). In addition, further new molecules are currently being studied in research laboratories.

2. If ultrasound did not bring about any new notions concerning contrast media, the same cannot be said of X-ray digitalized imagery, which, be it scanner or conventional radiology, has increased the use of contrast media and been responsible for the evolution of a number of ideas on the subject. Thus we analyze the intravascular and extravascular phases of various contrast media, study the partition coefficients between the parenchyma and vessels of various organs, and utilize the physical properties of iodine (Kedge example) – all with a view to developing contrast media better adapted to and more specific for the different tissues studied and examinations employed.

The first European symposium also increased the ties between the scientific communities intensely interested in these "image making" drugs and stimulated them to meet regularly to exchange their ideas and results concerning this research topic so full of promise.

M. Amiel

# Contents

Opening Address . . . . . . . . . . . . . . . . . . . . . . . . . . . . . V

Preface . . . . . . . . . . . . . . . . . . . . . . . . . . . . . . . . . . VII

**Section A:**
**General Toxicity**

Contrast Material Reactors: Pathogenicity and Clinical Aspects in 1981 (E.C. Lasser) . . . . . . . . . . . . . . . . . . . . . . . . . . 3

Risk Factors for Adverse Reactions in Intravenous Urography (G. Ansell, Mck. Tweedie, C.R. West, and D.A. Price Evans) . . . 7

Prevention of Shocks Induced by Intravenous Urography (J.R. Michel) . . . . . . . . . . . . . . . . . . . . . . . . . . . . . . . . 11

Adverse Reactions to Intravenous Contrast Media in Urography – Results of a National Survey (A. Pinet, D. Lyonnet, P. Maillet, and J.M. Groleau) . . . . . . . . . . . . . . . . . . . . . . . . . . . 14

Allergy to Radiographic Contrast Media: Accumulated Evidence for Antibody-mediated Human Toxicity and a New Animal Model (R.C. Brasch, J. Kay, S. Mark, and D. Nitecki) . . . . . . . 16

Immunobiological Effects of Contrast Media with Special Reference to "Nonsequential Activation" of Complement (J.L. Touraine, A.M. Freyria, A. Pinet, P. Thevenin, and M. Amiel) 20

Contrast Media and Immediate Hypersensitivity (M.Ch. Plainfosse, J. Sainte-Laudy, D. Sirinelli, and P.H. Bor). . . . . . . . . . . . . . 25

Iodinated Contrast Agents: Effect on ATP: Creatine N-Phosphotransferase Isoenzymes in the Arterial Wall (J. Guidollet, O. Gateau, F. Borson, C. Canillot, O. Gourdol, J. Etienne, M. Amiel, and P. Louisot) . . . . . . . . . . . . . . . . . . . . . . . . . 28

The Effect of Radiographic Iodized Contrast Media on Coagulation, Fibrinolysis, and Complement System (B. Schulze and H.K. Beyer) . . . . . . . . . . . . . . . . . . . . . . . . . . . . . . . 31

In Vivo and in Vitro Modifications of Platelet Aggregation and Release of ATP by Ionic and Nonionic Contrast Media Used in Angiography (R. Eloy, J. Belleville, B. Cornillon, A.M. Freyria, M. Amiel, and A. Pinet) . . . . . . . . . . . . . . . . . . . . . . . . . . 40

Toxicity of New Contrast Media in Cell Cultures (M. Kormano and H. Frey) . . . . . . . . . . . . . . . . . . . . . . . . . . . . . . . . . 44

Effects of Contrast Media on Cell Cultures (D. Christmann and A. Wackenheim) . . . . . . . . . . . . . . . . . . . . . . . . . . . . . . 49

The Comparative Effect of Ionic and Nonionic Contrast Media on the Sickling Phenomenon (V.M. Rao, A.K. Rao, R.M. Steiner, E.R. Burka, R.G. Grainger, and S.K. Ballas) . . . . 52

Summary of the Discussion (J.F. Moreau) . . . . . . . . . . . . . . . 54

## Section B:
## Effect on the Heart

Considerations of Pathogenicity and Clinical Aspects of Contrast Media Toxicity on the Heart in 1981 (Ch.B. Higgins) 59

Effects on Cardiac Function of Contrast Media Used in Angiography: An Experimental Study (P. Besse, M. Sicart, S. Bonoron-Adele, L. Tariosse, Ph. D'Agatha, and G. Delorme) . . . . . . . . . 70

Comparison of Iopamidol, Ioxaglate, and Diatrizoate During Coronary Angiography in Dogs (C.A. Evill, G.T. Benness, and R. Hassam) . . . . . . . . . . . . . . . . . . . . . . . . . . . . . . . . . 76

Effects of Iohexol on Heart Functions During Coronary Arteriography in Dogs (B. Trägårdh and P. Lynch) . . . . . . . . . . . . . . 79

The Importance of Electrolyte Shifts and Calcium Binding on Cardiotoxicity of Contrast Media (G. Hellige, D. Baller, A. Hoeft, H. Korb, H.G. Wolpers, and J. Zipfel) . . . . . . . . . . . 80

Regional Myocardial Hemodynamic and Metabolic Effects of Ionic and Nonionic Contrast Media in the Normal and Ischemic State (Ch.B. Higgins and K.H. Gerber) . . . . . . . . . . . . . . . . . 84

Modifications in Coronary Flow After Injection of Contrast Media (M.E. Bertrand, M.R. Delforge, J.M. Lablanche, P.Y. Tilmant, and F.A. Thieuleux) . . . . . . . . . . . . . . . . . . . . 91

Changes in Left Ventricular Preload and Afterload Induced by Coronary Angiography: Influence of Contrast Medium Osmolality (H. Petitier, D. Crochet, P. Wanglin, J. de Laguerenne, and D. Krause) . . . . . . . . . . . . . . . . . . . . . . . . . . . . . . . . 92

Influence of Ioxaglix Acid on Hemoglobin Affinity During Selective Coronarography (M. Seurot, F. Volter, M. Paris, B. Teissere, A. Raynaud, V. Bismuth, and J.C. Gaux) ....... 98

The Use of Amipaque in Pediatric Angiocardiography (H.A. Baltaxe, P. Mooring, P. Hofschire, J. Kugler, W. Pinsky, and W. Chu) .................................. 101

Comparative Study in Small Infants of the Hemodynamic Effects of Ioxaglate and Diatrizoate Contrast Media in Left Ventriculography (V.H. de Villeneuve, M. Meradji, A. Penning, and A. van de Wiel) ................................ 104

A Comparison Between the New Low Osmolality Contrast Agent, Hexabrix, and a Conventional One (F.D.M. Haagen, M.L.F. Landsman, L.E.J.M. Schrijvers, and J.H. Pasteuning) ... 108

Summary of the Discussion ......................... 111

## Section C:
## Effects on the Nervous System

The Neurotoxicity of Water-soluble Contrast Media: Actual Concepts and Future (R.E. Gonsette) ................. 115

A Nonionic, Isotonic Dimer Iotrol: A New Contrast Medium for the Intrathecal Space. A Review of Pharmacological Evaluation (A. Sovak, R. Ranganathan, and C. Kerber) ...... 123

Excretion of Aqueous Contrast Media From the Subarachnoid Space of Primates (V.M. Haughton, O.P. Eldevik, E.A. Sasse, and B.T. Lipman) ............................... 129

Experimental Model of Neurotoxicity Study of Water-soluble Contrast Media (M. Gioux, P. Arne, J. Paty, and J.M. Caille) ... 134

Immediate and Delayed Neurotoxicity of Newly Synthesized Contrast Media Demonstrated by EEG Sequential Analysis (R.E. Gonsette) .............................. 141

The Effect of Myelographic Contrast Media on the Arachnoid (V.M. Haughton) ............................... 149

Comparative Experimental Study of Contrast Media in Neuroradiology (J. Cahn, M.G. Borzeix, R. Cahn, J.P. Akimjak, M. Labos, J. Angignard, and J.P. Brizard) ............... 154

Changes in the Cerebrospinal Fluid Pressure After Intrathecal Injection of Contrast Media in Rabbits (B. Carlborg, P. Maly, K. Golman, T. Almén, and C. Lindqvist) ................ 159

Adverse Effects From Contrast Media: Preliminary Results Obtained with an Experimental Model (U. Salvolini, U. Pasquini, A. Molinari, and P. Tirone) . . . . . . . . . . . . . . . . . . . . . . . . . 164

First Round Table: Concluding Remarks (R.E. Gonsette) . . . . . 169

The Stream of Metrizamide in the Subarachnoid Spaces in Relation to Adverse Effects of Cisternography (N. Kobayashi, Y. Saito, and T. Miyashita) . . . . . . . . . . . . . . . . . . . . . . . . . 170

Use of the New Hydrosoluble Contrast Materials (Metrizamide and Iopamidol) in Tomodensitometric Exploration of the Subarachnoid Spaces and Cisterns (C. Manelfe, A. Bonafe, and J. Prere) . . . . . . . . . . . . . . . . . . . . . . . . . . . . . . . . . 174

Adverse Reactions to Myelography with Metrizamide in Children (H. Petterson, Ch.R. Fitz, D.C.F. Harwood-Nash, S.H. Chuang, and E. Armstrong) . . . . . . . . . . . . . . . . . . . . . . . . . . . . 175

Iopamidol, a New Nonionic Contrast Medium for Myelography and Sacculoradiculography: A Review of 800 Cases (E. Signorini, E. Ciorba, and N. Caputo) . . . . . . . . . . . . . . . . 179

Ioglunide: A New Contrast Medium for Myelography and Cisternography (Animal Experiments and Preliminary Clinical Experience) (R.E. Gonsette and L. Liesenborgh) . . . . . . . . . . 182

Second Round Table: Discussion (J.M. Caille) . . . . . . . . . . . . 188

## Section D:
## Effects on the Kidney

Kidney: Pharmacology of Contrast Media (G.T. Benness) . . . . . 191

Nephrotoxicity of Uroangiographic Contrast Media (J.F. Moreau) 195

The Urinary Concentration of Urographic Radiocontrast Drugs: The Role of Sodium Chloride Excretion and Free-Water-Production (G.H. Mudge) . . . . . . . . . . . . . . . . . . . . . . . . . 201

Variations of Urinary Sodium Concentration After Contrast Media with Different Osmolality (J. Dupuy, J. Pengloan, P. Thienpont, J.L. Jourdan, H. Nivet, and Ph. Rouleau) . . . . . . 207

Nephrotoxicity of Iodinated Contrast Media: A Preliminary Report on Five Compounds Used for Urography (A. Pinet, C. Vincent, J.P. Revillard, N. Pozet, and J. Bertrand) . . . . . . . . 211

Acute Renal Failure Initiated by Contrast Media (K. Golman, Å. Aulie, C. Tørnquist, and T. Almén) . . . . . . . . . . . . . . . . 215

Summary of the Discussion (J.F. Moreau) . . . . . . . . . . . . . . . 218

## Section E:
## Various Topics


The Effect of X-ray Contrast Media on the Endothelium of the Aorta and Vena Cava in Rats (Ch. Gospos, N. Freudenberg, J. Staubesand, and H. Koch) . . . . . . . . . . . . . . . . . . . . . . . . 223

Rapid Injection of a Cold Water-soluble Triiodide for Cardiovascular Investigation. Physicochemical Basis, Injection Technique, Tolerance, Prospects of Utilization (M. Ducos de Lahitte, C. Manelfe, A. Bonafe, and J.P. Marc-Vergnes) . . . . . . . . . . . . . . . . . . . . . . . . . . . . . . . . . 227

Comparison of Hexabrix and Urografin in the Study of Post-phlebographic Thrombotic Side Effects (A. Hørup, B. Eliasen, A. Reimer-Jensen, and J. Praestholm) . . . . . . . . . . . . . . . . . 231

Effects of Contrast Material on Blood Volume (Y. Huet, E. Wirquin, H. Geschwind, and J. Loiret) . . . . . . . . . . . . . . . 233

Labeling of Embolizing Substances with Contrast Agents (D. Novak) . . . . . . . . . . . . . . . . . . . . . . . . . . . . . . . . . 237

Contrast Media in Arthrography. Experimental Study (G. Pallardy, R. Abelanet, G. Correas, B. Gerardin, and J.C. Zenny) . . . . . . . . . . . . . . . . . . . . . . . . . . . . . . . . . 241

Iodinated Compound and Thyroid Status (A. Piffanelli, P.B. Romelli, G. Giovannini, A. Caputo, R. Rossi, D. Pelizzola, L. Ricci, G. Camerini, and A. Toti) . . . . . . . . . . 244

Binding of Contrast Media to Human Prealbumin: Another Cause of Thyroid Hormonal Disorder (J. Mathieu, Y. Looze, M. Deconinck, and R. Potvliege). . . . . . . . . . . . . . . . . . . . . . 251

Summary of the Discussion (J.F. Moreau) . . . . . . . . . . . . . . 254


## Section F:
## Various Topics


Angiography in Lower Extremities with New Contrast Media: Review of Double-blind Studies (E. Zeitler, M. Georgi-Tönnesen, H.G. Hinski, H. Mader, and E.-I. Richter). . . . . . . . . . . . . . . . 257

Patient Reactions During Hexabrix, Iopamidol and Conray Angiography (R.G. Grainger) . . . . . . . . . . . . . . . . . . . . . 265

Experience of Cerebral Arteriography with Iopamidol: Clinical Data (P. Dettori) . . . . . . . . . . . . . . . . . . . . . . . . . . . . . . 269

Painless Angiography with Newer Contrast Media (K. Mathias, P. Billmann, and E. Schmiedel) . . . . . . . . . . . . . . . . . . . . . . 274

Hemodynamic Changes During Aortic Arch Angiography. A Comparative Study Using Two Contrast Media: Telebrix 30 (Ioxitalamate) and Hexabrix (Ioxaglate) (J.M. Caillé, A.M. Bidabé, P. Floras, and F. Guibert-Tranier) . . . . . . . . . . . 276

B 15 000: A Nonionic Contrast Medium in Peripheral Angiography (P. Falappa, M. Rossi, A.R. Cotroneo, F.M. Danza, and R.F. Baici) . . . . . . . . . . . . . . . . . . . . . . . . . . . . . . . . . . 279

First Part: Discussion (E. Zeitler) . . . . . . . . . . . . . . . . . . . . . . 280

Compared Effects on Various Blood Parameters of Iopamidol and Iodamide in Man During Infusion Urography (G. Cittadini, G.A. Gambaro, G.A. Rollandi, and F. Romanzi) . . . . . . . . . . . 281

Conventional Versus Low Osmolality Nonionic and Dimeric Intravenous Contrast Media: Noninvasive Evaluation of Hemodynamic Effects (P. Vock and W.A. Fuchs) . . . . . . . . . . . . . . 285

Comparative Study of the Effects of Two Contrast Media of Different Osmolarity on Pulmonary Hemodynamics and Lung Function (J.P. Senac, Ch. Prefaut, M. Adda, F.B. Michel, J. Lautrou, and V. Laporte). . . . . . . . . . . . . . . . . . . . . . . . . 288

Synergism of Radiographic Contrast Media and X-Irradiation (D. Carr, A.C. Walker, and R.G. White) . . . . . . . . . . . . . . . . . 291

Design and Synthesis of New Compounds for Hepatobiliary Imaging (C.A. Evill, M.J. Thompson, P. Habel, and G.T. Benness) 292

Comparative Double-blind Study of Three Different Oral Contrast Media in Cholecystography (D. Doyon, A. Spira, F. Kunstlinger, H. Farah, Ch. Sassoon, A. Roche, and B. Ducot) 295

Can We Improve Cholecystography? A Multiple Factor Experiment (G. Cittadini, S. Cantoni, G.A. Gambaro, and F. Romanzi) . . . . . . . . . . . . . . . . . . . . . . . . . . . . . . . . . 299

Choice of Radiologic Contrast Medium: The Medico-legal Point of View (D. Fierro and M. Canale) . . . . . . . . . . . . . . . . . . . . 302

## Section G: Contrast Media and CT

Optimal Contrast Media for CT: Ionic or Nonionic, Monomer or Dimer? (P.B. Dean) . . . . . . . . . . . . . . . . . . . . . . . . . . 307

The Value of Nonionic Contrast Media in CT (P. Rossi, S. D'Auria, P. Pavone, S. Minucci, L. Tipaldi, and K. McBride) 311

Comparison of Contrast Enhancement Pharmacokinetics of Contrast Media in Clinical Patients (M. Kormano, R.F. Spataro, S. Soimakallio, and M. Wiljasalo) . . . . . . . . . . . . . . . . . . . . . 314

Contrast Materials and the Liver: Application to Scanography X (J.L. Lamarque, J.M. Bruel, J.P. Rouanet, X. Triby, P. Lopez, and F. Jauvion). . . . . . . . . . . . . . . . . . . . . . . . . . . . . . . . 319

Water-soluble Contrast Agents for Computed Tomography of the Liver: Experimental Studies in Dog (W. Mützel, O.H. Wegener, R. Souchon, and H.-J. Weinmann) . . . . . . . . . . . . . . . . . . . . 320

Contrast Enhancement Pharmacokinetics of Ionic and Nonionic Contrast Agents (L. Kivisaari, P.B. Dean, and M. Kormano) . . . 324

## Section H: New Molecules and New Images

Futurology of Contrast Media: A Partially Warranted Prophecy (M. Sovak) . . . . . . . . . . . . . . . . . . . . . . . . . . . . . . . . . 329

Two New Classes of Low-Osmotic Contrast Agents: Triiodinated Cations and Nonionic Dimers (U. Speck and W. Mützel) . . . . . . 335

Experiences of Dimeric and Polymeric Contrast Agents (U. Erikson, B. Ingelman, and L. Björk) . . . . . . . . . . . . . . . . 340

Corporeal Distribution of Iodinated Lipid Emulsions in Terms of Particle Size (M. Laval-Jeantet and A.M. Laval-Jeantet). . . . . 344

Contrast Media for Long-term (Blood Pool) Opacification of the Vascular System (L. Björk) . . . . . . . . . . . . . . . . . . . . . . . . . 348

Summary of the Round Table (M. Sovak) . . . . . . . . . . . . . . . . 351

Subject Index . . . . . . . . . . . . . . . . . . . . . . . . . . . . . . . . 353

# List of Senior Authors


Amiel, M., Prof. Dr., Service de Radiologie, Hôpital Cardio-Vasculaire, B.P. Lyon Montchat, F-69394 Lyon Cédex 3, France

Ansell, G., Dr., 101, Childwall Park Avenue, Liverpool L16 OJF, Great Britain

Baltaxe, H.A., Prof. MD, Professor and Chairman, Radiology Department, University of California, Davis, 4301 X Street, Sacramento, CA 95817, USA

Belleville, J., Dr., INSERM-U37, 18, Avenue Doyen Lepine, F-69500 Bron, France

Benness, G., Dr., Flinders Medical Center, Adelaide 5046, South Australia

Bertrand, M., Prof. Dr., Hôpital Cardiologique, Bd. du Prof. J. Leclercq, F-59037 Lille Cédex, France

Besse, P., Prof. Dr., Service de Cardiologie et unité INSERM, Hôpital Cardiologique, Bordeaux, France

Björk, L., Prof. Dr., Dept. of Diagnostic Radiology, University of Göteborg, Sahlgren's Hospital, S-41345 Göteborg, Sweden

Brasch, R., MD, Assistant Prof. of Radiology and Pediatrics, School of Medicine, Dept. of Radiology, University of California, San Francisco, CA 94143, USA

Cahn, J., Prof. Dr., ITERC, 6, Rue Blanche, F-92120 Montrouge, France

Caille, J.M., Prof. Dr., Service de Neuro-Radiologie, Hôpital Pellegrin-Tripode, Place Amélie Raba-Léon, F-33076 Bordeaux Cédex, France

Carlborg, B., Dr., Dept. of Experimental Research, University of Lund, General Hospital Malmö, S-21401 Malmö, Sweden

Carr, D., Dr., 14, Matherton Avenue, Newton Mearns, Glasgow G 775 EY, Great Britain

Christmann, D., Dr., Service de Radiologie I, C.H.R., B.P. no. 426, F-67091 Strasbourg, France

Cittadini, G., Prof. Dr., Cattedra di Radiologia "R", Universita di Genova, Viale Benedetto XV 10, I-16132 Genova, Italy

Crochet, D., Dr., Centre Hémodynamique, Hôtel Dieu, Place Alexis Ricardeau, F-44000 Nantes, France

Dean, P.B., Dr., Dept. of Diagnostic Radiology, The University Central Hospital of Turku, SF-20520 Turku 52, Finland

Dettori, P., Dr., Via Fra' Paolo Sarpi 4, Vicenza, Italy

De Villeneuve, V.H., Prof. Dr., Dept. of Pediatric Cardiology and Pediatric Radiology, Sophia Children's Hospital, Medical Faculty, Erasmus University, Rotterdam, The Netherlands

Donato, F., Dr., Via Cesare Rossi, 5–12, I-16100 Genova, Italy

Doyon, D., Prof. Dr., Service de Radiologie, Hôpital Bicetre, 78, Rue Gal Leclerc, F-94270 Kremlin-Bicêtre, France

Ducos de Lahitte, M., Dr., INSERM FRA no. 40, Hémodynamique et Energétique Cérébrales, Service de Neurologie, C.H.U. Purpan, F-31052 Toulouse Cédex, France

Dupuy, J., Prof. Dr., Service de Radiologie, C.H.U. Bretonneau, 2, Bd. Tonnelé, F-37000 Tours, France

Eloy, R., Dr. MD, Directeur unité INSERM, U 37, 18, Avenue Doyon Lépine, F-69500 Bron, France

Erikson, U., Prof. Dr., Dept. of Diagnostic Radiology, University Hospital, S-75014 Uppsala 14, Sweden

Evill, C., Ph. D., Radiology Department, Flinders Medical Center, Bedford Park 5042, Adelaide, Australia

Falappa, P.G., Dr., Universita Cattolica del S. Cuore, Via Pinetta Sacchetti 526, I-00168 Roma, Italy

Geschwind, H., Dr., Service d'Explorations Fonctionnelles, C.H.U. Henri Mondor, 51, Avenue Maréchal de Lattre de Tassigny, F-94010 Creteil, France

Gioux, M., Dr., Service d'Explorations Fonctionnelles du Système Nerveux, Hôpital Pellegrin Tripode, Plateau Technique, 2ème ét, F-33076 Bordeaux, France

Golman, K., Dr., Dept. of Experimental Research, University of Lund, MAS, S-21401 Malmö, Sweden

Gonsette, R., Prof. Dr., Université Catholique de Louvain, 76, Bd. Saint-Michel, B-1040 Bruxelles, Belgium

Gospos, Ch., Dr., Kronenstr. 6, D-7809 Deuzlingen, Federal Republic of Germany

Grainger, R.G., Dr., Consultant Radiologist, X-Ray-Dept., Royal Hallamshire Hospital, Glossop Road, GB-Sheffield S10 2JF, Great Britain

Guidollet, J., Dr., Laboratoire de Biochimie, Hôpital Cardiologique, B.P. Lyon Montchat, F-69394 Lyon Cédex 3, France

Haagen, F., Dr., Dept. of Radiology, University of Groningen, Groningen, The Netherlands

Haughton, V.M., Prof. Dr., Dept. of Neuroradiology, The Medical College of Wisconsin, 9200 West Wisconsin Avenue, Milwaukee, WI 53226, USA

Hellige, G., Dr., Physiologisches Institut, Humboldtallee 7, D-3400 Göttingen, Federal Republic of Germany

Higgins, C., Prof. Dr. MD, University of California Medical Center, 225, Dickinson Street, San Diego, CA 92103, USA

Hørup, A., Dr., Radiology Dept. 1, Bispebjarb Hospital, DK-2400 Copenhagen, Denmark

Huet, Y., Dr., Dept. of Clinical Investigation and the Dept. of Nuclear Medicine, University Hospital Henri Mondor, F-94010 Créteil, France

Kivisaari, L., Dr., Associate Chief Radiologist, Dept. of Radiology 2, Helsinki University Central Hospital, Haartmaninkatu 4, SF-00290 Helsinki 29, Finland

Kobayashi, N., Prof. Dr., Dept. of Neuroradiology, Neurological Insitute, Tokyo Women's Medical College, Kawada-Cho, 10 Shinjuku-Ku, Tokyo, Japan

Kormano, M., Prof. Dr., University Hospital of Turku, Dept. of Radiology, SF-20520 Turku 52, Finland

Lamarque, J.L., Prof. Dr., Service de Radiologie, Hôpital Saint Eloi, 4, Avenue Bertin Sans, F-34000 Montpellier, France

Lasser, E., Prof. Dr., Radiology Research, University of California, San Diego, La Jolla, CA 92093, USA

Laval-Jeantet, M., Prof. Dr., 24, Rue de la Véga, F-75012 Paris, France

Manelfe, C., Prof. Dr., Hôpital Purpau, Dept. de Neuroradiologie, Place du Docteur Baylac, F-31059 Toulouse Cédex, France

Mathias, K., Dr., Abt. für Röntgendiagnostik der Universität Freiburg, Hugstetterstr. 55, D-7800 Freiburg, Federal Republic of Germany

Mathieu, J., Dr., Service de Radiologie, Hôpital Universitaire de Brugmann, Place A Van Gehuchten 4, B-1020 Bruxelles, Belgium

Michel, J.R., Prof. Dr., Service de Radiologie, Hôpital Necker, 149, Rue de Sèvres, F-75015 Paris, France

Moreau, J.F., Prof. Dr., Service de Radiologie Urinaire, Hôpital Necker, 161, Rue de Sèvres, F-75743 Paris Cédex 15, France

Mudge, H., Prof. Dr. MD, Dept. of Pharmacology and Toxicity, Dartmouth Medical School Hanover, NH 03755, USA

Mützel, W., Dr., Schering AG, D Kontrastmittel-Pharmakologie, Postfach 65 03 11, D-1000 Berlin 65

Novak, D., Prof. Dr., Baumschulallee 12–14, D-5300 Bonn 1, Federal Republic of Germany

Pallardy, G., Prof. Dr., Radiologie B, Hôpital Cochin, 27, Rue de Faubourg St. Jacques, F-75674 Paris Cédex 14, France

Petitier, H., Prof. Dr., Service de Radiologie, Hôpital Hotel Dieu, Place Alexis Ricardeau, F-44000 Nantes, France

Pettersson, H., Dr., Dept. of Radiology, General Hospital, S-21401 Malmö, Sweden

Piffanelli, A., Dr., Istituto di Radiologia dell'Universita, Corso Giovecca 203, I-44100 Ferrara, Italy

Pinet, A., Prof. Dr., Service de Radiologie, Hôpital E. Herriot, 5, Place d'Arsonval, F-69374 Lyon Cédex 2, France

Plainfosse, M. Ch., Prof. Dr., Service de Radiologie, Hôpital Broussais, Paris, France

Rao, U.M., Dr., Service Pr. R.G. Grainger, Consultant Radiologist, Hallamshire Hospital, Glossop Road, Sheffield S10 2JF, Great Britain

Rossi, P., Prof. Dr., Universita Degli Studi di Roma, Istituto de Radiologia, Cattedra II, Policlinico Umberto I, Roma, Italy

Sainte-Laudy, J.L., Dr., 5, Bd. de Montparnasse, F-75006 Paris, France

Salvolini, U., Dr., Corso Stamira 49, I-60100 Ancona, Italy

Schulze, B., Dr., Abt. für Röntgendiagnostik, Städt. Krankenanstalten, D-7300 Esslingen, Federal Republic of Germany

Senac, J.P., Prof. Dr., Service Central de Radiodiagnostic, Hôpital Saint Charles, F-34059 Montpellier Cédex, France

Seurot, M., Dr., Service du Prof. Gaux, Hôpital Broussais, 96, Ure Didot, F-75674 Paris Cédex 14, France

Sicart, M., Dr., Service d'Electroradiologie, Hôpital Pellegrin, Place Amélie Raba-Léon, F-33076 Bordeaux Cédex, France

Signorini, E., Prof. Dr., Ospedale Generale Regionale, Servizio di Neuroradiologia, I-06100 Perugia, Italy

Sovak, M., Prof. Dr., UCSD, Dept. of Radiology, S 004 La Jolla, CA 92093, USA

Speck, U., Dr., Schering AG, HD Biodynamik, Müllerstr. 170–178, D-1000 Berlin 65

Trägårdh, B., Dr., Allmanna Sjukhuset, Rontgeñard, S-21401 Malmö, Sweden

Touraine, J.L., Prof. Dr., Pavillon P, Hôpital E. Herriot, 5, Place d'Arsonval, F-69374 Lyon Cédex 2, France

Vock, P., Dr., Universität Bern, Institut für Diagnostische Radiologie, Inselspital, CH-3010 Bern, Switzerland

Zeitler, E., Prof. Dr., Radiologisches Zentrum, Klinikum Nürnberg, Flurstr. 17, D-8500 Nürnberg, Federal Republic of Germany

# Section A: General Toxicity

# Contrast Material Reactors: Pathogenicity and Clinical Aspects in 1981

E.C. Lasser*

While the overall incidence of adverse reactions to injectable contrast media is remarkably small, the extensive utilization of these substances, and the dramatic increase in utilization in recent years, create a situation in which the total scope of the problem is not commensurately small. I should like to point out at the outset, however, that these statements apply to the use of the ionic media currently available in the United States and elsewhere, and my remarks will be confined to the pathogenesis of adverse reactions engendered solely by the ionic media. The situation with the injectable nonionic media has not yet been sufficiently crystallized, but all indications are that the incidence of systemic reactions will be considerably below those attributed to the ionic substances.

Adverse effects resulting from contrast media injections can be considered in two major categories: (1) chemotoxic or local reactions and (2) systemic or idiosyncratic or anaphylactoid reactions. Local adverse reactions have, in general, been attributed to some chemical property of the injected material and result when high concentrations and/or quantities of contrast media are injected into a vessel supplying a critical organ or tissue. In this light, concentration and application time of the injected material become important parameters. In spite of the fact that there has been an astounding acceleration in basic research applied to these areas in recent years, we are still uncertain of the precise pathogenesis of local reactions. In general, however, it is believed that the two major contributing factors are the hyperosmolarity of the triiodinated compounds and the hydrophobic nature of these substances. This latter correlates in our own studies with the enzyme inhibitory potential of the various media.

Systemic toxicity, on the other hand, may result from the introduction of even very small quantities of contrast material into any vessel in the body. At the same time, it is important to realize that idiosyncratic reactions resulting from very small quantities of contrast material are the exception rather than the rule, and I believe you will hear later this morning that there is in fact some evidence that systemic reactions increase in incidence with increasing quantities of injected material.

For convenience of discussion, one can consider idiosyncratic contrast reactions under four major headings: (1) mediator release; (2) antibody-antigen reactions; (3) psychogenic factors; (4) involvement of acute activation systems (these include the complement system, the coagulation system, the kinin system, and the fibrinolytic

*Supported by grant PHS GM 22794-05 from the National Institutes of Health, Bethesda, Maryland 20205

system). It is our belief that one or all of these factors may be involved in any individual anaphylactoid reaction. We also believe that, regardless of the primary event, most reactions can be characterized by some degree of mediator release and some involvement of the acute activation systems. The principal and best known of the released mediators is of course histamine. The in vitro incubation of mast cells with contrast media will result in the direct release of histamine [1]. If serum is present, there is augmentation of this release presumably due to the participation of the third component of the complement system. It is also well-appreciated that contrast injections will produce histamine release in experimental animals and in man [2]. Some correlation appears to exist between the occurrence of reactions and the potential of contrast media to induce histamine release in vitro. However, no direct correlation has been shown between the extent of in vivo histamine release in the presence or absence of reactions.

The role to be assigned to true hypersensitivity or antibody-antigen reactions will be discussed at length by another speaker. Our own belief in this regard is that one cannot exclude the occurrence of a true contrast allergy, but we believe that these reactions, when they occur, are more likely to be associated with the injection of a cholangiographic substance, or some other contrast molecule having a dimer structure, rather than the monomer structure of the media currently available in the United States.

Recently, a role of the so-called activation systems in contrast idiosyncrasy has been suggested [3]. Work done in our laboratory and elsewhere has shown that the complement system can be activated by incubation with contrast media [4]. Activation of the complement system has also been noted in both experimental animals and in man, following reactions induced by contrast media [5, 6]. It is important to point out at this juncture that the degree of complement activation in these cases is considerably greater than that which could be postulated on the basis of the circulating concentrations of contrast media present. Clearly, some other factors must then come into play. Activation of the coagulation system and elevation of circulating fibrinolysis have also been noted in animals and in man having idiosyncratic reactions [6, 7]. The series of events that are believed to occur following contrast injections is predicated upon the initial activation of factor XII of the intrinsic coagulation system. High concentrations of contrast media are known to disrupt vascular endothelium, and it has been shown by cell culture and other studies that endothelium contains substances that are capable of activating factor XII when released into the circulation [8]. Activation of factor XII, in turn, can initiate the coagulation, the kinin, the fibrinolysin, and, indirectly, the complement cascades. Powerful feedback amplification systems from downstream factors considerably amplify the initiating protease [9]. The CT-esterase inhibitor has a critical, controlling role in this cascade. The inhibitor exerts a stoichiometric influence on the activated proteases. Hence, activation of one molecule of a protease produces an interaction that ultimately results in the consumption of one molecule of the inhibitor. In examining a group of confirmed reactors, we found that the mean inhibitor concentration as well as the mean total hemolytic complement was statistically lower than in a control group of confirmed nonreactors [10].

On the other hand, we found that elevated inhibitor levels protected rabbit models against a lethal dose-range challenge with cholangiographic contrast material [11]. Utilizing the same rabbit model, we also noted that adrenalcorticosteroid injections elevated inhibitor concentrations, and that this elevation did not occur for at least 7 hours post-steroid injection. Follow-up studies indicated that elevation of the inhibitor level in the rabbit was preceded by a progressive increase in endogenous heparin levels following the steroid injection (E.C. Lasser, J.H. Lang, W. Funk et al., Glucocorticoids and radiation induce endogenous heparin mobilization and elevate CT-esterase inhibitor concentrations; abrupt inhibitor elevations effect white blood cell dynamics, submitted for publication.) This has suggested that endogenous mobilization of heparin conditions the subsequent elevation in inhibitor level. This could be accomplished in the following way: In normal circumstances, activation of factor XII is known to be inhibited solely by the CT-esterase inhibitor. When heparin is present, however, two additional factors come into play – the first is a potentiation of the inhibitor capacity of the CT-esterase inhibitor [12], and the second is the mobilization of heparin that, together with antithrombin III acting as a cofactor, exerts an additional inhibitory influence on activated factor XII [13]. If one then assumes there is a constant low-level ongoing activation of factor XII and subsequent proteases that would result in a continuous consumption of CT-esterase inhibitor, it is obvious that the blunting of XII activation by virtue of heparin mobilization would eventually result in elevated levels of both XII and the inhibitor. We should also like to point out that, in recent studies, we have found that epsilonaminocaproic acid (EACA) appears to increase the expressivity of heparin in some yet undiscovered fashion. This raises the possibility that the protective effects of epsilonaminocaproic acid against contrast reactions, and its effectiveness in general allergy, might be related to a braking effect on contact system and complement system components.

Finally, we should like to point out that an in vitro test to screen potential reactors, based on the concepts mentioned earlier, has been developed [14]. In this test, we simulate factor XII activation in vivo by providing a soluble contact activator, dextran sulfate in vitro. By simply incubating plasma with dextran sulfate at 0 °C to minimize inhibitor influences, we can determine the rate of conversion of prekallikrein to kallikrein at specified time periods. Utilizing this test, we have found that a group of confirmed reactors exhibits a significantly higher mean level of prekallikrein conversion than does a control group of nonreactors [14]. In vivo, the production of kallikrein results in the release of bradykinin from high molecular weight kininogen. Bradykinin is a vasoactive substance that has the same general actions as histamine, but is considerably more potent. It is also of interest that, on testing a group of confirmed atopic asthmatics, a similar acceleration of prekallikrein conversion was noted (E.C. Lasser, J.H. Lang, J.H. Curd et al., Contact factor-associated conversion of prekallikrein to kallikrein is elevated in atopic asthma: a possible role for endogenous heparin, submitted for publication). It appears as if we are testing in both groups an index of contact system activation rate potential against endogenous challenge. The challenge could be either that resulting from the endogenous release of known contact activators, such as are present in endothelium, or could be that resulting from antibody-antigen reactions. In this light, the test may be illustrating a "final common pathway" for anaphylaxis from diverse origins.

## References


1. Rockoff SD, King C, Creplyvy M (1972) Contrast media as histamine liberators. V. Comparison of in vitro mast cell histamine release by sodium and methylglucamine salts. Invest Radiol 7: 177–181
2. Lasser EC, Walters AJ, Reuter SR, et al. (1971) Histamine release by contrast media. Radiology 100:683–686

3. Lasser EC, Lang JH, Lyon SG, et al. (1980) Activation systems in contrast idiosyncrasy. Invest Radiol [suppl] 15:S2–S5
4. Kolb WP, Lang JH, Lasser EC (1978) Nonimmunologic complement activation in normal human serum induced by x-ray contrast media. J Immunol 121:1232–1238
5. Lasser EC, Slivka J, Lang JH, et al. (1979) Complement and coagulation – causative considerations in contrast catastrophies. AJR 132:171–176
6. Lasser EC, Lang JH, Lyon SG et al. (1980) Changes in complement and coagulation factors in a patient suffering a severe anaphylactoid reaction to injected contrast material: some considerations of pathogenesis. Invest Radiol [suppl] 15:S6–S12
7. Lasser EC (1968) Basic mechanisms of contrast media reactions. Radiology 91:63–65
8. Wiggins RC, Loskutoff DJ, Cochrane CG, et al. (1980) Activation of rabbit Hageman Factor by homogenates of cultured rabbit endothelial cells. J Clin Invest 65:197–206
9. Cochrane CG, Revak SD (1980) Dissemination of contact activation in plasma by plasma kallikrein. J Exp Med 152:608–619
10. Lasser EC, Lang JH, Lyon SG, et al. (1979) Complement and contrast material reactors. J Allergy Clin Immunol 64:105–112
11. Lasser EC, Lang JH, Lyon SG, et al. (1981) Glucocorticoid-induced elevations of CT-esterase inhibitor: a mechanism for protection against lethal dose-range contrast challenge in rabbits. Invest Radiol 16:20–23
12. Rent R, Myhrman R, Fiedel BA, et al. (1976) Potentiation of CT-esterase inhibitor activity by heparin. Clin Exp Immunol 23:264–271
13. Stead N, Kaplan AT, Rosenberg RD (1976) Inhibition of activated Factor XII by antithrombin-heparin cofactor. J Biol Chem 251:6481–6488
14. Lasser EC, Lang JH, Lyon SG, et al. (1981) Prekallikrein-kallikrein conversion: conversion rates as a predictor for contrast catastrophies. Radiology 140:11–15

# Risk Factors for Adverse Reactions in Intravenous Urography*

G. Ansell, MCK. Tweedie, C.R. West, and D.A. Price Evans

To accumulate data about rare severe and fatal reactions, it is necessary to undertake a large scale survey [1–5]. In this communication we shall present brief results from a recent survey in the U.K. involving 272 hospitals. More detailed information on the survey is given elsewhere [6].

From a clinical point of view, it is important to try to define those groups of patients who may be at increased risk of a reaction to contrast media. Table 1 shows data from our recent survey.

## History of Allergy

It is well known that patients with a history of allergy have an increased risk of a reaction to contrast media. The calculated risk ratios show that these patients have approximately a fourfold increased risk of a severe reaction. Patients with a history of asthma have a fivefold increased risk of a severe reaction. There is also an increased risk of moderate reactions, but no appreciable effect on minor reactions.

In patients with a previous reaction to contrast medium, there is an 11-fold increased risk of a severe reaction. Approximately 40% of patients who have had a previous reac-

**Table 1.** IV urograms: risk ratios related to clinical history

| History | Minor reactions | Intermediate reactions | Severe reactions | Death |
|---|---|---|---|---|
| Allergy (all types) | 1.6 | 2.6 | 3.9 | |
| Hay fever | 1.7 | 1.8 | 2.3 | |
| Urticaria | 1.5 | 4.8 | 2 | |
| Asthma | 1.2 | 2.7 | 5.1 | |
| Previous reaction to contrast medium | 6.9 | 8.7 | 10.9 | |
| Previous reaction to other drugs | 1.8 | 2 | 3.2 | |
| Heart disease | 1.1 | 0.9 | 4.5 | 8.5 |

*Abridged for Publication

tion to contrast medium may be expected to have a reaction on re-challenge, but the majority of these repeat reactions are, of course, only minor or intermediate in severity.

Patients with a previous history of adverse reactions to other drugs also show an increased risk.

## Cardiac History

The risk ratio for severe reactions in patients with a history of cardiac disease is 4.5. For fatal reactions, the risk ratio is 8.5.

There was an increased risk of severe reactions with all types of cardiac disease and particularly in patients with coronary disease, but there was no significant effect on the incidence of minor or intermediate reactions.

## Dose

The scatter diagram (Fig. 1) shows the doses received in the severe and fatal IVU reactions related to age dose, and to various predisposing factors. The doses under 5 g in

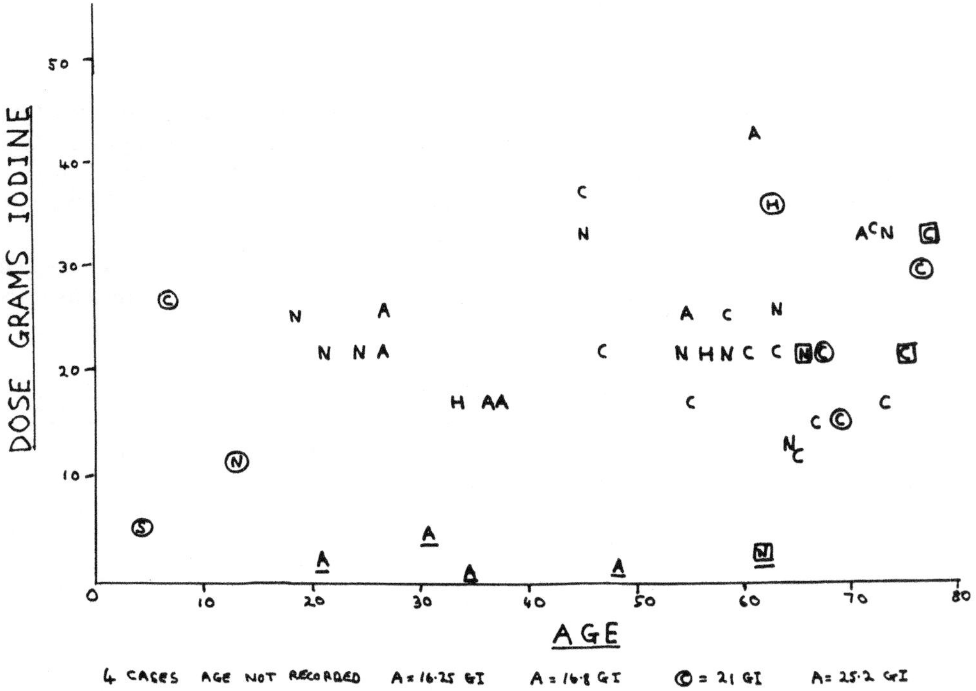


**Fig. 1.** Individual severe and fatal IVU reactions related to dose, age and other predisposing factors. *A*, allergy, previous reaction to contrast media or other drugs; *C*, cardiac disease; *H*, hypertension; *N*, three no history of A, C or H; *S*, previous IVUs with no reaction; –, premature termination of injection; ○, cardiac arrest; □, death

**Table 2.** IV urograms (age 15+): dose of contrast medium

| Dose (g Iodine) | 5–19.9 | 20–29.9 | 30+ |
|---|---|---|---|
| Total IVUs[a] | 67 574 | 62 816 | 20 332 |
| Severe and fatal reactions | 8 | 16 | 9 |
| | 1/8447 | 1/3926 | 1/2259 |

[a] Estimated for 52 weeks
$\chi^2$ for trend = 5.46 ($P < 0.05$)

adults were due to interrupted injections and these were mainly in patients with a previous history of allergy. If one takes a dividing line at 20 g, there are fewer cases of severe reactions below this level, and most of these are in patients with a history of cardiac disease or allergy.

The majority of the severe reactions occurred in the older age group. This is partly due to the higher number of IVUs performed in this age group. There were eight cases of cardiac arrest with recovery. Most of these were in patients with a history of cardiovascular disease.

The association between the dose of contrast medium and the incidence of severe and fatal reactions in adults is shown more clearly in Table 2. If one excludes the abandoned injections in patients who received less than 5 g iodine, we find a very suggestive relationship with dose. The incidence increased progressively from approximately 1/8000 when the dose range was 5–19.9 g iodine to approximately 1/2000 with doses above 30 g iodine. This trend is statistically significant.

## Preceding Drug Therapy

It is of interest to know if preceding drug therapy affects the risk of reactions to contrast media.

Beta-adrenergic blocking drugs such as propranolol are known to precipitate bronchospasm in susceptible patients.

Bronchospasm was present in 16 of the severe reactions, and four of these patients were receiving beta-blockers, whereas the expected number should have been 1.36.

This difference is statistically significant and suggests that there may be a synergic action between beta-blockers and contrast medium in causing bronchospasm. We also had an isolated case of bronchospasm in a patient receiving indomethacin.

There are theoretical reasons for believing that sodium cromoglycate (Intal) might be of prophylactic value in contrast medium reactions. Data from sample weeks indicated that 5.9% of patients with a reported history of asthma were receiving Intal.

During the survey, there were 22 reports of moderate or severe reactions in patients with a history of asthma. None of these patients with reactions was receiving Intal, whereas the expected number should have been 1.3.

The number of cases involved is too small to exclude a chance finding, but the trend is suggestive and it would be rational to consider the use of Intal in prophylaxis, particularly in the asthmatic patient.

## References


1. Pendergrass HP, Tondreau L, Pendergrass EP, et al. (1958) Reactions associated with intravenous urography: historical and statistical review. Radiology 71:1–12
2. Wolfromm R, Dehouve A, Degand F, et al. (1966) Les accidents graves par injection intraveineuse de substances iodees pour urographie. J Radiol Electrol 47:346–357
3. Ansell G (1970) Adverse reactions to contrast agents. Scope of problem. Invest Radiol 5:374–384
4. Witten DM, Hirsch FD, Hartman GW (1973) Acute reactions to urographic contrast medium. Incidence, clinical characteristics and relationship to history of hypersensitivity states. AJR 119:832–840
5. Shehadi WH, Toniolo G (1980) Adverse reactions to contrast media. A report from the committee on safety of contrast media of the international society of radiology. Radiology 137: 299–302
6. Ansell G, Tweedie MCK, West CR, et al. (1980) The current status of reactions to intravenous contrast media. Invest Radiol 15:S32–S38

# Prevention of Shocks Induced by Intravenous Urography

J.R. Michel

## Case Material and Method

The present paper is based on a survey of 80 339 IVUs, performed in the department of Uroradiology from January 1965 to July 1981.

### The Premedication

The prevention of severe adverse reactions, mainly shocks, is by the intravenous injection of a mixture of steroids (dexamethasone) and antifibrinolytic drug (epsilon aminocaproic acid). The doses injected for an adult are usually 8 mg dexamethasone (Soludecadron) and 4 g caproic acid (Hemocaprol). The mixture is injected about 5 min before the injection of contrast medium.

From 1965 to the end of December 1978, only "high risk" patients were submitted for a premedication. This group comprised all the patients who had previously developed adverse reactions against contrast media and/or all the patients with any types of allergic backgrounds. Out of 66 829 IVUs performed during that period, 8046 IVUs were performed under premedication (12%). The second period started on 1 January 1979. All the patients submitted for an IVU were premedicated systematically, because the accuracy and the efficiency of the pretreatment had been considered as demonstrated during the first period. This group consists of 13 447 IVUs.

### Classification of the Accidents

The present topic involves shocks only. Benign accidents, such as skin reactions, superficial edema, headache and transient dyspnea are excluded (Table 1). The diagnosis of shock was established on systemic hypotension, tachycardia, eventually associated cardiovascular and/or respiratory and/or digestive, and/or neurologic troubles. Vagal accidents, assessed by hypotension, bradycardia, sweat, fast recovery after intravenous injection of atropin sulfate, were excluded, despite of their frequency (84 cases).

Shocks were classified in one of the following three groups, according to the severity of the collapses. Group 1 is made of *mild shocks* characterized by a decrease in the systolic blood pressure near 7 mmHg. The renal excretion of contrast medium remained normal or vanished very transiently. The urographic procedure was not stopped during the course of the shock. The treatment was short and light (drip infusion, steroids, cardiovascular analeptic drugs). Group 2 is made of *moderate shocks* characterized

**Table 1.** Survey of adverse reactions following IVU at the Necker Hospital of Paris

| | | Group of nonpremedicated patients 1965–1978 | 1979–1981 | Group of premedicated pat. 1965–1978 | 1979–1981 |
|---|---|---|---|---|---|
| IVU | | 58 846 | 0 | 8046 | 13 447 |
| Shocks | Mild | 18 | – | 2 | 7 |
| | Moderate | 9 | – | 0 | 0 |
| | Severe | 8 (1 death) | – | 0 | 0 |
| Vagal reactions | | 23 known cases | | | 62 |
| Skin eruptions | | 155 known cases | | | 123 |
| Cutaneous or mucosal edema | | 45 known cases | | | 38 |
| Hyperventilation tetany | | 14 | | | 2 |
| Phlebitis | | 16 | | | 22 |

by a decrease in the systemic blood pressure below 7 mmHg. The renal excretion was suppressed. This led us to stop the IVU procedure. A fast recovery occurred under emergency treatment. That kind of shock was benign enough for avoiding the hospitalization of outpatients. Group 3 is made of *severe shocks*. Blood pressure and pulse were not measurable by clinical means. These shocks had to be treated by prolonged intensive cares. Outpatients had to be hospitalized, sometimes for several days.

## Results

### Period 1965–1978

Out of 66 892 IVUs, 8046 were performed under premedication. Out of 58 846 IVUs performed without premedication, 35 shocks were observed: 18 mild, 9 moderate, 8 severe. Out of these severe shocks, one patient died because of a bronchopasm: the IVU had been performed in spite of preexisting severe respiratory troubles and general ill-health. Out of 8046 premedicated IVUs performed in high-risk patients, only two mild shocks occurred.

**Second Period 1979–1981**

Out of 13 347 systematically pretreated IVUs, six mild shocks occurred in four patients. One patient had been submitted for three IVUs within several weeks; a shock occurred each time; the second shock was moderate; the other two were mild; the first two IVUs were done with a conventional medium (ioxathalamic acid); the third was done with ioxaglic acid.

Whatever the period, all the shocks observed in this survey always occurred after the first injection of contrast medium. (The dose of contrast medium is routinely administered several times.) In all cases of mild shock, the second dose could be injected without further trouble.

## Comments

The premedication with steroid + caproic acid allows us to prevent "allergic-anaphylactoid" shocks or to diminish their severity. That premedication fails to prevent other adverse effects such as cutaneous eruptions and vagal reactions.

The original case of the patient developing a shock after each IVU leads us to discuss two problems: (1) the rate of adverse reactions in patients who have previously demonstrated their sensibility to contrast media and have had to be submitted for further IVU; (2) the adequacy of the doses of the drugs used for the premedication. The same patient received similar doses each time. A better prevention could result from a progressive increase in doses of both drugs or from a longer delay of time separating the injections of drugs and of medium. One can emphasize that the rate of mild shock occurring in the premedicated patient group is almost similar to that of the added moderate and severe shocks observed in the group of nonpremedicated patients. This could signify that the premedication used at the Necker Hospital efficiently prevents the mild shocks and/or decreases the severity of collapses. A better efficiency might be expected from larger doses than those used routinely until now.

Numerous studies have proven the efficiency of steroids and caproic acid in preventing different kinds of shock. The mechanisms by which they are efficent remain poorly known. According to our 16 years of experience the mixture of steroids and caproic acid should be considered as an efficient and safe method for preventing severe urographic adverse reactions. Such a pretreatment is likely to be perfectible. However, the method now gives such reliable effects that we can accept the use of IVUs in spite of allergic backgrounds and/or former adverse reactions against contrast media which are usually considered as contraindications. The question of whether a systematic premedication of all patients submitted for IVUs is advisable depends on the unpredictability of the shocks induced by contrast medium injections.

# Adverse Reactions to Intravenous Contrast Media in Urography - Results of a National Survey

A. Pinet, D. Lyonnet, P. Maillet, and J.M. Groleau

A retrospective study was performed in France, Belgium, Luxembourg, and Switzerland to determine the incidence of adverse reactions after intravenous pyelography (IVP).

Of the 3489 forms which were sent to radiologists, we received 850 answers (24.3%). A similar study [4] in France obtained 24.2% answers, while Pendergrass [3] in the United States received. 41%.

Over a 10-year survey from 1970 to 1980, we pooled 4 million IVPs and at the same time in France, the total number of IVPs was estimated at about 8–9 million.

A systematic premedication is made in France in 23.3% of cases, mainly in private practice; it is rarely made in Belgium and Switzerland. Corticosteroids are used in 75% of cases less than 1 h before IVP.

An iodine test is still made in 5% of cases, mainly by radiologists performing less than 400 IVPs a year; most of the time the test is made intravenously. Acute reactions occurred 13 times after the test, with two severe reactions.

Minor reactions (nausea, vomiting, lipothymy) occurred in 6% of cases. Severe reactions were observed with an incidence of 1 in 2783 IVPs. Radiologists who performed less than 200 IVPs a year observed more adverse reactions.

Among these patients, previous history of allergy was noticed in 19.6% of cases. Cardiovascular and renal previous diseases were repeated in 38% of cases. A previous iodine contact was noticed in 24.6%. Twenty-seven percent of patients received premedication; 88.7% had been fasting for at least 10 h and 45% were anxious.

First symptoms occurred for 26.2% of adverse reactions during contrast medium injection, 61.8% between 1 and 60 min after injection; so 88% of acute reactions appeared during the first hour. Collapse and urticaria were the most frequent symptoms.

No correlation was observed between the age of patient and severity of reactions; only death rate increased with age. Forty-four deaths were reported in that period (1 in 91 000 IVPs). Only 34 have been clinically well described; 13 deaths occurred after bolus injection, 15 after a slow injection, and six after a drip infusion. Eight out of the 34 patients were pretreated, four with corticosteroids, four with corticosteroids and epsilon aminocaproic acid. Eighty percent of patients who died were over 50 years old. Mean age was 58.

Death was caused by anaphylactic shock in seven cases (20.5%), cardiovascular diseases in 13 cases (38.2%), and anuria in seven cases (20.5%); among the seven patients, four were diabetics). On that point, we agree with Ansari [1] and Kanfer's studies [2], who reported 60% of diabetics among the patients with fatal anuria.

Asthma people are high-risk patients. Two patients with asthma died after a bronchospasm.

Conclusion. Anaphylactic reactions are involved in only 20% of deaths. Cardiac and renal failures occur in 80% of the cases. Asthma and diabetes are high-risk factors. Prehydration and use of low osmolality contrast agents in the high-risk patients should reduce adverse reaction incidence.

## References


1. Ansari Z, Baldwin DS (1976) Acute renal failure due to radio contrast agents. Nephron 17: 28–40
2. Kanfer A, Mery JP (1978) Accidents des explorations nephrologiques. Concours Med [Suppl] 10:124–129
3. Pendergrasse EP, Chamberlin GW, Godfrey EW, Burdick ED (1955) Survey of deaths and unfavorable sequelas following the administration of contrast media. AJR 74:262–287
4. Wolfrom R, Dehouve A, Degand F, Wattez E, Lange R, Grehalet A (1966) Les accidents graves par injection intraveineuse de substances iodees pour urographie. J Radiol Electrol 47:346–357

# Allergy to Radiographic Contrast Media: Accumulated Evidence for Antibody-mediated Human Toxicity and a New Animal Model

R.C. Brasch, J. Kay, S. Mark, and D. Nitecki

## Review of Existing Data Supporting an Antibody Mediation of Certain Contrast Media Reactions

The wide spectrum of radiographic contrast media (RCM) reactivity includes reactions which are also seen to occur with other drugs and are known to be mediated by antibody-antigen interaction. It is specifically the idiosyncratic, non-dose-dependent RCM reactions which are similar to the Type I allergic reactions that have been long-studied in man and animals. These reactions include sneezing, angioedema, urticaria, and more dread responses such as bronchospasm, laryngeal edema, cardiovascular collapse, and death.

Epidemiologic studies of RCM reactions have invariably shown that reacting patients tend to be allergic to environmental substances and drugs more often than nonreactors. Asthma appears particularly to be a risk factor for an unfavorable RCM response.

These clinical observations, although consistent with an antibody-mediated hypotheses of certain RCM toxicity, provide only indirect support of the allergic theory.

More direct evidence derives from several independent investigators who have demonstrated by *in vitro* testing antibodies specific to RCM from the sera of patients suffering severe or fatal RCM reactions [1–3]. The antibodies have been identified by a variety of immunologic techniques including the Prausnitz-Küstner reaction for IgE [1], antiglobulin, hemagglutinating, and hemolytic assays for IgM [2] and radioimmunoassay for IgM [3].

Additionally, our laboratory has studied the antibody activity in the sera of reacting patients. Analysis of sera from 27 patients suffering severe RCM reactions as compared to control sera from 37 nonreacting patients demonstrated a significant elevation ($P < 0.01$) of binding of radiolabeled diatrizoate by the globulin fraction of reacting patients' sera [4]. This study suggests that antibody mediation of severe adverse reactions to RCM may be a relatively common mechanism. The data also suggests that anti-contrast media antibodies may not always produce an overt clinical reaction. Some patients appear to have antibody activity *in vitro* but the antibody type or amount was such that there was no clinical consequence from contrast media administration.

Antibodies to RCM have also been induced in our laboratory in experimental animals. Haptenicity of RCM is a virtual requisite of the allergic theory. Depending upon the method of immunization, antibodies of either the IgG or IgE classes can be induced to RCM analogues covalently linked to carrier proteins [5]. Independent investigations by Siegle and colleagues, using actual RCM molecules rather than RCM analogues, have also induced anti-RCM antibodies in animals [6].

## Type I Anaphylactic Reactions to Contrast Media in Guinea Pigs

Although anti-RCM antibodies have been experimentally induced and demonstrated by *in vitro* assays, clinical significance of anti-RCM antibodies in animals has not been described. We utilized systemic anaphylaxis in the guinea pig, a classic example of Type I antibody-mediated reactivity, and employed RCM as the hapten.

Adult male guinea pigs, each weighing 300–350 g, were sensitized by a single intraperitoneal injection of 0.5 mg diatrizoate-keyhole limpet hemocyanin (KLH). Twenty-one moles of diatrizoate were covalently linked to each mole of KLH. Control animals were sensitized to KLH alone without the diatrizoate hapten attached. A 0.5-ml aliquot of the sensitizing conjugate was emulsified in a equal volume of aluminum hydroxide gel before injection.

Allowing 8–10 days for the development of anti-RCM antibodies, the animals were challenged by intravenous injection of 2.5 mg bovine serum albumin (BSA) or of diatrizoate-BSA conjugates, or with 0.1 ml of commercially available RCM. For all challenge injections the volume was 0.1 ml and the dose of RCM was less than 0.5 mg. Animals were excluded from the study when the injection was subcutaneous rather than intravenous as intended.

The results are shown in Table 1. Only fatal reactions occurring within 5 min of the challenge injection were considered positive. Of the animals sensitized with diatrizoate-KLH, 100% (14/14) had a fatal anaphylactic reaction when challenged with diatrizoate-BSA. Control animals sensitized only with KLH and challenged with diatrizoate-BSA had no reactions (0/4). Control animals sensitized with diatrizoate-KLH and challenged with BSA alone also had no reactions (0/2). Control animals sensitized with KLH con-

**Table 1.** Results of guinea pig anaphylaxis study

| Sensitizing compounds – dose (mg)[a] | | Challenging compounds – dose (mg) | | Number with systemic anaphylaxis |
|---|---|---|---|---|
| | | *Multivalent* | | |
| Diatrizoate-KLH[b] | 0.5 | Diatrizoate-BSA[c] | 2.5 | 14/14 |
| Diatrizoate-KLH | 0.5 | Iodipamide | 0.5 | 6/6 |
| | | *Univalent* | | |
| Diatrizoate-KLH | 0.5 | Diatrizoate | 0.6–600 | 0/8 |
| Diatrizoate-KLH | 0.5 | Iothalamate | 6.0–60 | 0/4 |
| | | *Controls* | | |
| Diatrizoate-KLH | 0.5 | BSA | 2.5 | 0/4 |
| Ioxynil-KLH[d] | 0.5 | Diatrizoate-BSA | 2.5 | 0/2 |
| KLH | 0.5 | Diatrizoate-BSA | 2.5 | 0/4 |

[a] Sensitizing compounds were emulsified in 0.5 ml aluminum hydroxide gel, 60 mg/ml, before intraperitoneal injection

[b] An average of 21 mol of diatrizoate were conjugated to each mole of keyhole limpet hemocyanin (KLH) by a previously described method (5)

[c] An average of 15 mol of diatrizoate were conjugated to each mole of bovine serum albumin (BSA)

[d] An average of 20 mol of 3,5-diiodo-4-hydroxybenzonitrile, "ioxynil", were conjugated to each mole of KLH. Ioxynil is a commercially used pesticide

jugated to a noncontrast media hapten (3.5-diiodo-4-hydroxybenzonitrile, "Ioxynil") and challenged with diatrizoate-BSA had no reactions (0/4).

One hundred percent (6/6) of animals sensitized with diatrizoate-KLH and challenged by intravenous injection of 0.1 ml of the bivalent molecule, iodipamide, had a fatal anaphylactic reaction. Univalent RCM molecules, including diatrizoate and iothalamate, produced no fatal RCM reactions under the conditions of this experiment.

Prior immunologic studies indicate that multivalent haptens are required for anaphylactic reactions [7]. The multivalent hapten provides a bridge between two membrane-fixed antibody molecules which initiates a chain of events leading to the release of histamine and other vasoactive substances from macrophages [8]. Unconjugated iodipamide and diatrizoate-BSA conjugates are multivalent molecules which could provide such a bridge between membrane-fixed antibodies. Unconjugated diatrizoate and iothalamate are univalent haptens and would not be expected to initiate an anaphylactic reaction under usual circumstances. Our results indicate that in the clinical circumstances a bivalent biliary RCM molecule should be more toxic than a univalent RCM molecule such as diatrizoate. This prediction correlates well with observed RCM reactivity. Univalent RCM molecules may even be capable of eliciting anaphylactic reactions if spontaneous dimerization occurs. The investigation of this possibility is planned.

The sequence of clinical manifestations observed in the reacting guinea pigs was quite uniform. Generalized hyperactivity in the first minute was followed by scratching of the nose. The animals demonstrated labored respirations, collapse, convulsive movements, and finally respiratory arrest. Autopsy of guinea pigs dying following the injection of RCM and RCM conjugates showed profound pulmonary hyperinflation secondary to bronchospasm. In some instances, there were petechial hemorrhages on the lung surface which could be attributed to excessive negative intrathoracic pressure.

Type I anaphylaxis to RCM provides a unique model for the study of a phenomenon which clinically is unpredictable and exceedingly rare (approximately 1 in 17 000). This model is superior to $LD_{50}$ reactivity studies in several aspects. Idiosyncratic, human reactivity and Type I anaphylaxis are not dose dependent; fatal reactions may occur with doses less than 1 mg. $LD_{50}$ studies are by definition dose dependent and require RCM doses in the range of 10 000 mg/kg. The symptomatology, chronology of symptoms, and pathologic outcome of this animal model closely resemble severe clinical reactivity observed following RCM administration in humans.

Guinea pig anaphylaxis to RCM should prove useful in future investigations to evaluate preventive measures for RCM reactivity and potential therapeutic interventions. Heretofore, therapy and prevention of RCM reactions have been largely empirical.

## References


1. Wakkers-Garritsen BG, Houwerziji J, Nater JP, Wakkers PJM (1976) IgE-mediated adverse reactivity to a radiographic contrast medium – case report. Ann Allergy 36:122–126
2. Kleinknecht D, Deloux J, Homberg JC (1974) Acute renal failure after intravenous urography: detection of antibodies against contrast media. Clin Nephrol 2:116–119
3. Harboe M, Folling I, Haugen OA, Bauer K (1976) Sudden death caused by interaction between a macroglobulin and a divalent drug. Lancet 2:285–288

4. Brasch RC, Caldwell JL (1976) The allergic theory of radiocontrast agent toxicity: demonstration of antibody activity in sera of patients suffering major radiocontrast agent reactions. Invest Radiol 2:347–356
5. Brasch RC, Caldwell JL, Fudenberg HH (1976) Antibodies to radiographic contrast agents. Induction and characterization of rabbit antibody. Invest Radiol 2:1–9
6. Siegle RL, Lieberman P, Jennings BR, Rice MC (1980) Iodinated contrast material: studies relating to complement activation, atopy, cellular association, and antigenicity. Invest Radiol 15:513–517
7. Mossmann H, Meyer-Delius M, Vortisch U, Botho K, Hammer DK (1974) Experimental studies on the bridging hypothesis of anaphylaxis. J Exp Med 140:1468–1481
8. Fudenberg HH, Stites DP, Caldwell JL, Wells JV (1980) Basic and clinical immunology, 3rd edn. Lange Medical, Los Altos, CA p 193

# Immunobiological Effects of Contrast Media with Special Reference to "Nonsequential Activation" of Complement

J.L. Touraine, A.M. Freyria, A. Pinet, P. Thevenin, and M. Amiel

Injection of contrast media (CM) can be followed by adverse reactions of various types. Increasing evidence is accumulating to support the existence of several predisposing conditions and distinct pathophysiological mechanisms. Schematically one can distinguish minimal and severe reactions. The mild side effects following CM injection would appear as a consequence of nonspecifically induced histamine release. The explanations for more severe reactions are more speculative. Plasmin activators may be released as a result of endovenous hyperosmolarity. Anti-CM antibodies have occasionally been described [1] but cannot account for most of reactions. "Activation" of the complement system has been suggested to play a part in some of the side effects [2]. These mechanisms are not mutually exclusive and are not independent one from the other, many relationships linking the different systems of amplification mediators.

When activated, the complement system leads to endothelial cell injury, to recruitement of coagulation and kinin systems, and to release of several mediators with inflammatory activites (e.g., histamine, anaphylatoxins, SAS, chemotaxins, etc.). The complement system can be activated either by the classical or the alternative pathway. Dosage of the various complement components provides evidence for either type of activation. We have determined complement values in sera of patients submitted to IV urography and have found decreased levels during the minutes following CM injection, but these alterations could not be interpreted as the result of a typical activation by either of the two described pathways.

## Materials and Methods

### Patients

Sixty randomized patients undergoing excretory urography were investigated in this study.

### Radiographic Contrast Media

The following media were infused:

1. Sodium and meglumine diatrizoate (Radioselectan, Schering Laboratory) in 11 patients
2. Iopamidol 300 (Schering Laboratory) in 12 patients
3. Sodium and meglumine ioxaglate (Hexabrix, Guerbet Laboratory) in 10 patients

4. Sodium and meglumine ioxitalamate (Telebrix 38, Guerbet Laboratory) in 15 patients
5. Sodium amidotrizoate (Urografin, Schering Laboratory) in 12 patients

Low doses (60 ml) of CM were injected intravenously in one arm and venous blood samples were obtained by the same route after abundant rinsing of the catheter with a buffer solution. Three samples of blood were drawn: before, 90 s, and 30 min after the injection.

### Measurement of Complement Values

Whole complement tests (CH 50) were performed with a hemolytic microtiterplate assay. Dilutions of sera were made in gelatin veronal buffer by using microtiter dilutions and U-bottom microtiter plates. Assays were carried out in duplicate and results expressed as CH50 titers. Individual complement component C3, C4, and factor B, as well as C1s INA were determined either by radial immunodiffusion according to the Mancini technique [3] using plates from Behring Laboratory or by nephelometry using the Beckman immunochemistry system. C1q and C5 were quantitated with a 2% agarose plate containing monospecific antisera.

## Results

The variations of complement values over the 30 min following CM injections are shown in Fig. 1–5. After injection of ioxitalamic acid, the six proteins tested and the total complement activity were significantly decreased at 90 s, then tended to return to ini-

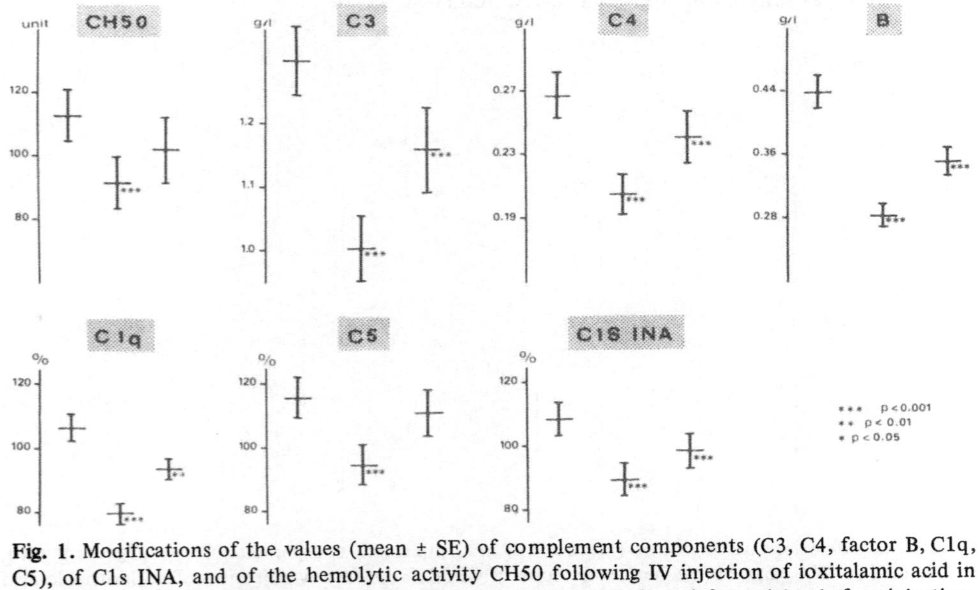


**Fig. 1.** Modifications of the values (mean ± SE) of complement components (C3, C4, factor B, C1q, C5), of C1s INA, and of the hemolytic activity CH50 following IV injection of ioxitalamic acid in 15 patients. For each protein or activity, three results are given from left to right: before injection, 90 s after injection, and 30 min after injection

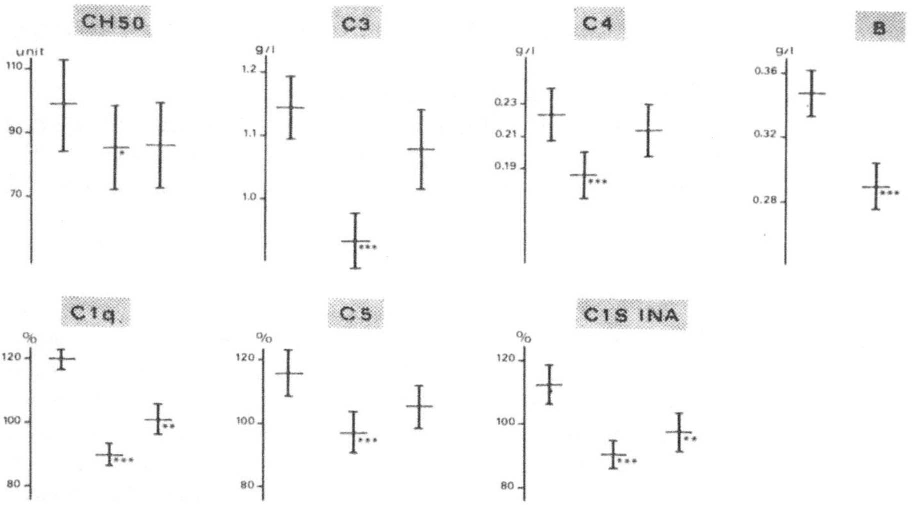


**Fig. 2.** Modifications of the values (mean ± SE) of complement components (C3, C4, factor B, C1q, C5), of C1s INA, and of the hemolytic activity CH50 following IV injection of diatrizoic acid in 11 patients. For each protein or activity, three results are given from left to right: before injection, 90 s after injection, and 30 min after injection

tial values although they were still significantly below preinjection levels (Fig. 1). Diatrizoic acid and amidotrizoic acid, two very similar products, were also responsible for a significant decrease of complement at 90 s, followed by a progressive correction of the altered values (Figs. 2, 3). Iopamidol and ioxaglic acid also led to a significant decrease in several complement components, but this diminution appeared to be of a lesser magnitude and was fully compensated after 30 min (Figs. 4, 5).

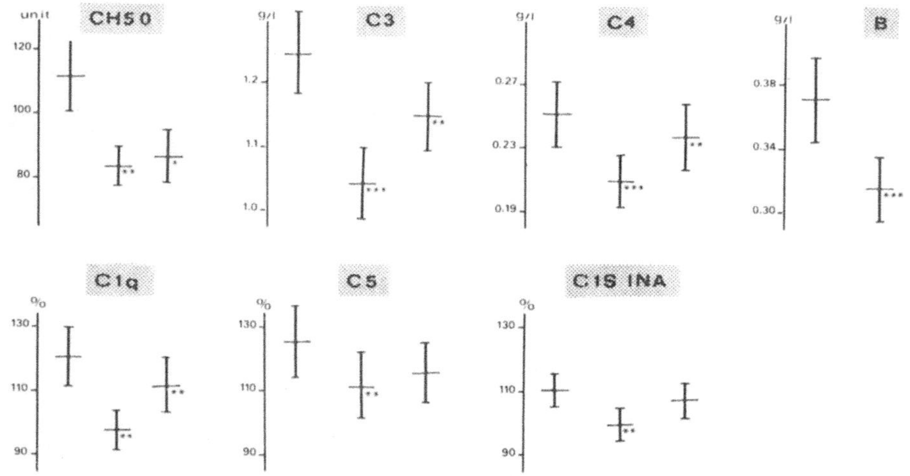


**Fig. 3.** Modifications of the values (mean ± SE) of complement components (C3, C4, factor B, C1q, C5), of C1s INA, and of the hemolytic activity CH50 following IV injection of amidotrizoic acid in 12 patients. For each protein or activity, three results are given from left to right: before injection, 90 s after injection, and 30 min after injection

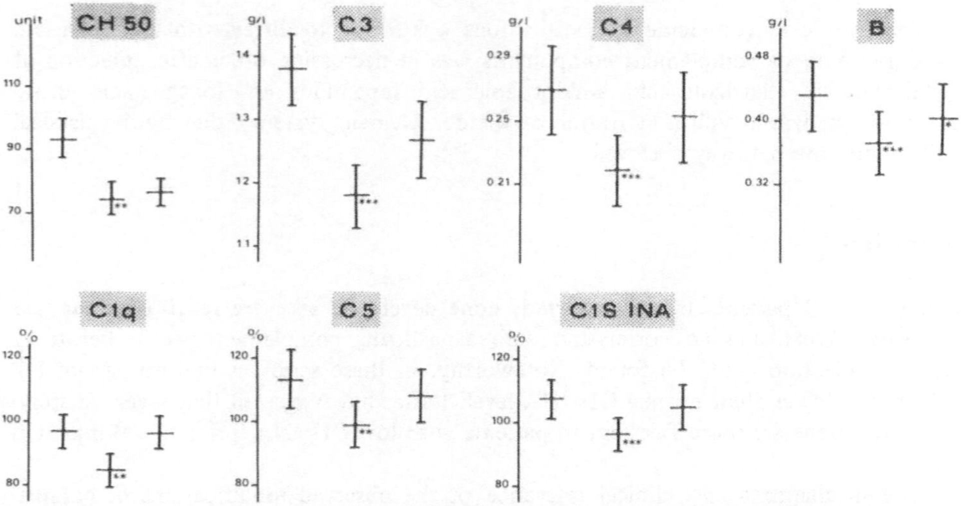


**Fig. 4.** Modifications of the values (mean ± SE) of complement components (C3, C4, factor B, C1q, C5) of C1s INA, and of the hemolytic activity CH50 following IV injection of iopamidol in 12 patients. For each protein or activity, three results are given from left to right: before injection, 90 s after injection, and 30 min after injection

Following the injection of any of the five tested compounds, most of the complement components were thus decreased. Factor B and C1q proteins were the most markedly decreased (drop of 34% of factor B with ioxitalamic acid and drop of 25% of C1q with diatrizoic acid). C3, C4, C5, and C1s INA were significantly decreased but to a lesser degree. The diminution of CH50 was less impressive.

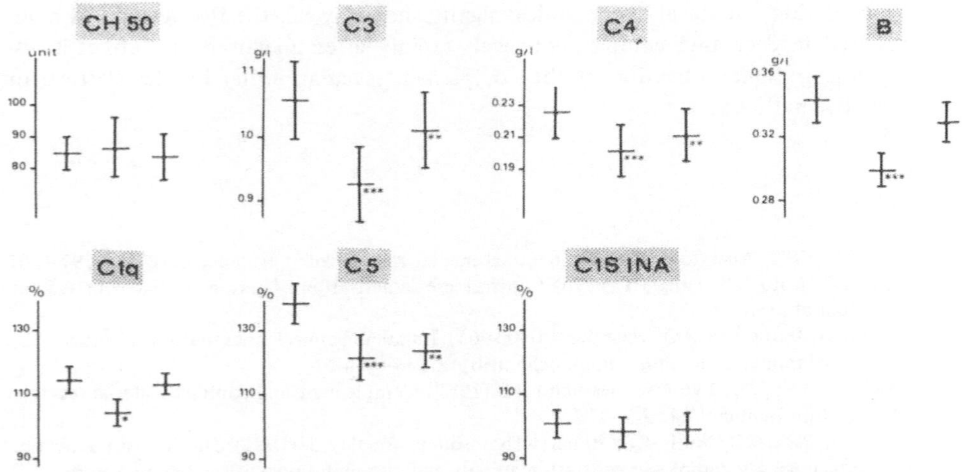


**Fig. 5.** Modifications of the values (mean ± SE) of complement components (C3, C4, factor B, C1q, C5), of C1s INA, and of the hemolytic activity CH50 following IV injection of ioxaglic acid in 10 patients. For each protein or activity, three results are given from left to right: before injection, 90 s after injection, and 30 min after injection

The profile of complement modifications was found to differ with the CM used. The diminution of complement components was in decreasing order after injection of ioxitalamic acid, diatrizoic acid, amidotrizoic acid, iopamidol, and ioxaglic acid. In no case, however, was a typical activation of the complement system either by the classical of the alternative pathway observed.

## Discussion

Among the 60 patients herein reported, none developed a severe reaction. Four had mild side effects, and no correlation with a particular complement profile before or after CM injection could be found. Noteworthy, in these series, is that no patient initially had a lower than normal C1s INA level. Lasser has suggested that severe anaphylactoid reactions are more frequent in patients with low C1s INA, prior to CM injection [4].

The mechanisms and clinical relevance of the observed modifications of complement after CM injection are still uncertain. A direct effect of CM on some proteins, including complement components, has been suggested by in vitro experiments [5]. The in vivo modifications are, however, unlikely to be the exact counterpart of this effect observed in vitro. The required doses are larger in vitro, the effect being dose dependent. In our patients, the serum concentration of CM was low (0.85–1.10% v/v) 90 s after CM injection. The effects of the five CM on complement system, both in vitro and in vivo, were of a different magnitude despite comparable concentrations. Attempts at correlating the degree of the transient complement alterations with the chemical structure and the physical properties of these five CM have not yet resulted in a simple explanation. In this regard, it has been demonstrated that the in vitro effects of several CM are different to an extent which should preclude considering them as members of a very homogeneous group [6].

In conclusion, whatever their clinical significance may be, the five tested CM regularly resulted in decreased complement levels rapidly after injection. This effect is distinct from a genuine activation of the complement system, either by the classical or the alternative pathway.

## References


1. Brash RC (1980) Allergic reactions to contrast media: Accumulated evidence. AJR 134:797–801
2. Lasser EC, Kolb WP, Lang JH (1974) Contrast media activation of serum complement system. Invest Radiol 9:6A
3. Mancini G, Carbonara AO, Heremans JF (1965) Immunochemical quantitation of antigens by single radial immunodiffusion. Immunochemistry 2:235–254
4. Lasser EC, Lang JH, Lyon SG, Hamblin AE (1979) Complement and contrast material reactors. J Allergy Clin Immunol 64:105–112
5. Neoh SH, Sage MR, Willis RB, Roberts-Thomson P, Bradley J (1981) The in vitro activation of complement by radiologic contrast materials and its inhibition with ϵ-Aminocaproic Acid. Invest Radiol 16:152–158
6. Hasselbacher P, Hahn J (1980) In vitro effects of radiographic contrast media on the complement system. J Allergy Clin Immunol 66:217–222

# Contrast Media and Immediate Hypersensitivity

J. Sainte-Laudy, M.Ch. Plainfosse, D. Sirinelli, and P.H. Bor

## Introduction

The analysis of allergic status due to iodinated contrast media is made difficult by the variety of clinical manifestations and pretreatment of all patients suspect of being allergic.

Because of our long and quite satisfactory experience of HBDT (Human Basophil Degranulation Test) in drug allergy we chose this technique for our study.

## Material and Methods

We used ioxithalamic and ioxaglic acid as haptens; they become antigenic when bound to a macromolecule.

A randomized study of 103 patients coming for intravenous urography (93%), cholecystography (3%), arteriography (2%), cholangiography (1%), and hysterography (1%) was made. Every patient was asked for any allergic antecedent and previous iodine contact.

Samples were taken before premedication and 13 patients were given an injection of contrast media before taking another sample. The HBDT was performed by counting the undegranulated basophils after contact with the tested allergen. Those basophils were stained in red by toluidin blue. The result was then expressed as maximum percentage of degranulation for a given dose of allergen. Successive dilutions were generally

**Table 1.** Patients with clinical reactions ($n = 5$)

| | HBDT+ $n = 2$ | HBDT− $n = 3$ |
|---|---|---|
| Iodine contact | 1 | 1 |
| Other allergies | Penicillin | |
| | Aspirin | Asthma |
| | Quinidine | |
| Clinical reactions | Rash | Nauseas |
| | Pruritus | Tachycardia |
| | Nauseas | ↙Blood pressure |

**Table 2.** Previous iodine contacts and allergic antecedents in 103 patients given the HBDT

| HBDT | + | – |
|---|---|---|
| $n$ = 103 | 11 | 92 |
| Previous iodine contacts<br>$n$ = 37 | 4 | 33 |
| Allergic antecedents<br>$n$ = 22 | 7 | 15 |

tested simultaneously by allergen from 100 μg/ml to 1 ng/ml. HBDT could be performed in whole blood or washed and resuspended in a mineral buffer solution in order to get rid of possible plasmatic-blocking agents.

## Results

Of the 103 patients studied, 37 had had previous iodine contacts. The HBDT proved positive in 11 patients and doubtful in four patients. Table 1 gives details of the five patients with clinical reactions, and Table 2 shows the previous iodine contacts and allergic antecedents of all 103 patients.

## Discussion

Basophil cell degranulation is related to mediator release, which is immunological and not toxic. The degranulation percentage curve for the six dilutions shows an antigen excess inhibition zone. For the compounds which induce a nonspecific degranulation there is a linear relations between dose and degranulation percentage. The degranulation is blocked by using a calcium-free buffer solution; this ion is necessary for the biochemical degranulation reaction.

Furthermore, HBDT is positive when washed blood is used, which means that complement fractions do not have a role in this reaction. We can say that this degranulation generally has no clinical expression. This might be due to the enormous quantity of iodinated media injected (in the excess antigen inhibition zone of the degranulation curve), to the premedication, or because there is no triggering of the anaphylactic reaction. Those positive HBDTs might be the result of a previous sensibilization by iodine, iodinated compound, or by the organic part of the molecule with a crossed reaction. We consider that when a patient has a positive HBDT, he must be considered as high-risk patient; so he must be closely monitored and premedicated.

## Conclusion

In practice, among the 103 patients, 10% must be considered as having a potential risk. At the present, HBDT is not a screening test because of technical reasons. However, we note that the actual risk is far inferior to the potential clinical risk.

We plan to go further and deeper into this study of those immunological reactions to iodinated contrast media thanks to HBDT.

## References


1. Benveniste J (1981) The human basophil degranulation test as an "in vitro" method for the diagnostic of allergies. Clin Allergy 11:1
2. Lang JH, Lasser EC, Kold WP (1976) Activition of serum complement by contrast media. Invest Radiol 11:303
3. Lieberman P, Siegle RL, Taylor WW (1978) Anaphylectoid reactions to iodinated contrast material. J Allergy Clin Immunol 62:473

# Iodinated Contrast Agents: Effect on ATP: Creatine N-Phosphotransferase Isoenzymes in the Arterial Wall

J. Guidollet, O. Gateau, F. Borson, C. Canillot, O. Gourdol, J. Etienne, M. Amiel, and P. Louisot

## Introduction

The present study concerns the iodinated contrast media used for arterial radiological exploration in man, and more exactly the problems posed by the toxicity of these agents on the vessel wall.

Previous studies have shown that the toxic effects of the compounds are related to a number of factors. Thus in the circulation, the in vivo injection of contrast agents causes hemodilution due to the hyperosmolarity of these molecules in blood, slowing of circulatory flow and endovascular cellular aggregation, disturbances in coagulation [1], histamine liberation and activation of complement components [2], and finally hemodynamic effects that are related to the particular vascular territory concerned. At tissue level, the toxic effects of contrast agents are very varied: the toxicity depends on the nature of the compound, the osmolarity of its solution, and its solubility in lipids. Their toxicity on aortic endothelium is related to the osmolarity of their solution.

The interactions of contrast agents with serum proteins, particularly enzymes, have been examined in a number of preliminary nondefinitively conclusive studies [3]. For this reason, in order to clarify the precise nature of their effect, we chose ATP: creatine N-phosphotransferase (CPK), an enzyme present in serum and a variety of tissues, a dimer resulting from the association of two protein subunits, M and B, thus creating the isoenzymes MM, MB, and BB. The distribution of these molecular variants in a number of organs is already partially known.

## Materials and Methods

The organs used were taken from dogs immediately after they were killed. The portion of the aorta between the arch and iliac bifurcation was opened longitudinally and washed rapidly in ice-cold physiological saline. The two layers intima-media and adventitia were separated from each other. They were weighed and homogenized in a Sorvall homogenizer in a 50 m*M* Tris-HC1 buffer (pH 7.4), 5 ml buffer being used per gram of fresh tissue. All these procedures were carried out at + 4°. The homogenates were then centrifuged for 20 min at 1000 g. The supernatant was collected for the following studies.

### Study of Isoenzyme Distribution in each Layer

For each layer, protein content was measured using Gornall's method [4].

Total CPK activity was measured by the CK-NAC test (Boehringer activated UV system) at 30 °C. The reaction was allowed to continue for 4–5 min: under these conditions kinetics were ordered zero. The wavelength chosen to avoid any spectrum interference from the contrast agents was 366 nm. Results are expressed in international units (IU).

Isoenzymes MM, MB, and BB were separated by ion-exchange chromatography, according to Mercer's method [5] on a DEAE Sephadex A 50 column. Isoenzymes MB and BB bind to the resin anions according to their electrostatic charges. The dimers MM, MB, and BB can be separated quantitatively by a discontinuous elution gradient. The purity of the eluate was verified by agarose gel electrophoresis.

### Study of the Effect to Contrast Agents on the Activity of CPK Isoenzymes

Six agents were used: iotalamic acid, diatrisoic acid, ioxitalamic acid, metrizamide, and iopamidol, at concentrations between 40 and 100 m*M*.

## Results and Discussion

The influence of diatrizoate, ionic compound, on CPK isoenzyme is shown in Table 1 (top); marked inhibition of all isoenzymes is observed in the arterial wall. The same results are observed under the effect of iotalamate, diatrizoate, and ioxitalamate. Ioxaglate (Table 1, middle) has only a weak inhibitory effect on the arterial wall. Furthermore, an important role is clearly played by the concentration of the compound, suggesting that the high osmolarity of certain solutions used in angiography constitutes a toxic factor on the arterial walls with which the compounds are in direct contact. Conversely, Table 1 (bottom), concerning nonionic compounds, shows that these are only very slightly toxic to the CPK isoenzymes in arterial wall. Activation of isoenzyme MB was even observed, particularly in the intima-media. Identical results are observed with iopamidol.

If the problem is examined from the point of view of structure-function relationships, it may be observed that the compounds in present use are solutions of one or several triiodinated organic acid salts, made up of an aromatic nucleus carrying:

An acid group in position 1

An iodine atom responsible for opacity to X-rays, in positions 2, 4, and 6

Side chains in positions 3 and 5; these chains are the only elements in the structure which differentiate the compounds from each other. The acid group is generally blocked in the form of a sodium, calcium, methyl-glucamine, or monoethanolamine salt. In solution these compounds are highly osmolar, which generally accounts for their side effects. The results of the present study show the sensitivity of CPK in different tissues to such effects. The fundamental importance of this enzyme in tissue energy metabolism justifies the undertaking of such studies. The finding that *nonionic* compounds have only a slight effect on CPK isoenzymes in the arterial wall supports the current practice of neutralizing the acid group in a stable amide bond; the absence of a negative effect by metrizamide or iopamidol argues incontrovertably in favor of the development of such compounds.

**Table 1.** Action of iodinated contrast media on ATP: creatine phosphotransferase (E.C. 2.7.3.2.) isoenzymes in the arterial wall

| | Diatrizoate | | | | | |
|---|---|---|---|---|---|---|
| | Intima-media | | | Adventitia | | |
| | MM | MB | BB | MM | MB | BB |
| 60 m*M* | 0% | −37% | −13% | −39% | −38% | −13% |
| 120 m*M* | 0% | −51% | −31% | −46% | −58% | −31% |

| | Ioxaglate | | | | | |
|---|---|---|---|---|---|---|
| | Intima-media | | | Adventitia | | |
| | MM | MB | BB | MM | MB | BB |
| 40 m*M* | 0% | −11% | −3% | −20% | −10% | −1% |
| 80 m*M* | 0% | −22% | −6% | −23% | −23% | −4% |

| | Metrizamide | | | | | |
|---|---|---|---|---|---|---|
| | Intima-Media | | | Adventitia | | |
| | MM | MB | BB | MM | MB | BB |
| 40 m*M* | 0% | +15% | 0% | −4% | +9% | +1% |
| 80 m*M* | 0% | +44% | 0% | +7% | +7% | 0% |

%, percentage of enzyme activation or inhibition compared to control

## References


1. Kutt H, Verebely F, Bang N, Streuli F, Mc Dowell F (1966) Possible mechanisms of complications of angiography. Acta Radiol 5:276
2. Lang J, Lasser EC, Kolb WF (1976) Activation of serum complement by contrast media. Invest Radiol 11:303
3. Salvesen S, Frey K (1973) Protein binding of metrizamide. Acta Radiol [Suppl] 335:247
4. Gornall AG, Bardawill CJ, David MM (1949) Determination of serum proteins by means of the biuret reaction. J Biol Chem 177:151
5. Mercer D (1975) Seperation of tissue and serum creatine kinase isoenzymes by ion exchange chromatography. Clin Chem 21:975

# The Effect of Radiographic Iodized Contrast Media on Coagulation, Fibrinolysis, and Complement System

B. Schulze and H.K. Beyer

The frequency of adverse reactions after intravascular application of radiographic iodized contrast media (RCM) amounts to 5%. The overall lethality of adverse reactions due to RCM is 1:14 000. Patients with a history of previous adverse reactions, atopics, and those undergoing intravenous cholegraphy run a risk of 10% of developing an adverse reaction.

Our investigations are concerned with the cause and pathogenesis of systemic anaphylactoid adverse reaction (SAR). The role of IgE cytophilic antibodies has not yet been conclusively established [4]. The differential histamine release concept [12] has likewise not proven to be of practical usefulness. We have summarized our previous experiments [10–11] as highly suggestive of serine proteases of coagulation, fibrinolysis, complement system, and kinin generating system being involved in SAR.

The following RCM were studied: (1) conventional nephrotropic CM: (diatrizoate, iothalamate, ioglicinate, ioxitalamate), (2) hepatotropic CM: (iodipamide, iodoxamate, ioglycamide, iotroxinate), (3) nonionic CM: (metrizamide, iopamidol), and (4) ionic dimer CM: (ioxaglate).

Scattered aspects of this concept have been verified experimentally [3, 5, 6]. Figure 1 gives a simplified scheme of the four systems with their interrelations. Special notice should be made of the rather unspecific inhibitors of these systems, e.g., antithrombin III not only inhibits thrombin but prothrombinase as well. Furthermore C-1-esterase inhibitor additionally inhibits activated Hageman factor and kallikrein. Theoretically, the clinical symptoms of SAR can be deduced from the function of activation products of these systems.

From a chemist's point of view, the crucial factors of RCM toxicity are: (1) osmolarity, (2) protein binding, (3) changes of membrane potential by RCM cations.

## Coagulation and RCM

### Global Tests

Thrombin time, reptilase time, partial thromboplastin time, calcium thromboplastin time, and thrombin coagulase time all show a dose-dependent lengthening of clotting time by RCM, hepatotropic RCM being by far the more effective. Further, at low concentrations, hepatotropic RCM cause a transient hypercoagulation, expecially well documented in the case of thrombin coagulase time (Fig. 2).

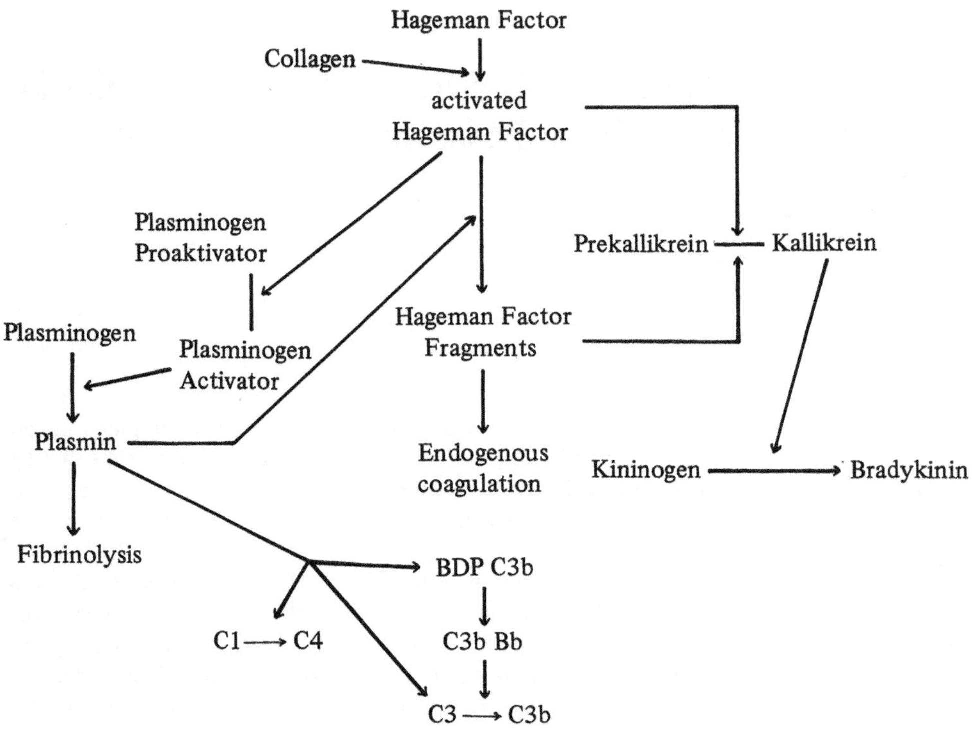


**Fig. 1.** Simplified diagram showing the four systems of coagulation, fibrinolysis, complement, and kinin system with their principal interrelations. *B, D, P* denote complement factors B, D and properdin, respectively

## EDTA Interference

Since EDTA is a constituent of commercial RCM preparations, lowering of ionized calcium may be responsible for the above-mentioned anticoagulant effects. Our results cannot affirm this possibility. The reasons are as follows:

1. Lengthening of clotting time is likewise caused by calcium independent global tests, e.g., thrombin coagulase time.
2. Prolongation of iodipamide induced recalcification time could not be reversed by subsequent addition of calcium ions.
3. EDTA-free RCM preparations triggered the same anticoagulant effects as their commercial EDTA-containing counterpart.

## Changes of Thrombin Activity by RCM

Fresh pool sera exhibit substantial thrombin activity. Incubation of these sera by rising concentrations of RCM resulted in no (nephrotopic) or only very delayed impairment of thrombin activity (hepatotropic RCM).

Parallel determinations of thrombin activity and thrombin time were made after a purified human fibrinogen solution (250 mg%) had been incubated with rising concen-

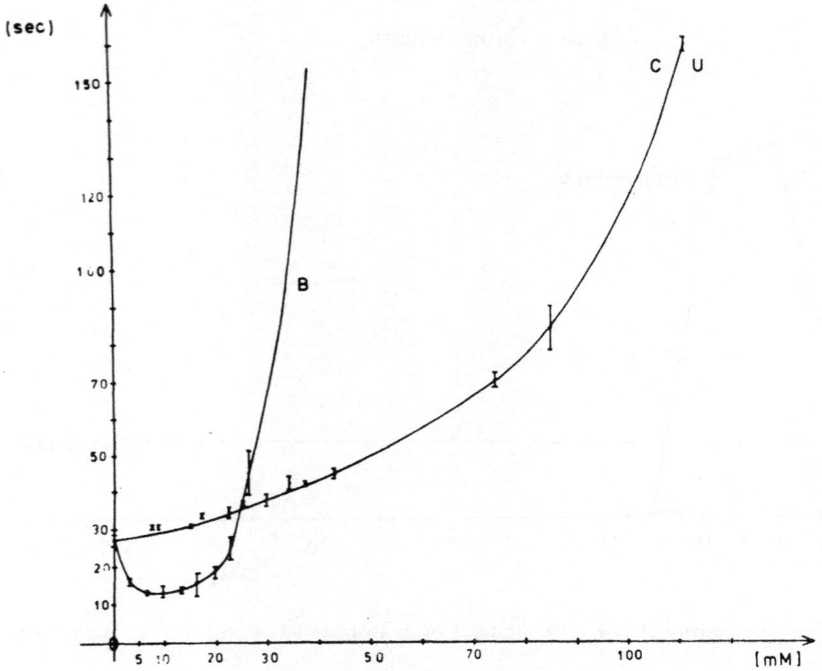


**Fig. 2.** Prolongation of thrombin coagulation time by RCM. *B*, iodipamide; *C*, iothalamate; *U*, diatrizoate. Note transient hypercoagulation of iodipamide in the range up to 30 m*M*

trations of iodipamide. Thrombin time was prolongated in a dose-dependent manner until complete anticoagulation. In contrast, thrombin activity was not impaired. Crossed immunoelectrophoresis of purified fibrinogen solutions (250 mg%) incubated with (1) no, (2) 17 m*M* (3) 35 m*M* iodipamide before and after addition of thrombin (3 IU/ml) revealed complete fibrinogen proteolysis to fibrin for (1) and (2). For iodipamide concentration of 35 m*M*, only incomplete fibrinogen/fibrin transition was noted. The results demonstrate that inhibition of the nonenzymatical fibrin polymerization step is the main cause of RCM-induced delay of clotting time. In addition, at very high concentrations of hepatotropic RCM, extensive protein denaturation of fibrinogen can be shown by crossed immunoelectrophoresis (CIE), resulting in impairment of thrombin/fibrinogen affinity with lower conversion rate of fibrinogen by thrombin.

Citrated pool plasma was incubated by rising concentrations of different hepatotropic and nephrotopic RCM. Extrinsic coagulation was subsequently triggered by further addition of calcium chloride and thromboplastin. After coagulation thrombin activity was measured. A remarkable rise in thrombin activity was found for hepatotropic RCM at low concentrations (Fig. 3). This increase in thrombin activity was followed by an abrupt drop of thrombin activity at only slightly higher RCM concentrations. Nephrotopic RCM did not show these changes of thrombin activity under the above conditions. Loss of thrombin activity by hepatotropic RCM was not restored by subsequent supply of calcium ions. The extent of enhancement of thrombin activity further varied with the amount of thromboplastin added to trigger coagulation. Since the direct

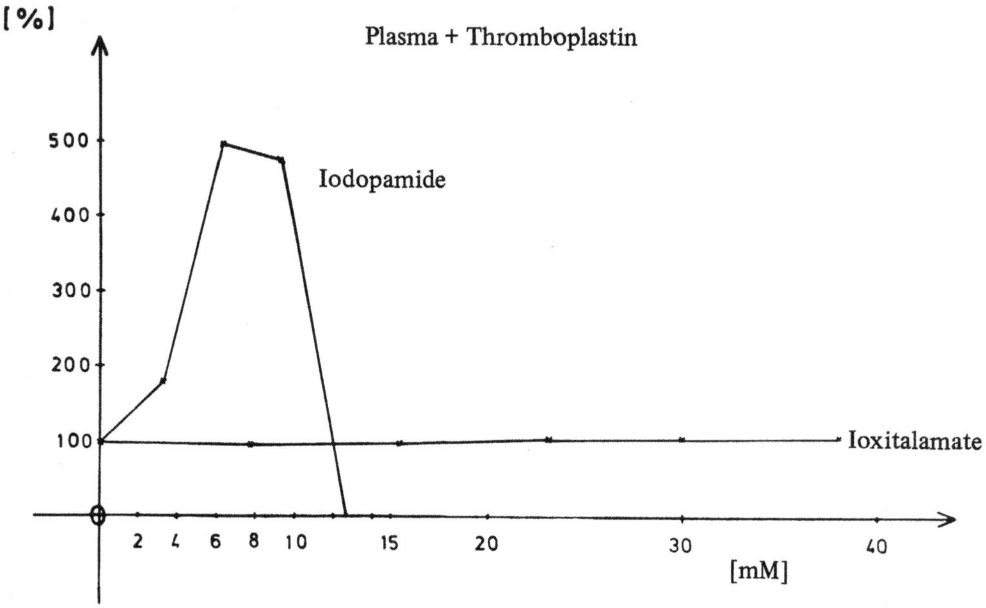


**Fig. 3.** Rise of thrombin activity at low concentrations of iodipamide in citrated plasma, as opposed to ioxitalamate

interaction of hepatotropic RCM with thrombin impaired thrombin activity only marginally, the observed rise in thrombin activity is explained by us as resulting from an activation of the prothrombinase complex.

## Effect of RCM on the Prothrombinase Complex

This complex, consisting of the clotting factors Xa, V, and prothrombin in addition to calcium and phospholipids, was generated by adding calcium thromboplastin to citrated pool plasma. We obtained two-thirds of the activity reported for the complex if generated by RVV. Hepatotropic RCM could not be investigated, since the chromogenic substrate for Xa was precipitated by these RCM. A gradual, dose-dependent decrease in activity was found after incubation by nephrotopic RCM, if these RCM were added after the generation of the prothrombinase complex. In contrast, addition of these RCM during the generation of prothrombinase complex reduced enzyme activity considerably (Fig. 4). We therefore propose RCM-induced interference with the formation of the prothrombinase complex, probably by disturbing composition of the phospholipid micelles. This would result in changes of spatial arrangements of the coagulation proteins at the surface of the phospholipid matrix.

## Aggregometry and RCM

Addition of thrombin to citrated plasma results in a reduction of light extinction at 546 nm (OD/546) in the aggregometer due to thrombocyte aggregation and fibrin for-

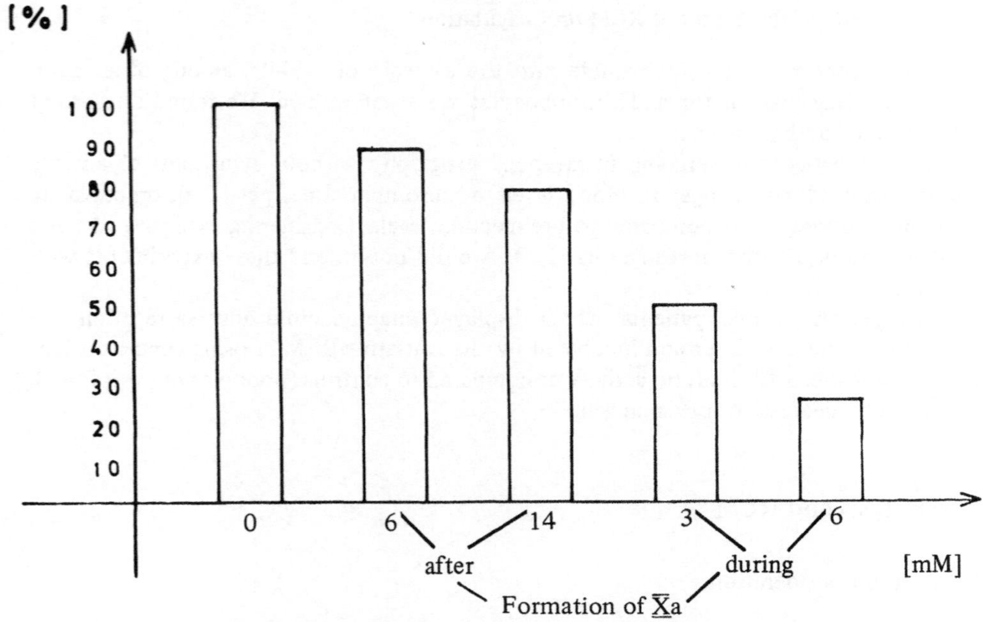


**Fig. 4.** Decrease of prothrombinase activity by nephrotopic RCM ioxitalamate. *Bar 1* is the control. *Bars 2, 3* show slight impairment of activity with rising RCM concentrations after prothrombinase complex had been generated. *Bars 4, 5* show considerable suppression of activity when RCM is added during formation of the prothrombinase complex

mation. In contrast, low concentrations of hepatotropic RCM cause an extensive increase of OD/546. Further, ADP-induced thrombocyte aggregation can be recorded by aggregometer tracings at 546 nm. Rising concentrations of hepatotropic RCM result in a reduction of amplitude and gradient of OD/546. These changes are suggestive of RCM-induced inhibition of ADP release from thrombocytes. In contrast, we found no interference of ADP-triggered thrombocyte aggregation by nephrotopic RCM. When we incubated platelet-rich plasma with rising concentrations of iodipamide, diatrizoate, and iothalamate (up to 15 m*M*), we found complete release of ADP from platelets by iodipamide and no release induction by the other two RCM. The results reflect, as interpreted by us, a profound RCM-induced change of responsiveness of platelets to ADP. Obviously, hepatotropic RCM change physical membrane characteristics by binding to the thrombocytes, destroying the fibrinogen receptors at the surface of platelets, or even denaturing fibrinogen so that it cannot further perform binding and aggregation of platelets.

### Sol-Gel Transition of Fibrinogen

In the context of the results described above, incubation of purified human fibrinogen (300–1000 mg%) with 30 m*M* iodipamide at 37 °C for 30 min results in sol-gel transition. Since CIE reveals extensive protein denaturation at these conditions by iodipamide, the results clearly demonstrate the chemical prerequisites of RCM toxicity: (1) protein binding, (2) dimeric proteins, (3) dimeric RCM.

### In Vivo Results of the Effect of RCM on Coagulation

After the injection of 1 g iodipamide into the ear vein of rabbits, among other parameters, the Hageman factor and thrombocytes were determined. We found a transient initial drop of both parameters.

Sixteen patients undergoing intravenous urography without symptoms of adverse reaction showed no changes in blood levels of thrombin time, partial thromboplastin time, and fibrinogen, as compared to preinjection levels. Considering extensive likewise negative results of other investigators [1, 9], we did not extend these experiments with nonreactors.

The plasma of two patients, which displayed anaphylactoid adverse reaction was withdrawn some days later and incubated by the causative RCM in rising concentrations in vitro. Enhanced fibrinolytic activity as compared to controls (pool plasma) was found, as assayed by decrease of plasminogen.

## Fibrinolysis and RCM

### Theoretical Considerations

Since plasmin is a suitable candidate for cross-linking coagulation, complement system, and kinin generating system, much effort has been spent to detect its generation after RCM application in vitro and in vivo.

In vivo activation of fibrinolysis has occasionally been reported [1, 3, 5, 8, 13]. The activation process was, however, not found in every case, except for the results of Albert et al. [1]. The latter author found the same shortening of euglobulin time in the course of other stress-inducing diagnostic procedures.

Our own preliminary results detected pit falls of fibrinolytic test systems in vitro, making the interpretation of in vitro results doubtful. We therefore decided to clarify the question of RCM-induced fibrinolysis by in vivo trials.

### In Vivo Results

Fibrinolytic split products (FSPs) and $\alpha_2$-antiplasmin were assayed before and several times after injection of substantial quantities of diatrizoate, ioxaglate, and iopamidol during arterial angiographies and phlebographies. Diatrizoate and iopamidol showed a transient decrease of $\alpha_2$-antiplasmin shortly after injection. Sixty-three patients were included in these series. For another group of 10 patients one leg was selectively perfused by diatrizoate and blood samples were withdrawn from the iliacal vein before and twice after perfusion.

FSPs were assayed, the lower level of detection being 12 μg/ml serum. No rise of FSP was detected with these ten nonreactors.

Another group of 16 patients undergoing intravenous urography without side reactions after injection of iothalamate also showed no rise of FSPs.

Finally mention must be made of two patients with anaphylactoid adverse reactions, whose plasma triggered enhanced fibrinolytic activity when incubated by the causative RCM.

## Complement System and RCM

### Evaluation of Previous In Vitro and In Vivo Results

Since the report of Lasser of a decrease of total hemolytic complement activity by RCM, this system has become the object of extensive and often contradictory research by many investigators of the field [2, 6, 7, 14]. In vitro results were compatible with a preferential activation of the alternate pathway of the complement system. CIEs showed factor C3 and B split products. Anaphylactoid biological activities were suppressed by anti-C5a antiserum.

Nevertheless, it was noted that EDTA did not prevent complement depletion by RCM. C4-depleted sera, Hagemann factor free plasma, prekallikrein-free plasma, and agammaglobulinemic serum all showed the same dose-dependent depression of total complement hemolytic activity by RCM. Lasser et al. [7] reported a close relation between intensity of adverse reaction and drop in hemolytic complement activity. Further he found a significantly lower C1-esterase inhibitor activity in reacting patients. Lieberman and Siegle [8] and Simon et al. [13] were not able to correlate complement activity decrease with immediate generalized reactions or with previously described clinical parameters.

### Own In Vitro Results

CIE was applied to detect C3 and B split products in vitro and in vivo as evidence of RCM-triggered activation of the complement sequence. Three hepatotropic, 3 nonionic, and five nephrotropic ionic RCM were tested in vitro over a wide range of concentrations and under vigorous conditions of incubation.

Metrizamide proved to be a strong activator of the alternate pathway of complement system, regardless of the presence or not of calcium EDTA. Iopamidol and iohexol likewise showed B and C3 split product formation to a lesser extent. EDTA of commercial preparations concealed split product formation.

Further, hepatotropic RCM induced dose-dependent peak deformation and diminution of factor B and C3 in CIE due to protein denaturation with subsequent loss of immunogenic determinants. Preincubation of serum by iodipamide did not suppress factor B split product formation by zymosan, nor did iodipamide change migratory characteristics of factor B and C3 in CIE. Prolonged dialysis of iodipamide-incubated serum did not reverse or restore iodipamide-induced peak deformation and diminution of factor B. Iodipamide showed complete C3 conversion at 35 m*M*, forming an anodal flying precipitate. This precipitate could not be reproduced by a solution of purified human C3 (gift of Prof. Vogt/Göttingen), incubated by comparable concentrations of iodipamide (35 m*M*). Even at relatively low concentrations (9 m*M*) iodipamide-incubated serum completely suppressed complement-induced hemolysis by sensitized sheep erythrocytes. In spite of this inhibition C3 anodal conversion product can be detected at 35 m*M* iodipamide. In contrast to EACA, metrizamide and iopamidol did not inhibit C3b inactivator. For iodipamide, the anodal conversion product migrated at the position of G3b without C3c shoulder. This leaves the possibility of inhibition of C3b inhibitor by iodipamide.

Another puzzling fact is the absence of complement hemolysis in the presence of C3 conversion by iodipamide. Either the conversion product is functionally defect, or the assembly of the membrane attack complex of complement is additionally impaired by iodipamide.

### In Vivo Results

#### *In Vivo Results with Nonreactors*

Sixteen patients undergoing intravenous urography without side reactions after injection of 18 g iothalamate showed no significant changes of total hemolytic complement activity in their sera, as compared to preinjection levels.

#### *In Vivo Results with Reactors*

The sera of 14 patients, who developed pronounced systemic anaphylactoid adverse reaction after application of iogycamide, iothalamate, diatrizoate, and ioxaglate, were analyzed for the presence of C3 split products. Of these, four could be shown to have developed C3b split product.

## Clinical Applications and Further Outlook

Since hepatotropic RCM cause transient hypercoagulation enhanced by thromboplastin, and also release of thromboplastins from platelets together with aggregation of corpuscular blood elements, patients with hyperviscosity syndrome are especially endangered by these agents. Myelomas, polycytemia, polyglobulism, exsiccosis, atherosclerosis, and hyperlipoproteinemia are examples of these considerations. Whereas these groups are mainly endangered by direct RCM toxicity, anaphylactoid side reactions seem not to be primarily triggered by an activation of the complement system. In this context emphasis should be made of RCM-triggered activation of Hagemann factor and prekallikrein mentioned by Lasser (1981) and Schulze (1978). Further, enhanced in vitro fibinolysis of reactor plasma by RCM deserves closer attention as a potential screening test for selecting high-risk patients.

## References


1. Albert JP, Bernsmeier R, Bruhn HD (1979) Einfluß von Röntgenkontrastmitteln auf das Blutgerinnungs- und Fibrinolysesystem. Med Klin 78:1811–1817
2. Arroyave CM, Bhat N, Crown R (1976) Activation of the alternative pathway of the complement system by radiographic contrast media. J Immunol 117:1866–1869
3. Bernstein EF, Gans H (1966) Anticoagulant activity of angiographic contrast media. Invest Radiol 1:162–168
4. Brasch RC, Caldwell JL (1976) The allergic theory of radiocontrast toxicity. Invest Radiol 10:347–356

5. Chandra R, Abraham J (1973) Preliminary studies on in vitro and in vivo effects of 50% Hypaque on coagulation in man. Angiology 24:199–203
6. Kolb WP, Lang JH, Lasser EC (1978) Nonimmunologic complement activation in normal human serum induced by radiographic contrast media. J Immunol 121:1232–1238
7. Lasser EC, Lang JH, Lyon SG, Hamblin AE (1979) Complement and contrast material reactors. J Allergy Clin Immunol 64:105–112

7a. Lasser EC, Lang JH, Hamblin AE, Lyon SG, Howard MM (1982) The Development of an in Vitro Assay to Screen Potential Contrast Material Reactors. In: Wackenheim and Salvolini (eds) Non Ionic Contrast Media. Interimages, Luxembourg

8. Lieberman P, Siegle RL (1979) Complement activation following intravenous contrast material administration. J Allergy Clin Immunol 64:13–17
9. Müller K, Hettler M, Gerhard R (1971) Blutgerinnungsveränderungen durch Röntgenkontrastmittel. Bruns Beitr Klin Chir 219:138–145
10. Schulze B (1980) Serine proteases as mediators of radiographic contrast media toxicity. Invest Radiol 15:S18–S20
11. Schulze B, Härting G, Blanke D, et al. (1978) In vivo and in vitro Versuche zur Wirkung trijodierter Röntgenkontrastmittel auf Gerinnung Fibrinolyse und Komplementsystem. Drug Res 28 I:755–764
12. Siegle RL, Lieberman P (1981) Leukocyte responses to contrast material relating to histamine release significance of iodine and surface receptors. In: Abstracts of the XVth international congress of radiology, Sect 1, Technics and physics TP 004, p 378
13. Simon RA, Schatz M, Stevenson DD, et al. (1979) Radiographic contrast media infusions. Measurement of histamine, complement, and fibrin split products and correlation with clinical parameters. J Allergy Clin Immunol 63:281–288
14. Till G, Rother U, Gemsa D (1978) Activation of Complement by radiographic contrast media: generation of chemotactic and anaphylatoxin activities. Int Arch Allergy Appl Immunol 56: 543–550

# In Vivo and in Vitro Modifications of Platelet Aggregation and Release of ATP by Ionic and Nonionic Contrast Media Used in Angiography

J. Belleville, B. Cornillon, A.M. Freyria, M. Amiel, A. Pinet, and R. Eloy

While the number of roentgenographic investigations using contrast media (RCM) is constantly increasing, it is necessary to know that adverse reactions of various nature and extent are observed in 5%–10% of these examinations [1].

The aim of the present report was to investigate the effects of RCM on hemostasis since after coronarography or excretory urography, myocardial infarction, coronary thrombosis, and/or consumption coagulopathy have been reported.

Since conflicting results have been reported concerning the effects of RCM on platelet function [4–7], this analytical study was conducted both in vitro and in vivo.

Five different RCM were tested: the sodium and meglumine salt of ioxitalamic acid (Telebrix, Guerbet) which is 30% sodium and 60% meglumine ioxitalamate, the sodium and meglumine salt of diatrizoic acid (Radioselectan, Schering), which is 66% methyl glucamine diatrizoate, the sodium and meglumine salt of ioxaglic acid (Hexabrix, Guerbet) which consisted of 20% sodium and 40% meglumine ioxaglate, the sodium amidotrizoate (Urografin, Schering), which is a 50% sodium diatrizoate, Iopamidol 300 (Schering), which consisted of *N-N'* Tris – (1,-3 dihydroxy-2-propyl) (5 lactoyl Amino 2, 4, 6-triiodo-isophtal diamide). One of them (Iopamidol 300) is of a nonionic nature whereas the four others are ionic. Three of them ioxitalamic acid, diatrizoic acid, and amidotrizoic acid are highly hyperosmolar, and their respective osmolality is 1800, 1500, and 1600 mosm/kg whereas Iopamidol 300 and ioxaglic acid are of lower osmolality (655 mosm/kg). Except for Iopamidol 300 the name of the corresponding acid will be used in this report.

## In Vitro Investigations

Platelet-rich plasma (PRP) was prepared by centrifuging citrated blood from control subjects. Platelet aggregation was investigated according to Born [2]. Three aggregating agents were used: Collagen Horm (2.5 $\mu$g/ml), ADP STAGO (5 $\mu M$/ml), and human purified thrombin Roche-Hoffman (0.1 UI/ml).

In addition the simultaneous and continuous monitoring of secretion of ATP and light transmission in the same sample was performed by the method of Detwiler and Feinman [3] using a chronolog Aggregometer Lumi 400 VS (Coultronics). The luminescent firefly Luciferase system was used for detection of secreted ATP, while 2.5 $\mu$g/ml collagen-induced aggregation was measured by the usual turbidimetric method.

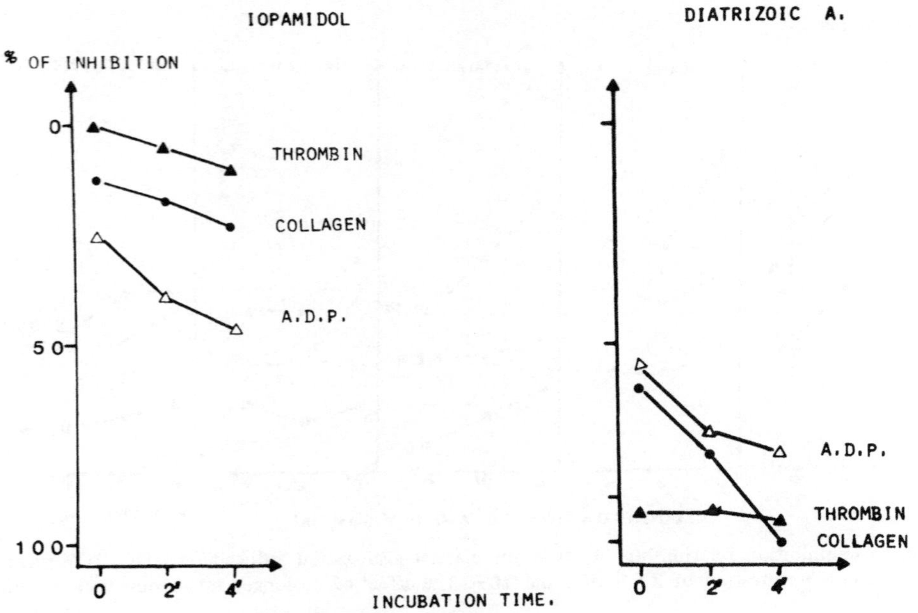


**Fig. 1.** Effect of two RCM, Iopamidol and diatrizoic acid (concentration, 5%) on platelet aggregation induced by thrombin (0.1 UI/ml), collagen (2.5 μg/ml), and ADP (5 μM/ml). Inhibition of platelet aggregation is related to the duration of incubation of platelets with RCM

After 5% RCM incubation (for 0, 2 and 4 min), the thrombin-, collagen-, and ADP-induced aggregation was inhibited. Platelet aggregation is impaired whichever inductor is tested and is time dependent. Thus the three pathways of platelet activation are impaired. Figure 1 represents the mean value of at least three different investigations of platelet aggregation induced by thrombin, collagen, and ADP after exposure of platelets to Iopamidol and diatrizoic acid. The effect of incubation time is also illustrated on Fig. 1. After 2.5, 5, or 10% RCM incubation for 0, 2 or 4 min, the impairment of platelet aggregation is dose and time dependent and variable according to the RCM tested. The results obtained after adjunction of ADP (2.5 *μM*/ml) are reported in Fig. 2.

Platelet release of ATP is also affected after RCM incubation, to various extent according to the different medium used. The washing of platelet (removing "plasmatic atmosphere") after RCM incubation does not fully restore platelet function: after 4 min incubation with 5% RCM, the inhibition of ATP release was still 35% with Iopamidol 300, 20% with ioxaglic acid, 50% with ioxitalamic acid, 35% with diatrizoic acid, and 65% with amidotrizoic acid.

## Clinical Investigations

The study was conducted on 65 patients submitted to excretory urography on a randomized basis (60–130 ml of one of the five RCM were injected intravenously). Blood collection was performed before (T0), at 90 s (T1), and 30 min (T2) after the injection.

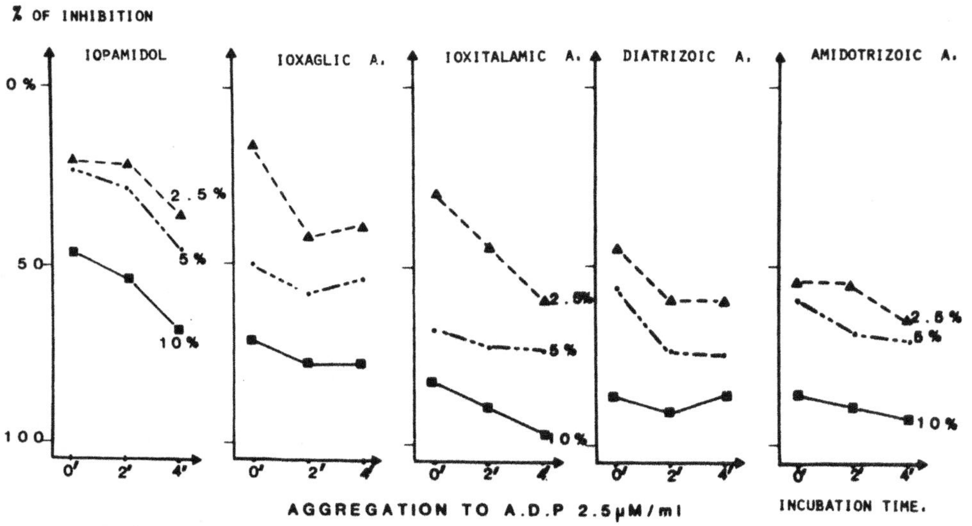


**Fig. 2.** Dose-inhibition relationship of RCM on platelet aggregation induced by ADP. RCM were tested at the concentration of 2.5%, 5%, and 10%. The effect of prolonged incubation time is also illustrated

In addition to the platelet aggregation and release of ATP, the following tests were performed: osmolality (determined on a FISKE osmometer), plasma RCM concentration (spectrophotometrically), evaluation of total calcemia and ionized calcium using a chelating method (EDTA) and an ion-selective electrode for $Ca^{++}$, respectively. The in vivo results of platelet aggregation and release of ATP confirm the in vitro results (Fig. 3):

At T1, platelet aggregation is impaired by about 20%–30% whichever inductor is tested.

For a given aggregating agent (collagen, thrombin or ADP) the impairment of platelet aggregation is variable according to the RCM tested.

The impairment of platelet aggregation observed 90 s after RCM injection is partly reversible 30 min after injection (T2).

The mean values of RCM concentration 90 s and 30 min following their injection ranged between 0.30% and 1.50%. No significant variation of systemic blood osmolality could be detected. There was a significant ionized calcium decrease only for diatrizoic acid, amidotrizoic acid, and ioxitalamic acid, whereas total calcemia was regularly decreased at T1 by about 7%–10% but returned toward normal value at T2.

By comparing in vitro and in vivo investigations of platelet function after exposure to RCM, which resulted in a decrease or even inhibition of platelet aggregation and release of ATP, the following ways of action of RCM might be discussed: (1) Hyperosmolality induced by RCM did not play a significant role, since in vivo there was no change of osmolality during excretory urography. Moreover hypertonic glucose or mannitol solutions did not modify platelet function in vitro in identical experimental conditions. (2) Divalent cation chelation has been evoked to occur after RCM exposure and might be responsible for platelet function inhibition. However, in vitro complementary studies showed that in the range of concentration tested, calcium chelation was low or even absent in plasma. In addition the chelating effect of RCM depended on their nature

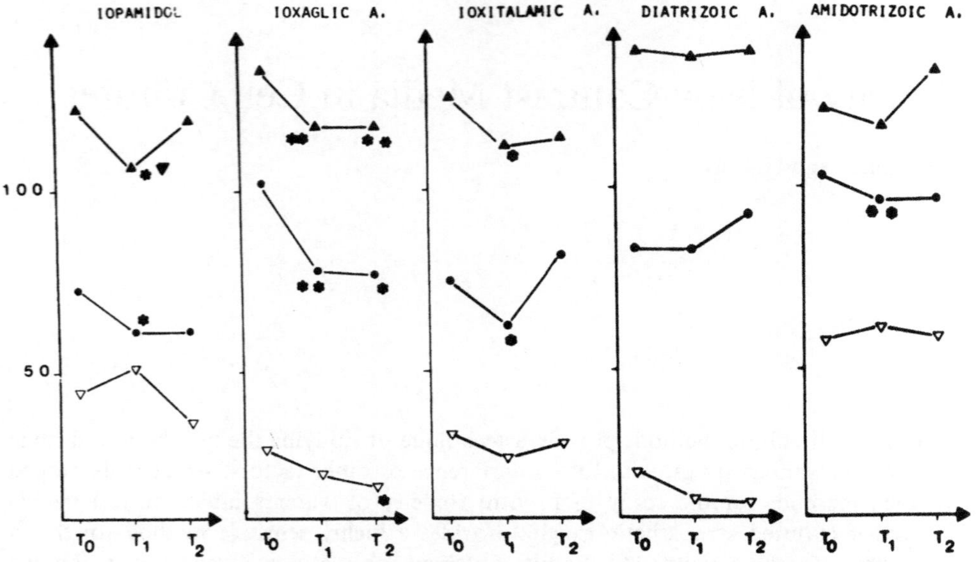


**Fig. 3.** In vivo effects of RCM during excretory urography on platelet aggregation. The extent of platelet aggregation is given in ordonate; T0 corresponds to blood sampling before injection of RCM; T1 and T2 correspond respectively to blood sampling 90 s and 30 min after the RCM injection. Statistical significance of T1 or T2 versus T0 is given: $*P < 0.05$, $**P < 0.01$. Platelet aggregation was induced by collagen 2.5 μg/ml (▲–▲–▲), ADP 5 μM/ml (●–●–●), or thrombin 0.1 UI/ml (△–△–△)

since in vivo ionized calcium was significantly decreased only for three RCM. Finally platelet aggregating agents are not all calcium dependent, and attempts to improve ADP-induced platelet aggregation by excess of calcium chloride. 0.25 *M*, were only partly successful. (3) It is therefore suggested that RCM may interact with the platelet membrane. This nonspecific interaction is not reversed completely by platelet washing, which otherwise removes plasmatic proteins associated with platelet membrane, i.e., Von Willebrand factor. Nevertheless the present results did not exclude other interactions between (a) plasmatic factors, (b) endothelial cells, and (c) contrast molecules modifying thus the normal ecology of platelets.

## References

1. Ansell G, Tweedi MCK, West CR, Price Evans DA, Couch L (1980) The current status of reactions to intravenous contrast media. Invest Radiol 15:32–39
2. Born GV, Cross MJ (1963) The aggregation of blood platelets. J Physiol (Lond) 168:178–195
3. Detwiler TC, Feinman RD (1973) Kinetics of the thrombin-induced release of adenosine triphosphate by platelets: Comparison with release of Calcium. Biochemistry 12:2462–2468
4. Fritzler MJ, Ring J, Arroyave M, Tan EM (1978) Human blood cells: ultrastructural changes and mediator release after exposure to roentgenographic contrast media. CMA Journal 119: 901–906
5. Gafter V, Creter D, Zevin D, Catz R, Djaldetti M (1979) Inhibition of platelet aggregation by contrast media. Radiology 132:341–342
6. Shapiro GA, Loch PM, Berk RN, Manton J, Ellzey B, Reynolds D (1977) Influence of cholografin and renografin 76 in Platelet function. Radiology 132:641–643
7. Zir LM, Carvalho AC, Harthorne JW, Colman RW, Lees RS (1974) Effect of contrast agents on platelet aggregation and $^{14}$C-serotonin release. N Engl J Med 291:134–135

# Toxicity of New Contrast Media in Cell Cultures

M. Kormano and H. Frey

Tissue and cell culture methods provide a technique of studying the metabolic and toxic influences of various drugs, with little interference of other factors. We have developed two such methods for the study of in vitro toxicity of water soluble contrast media. The use of cultured sympathetic ganglia provides a highly sensitive method for the in vitro study of neurotoxicity [1]. Results obtained show a close correlation to known clinical toxicity, but it is laborious for routine screening. Established cell lines provide a less sensitive but an easily reproducible and economical approach to study the cytotoxicity of substances being tested as potential contrast agents [2]. Furthermore, monolayer cell culture technique can be combined with electron microscopy and other methods to study the mechanisms of contrast-induced cell injury.

## Description of the Method

Three different cell types were used in the experiments: (1) human skin fibroblasts originating from embryos; (2) KHT, an astroglial cell line originating from a malignant human glioma (astrocytoma), that is GFA positive and has glial filaments in the cytoplasm; (3) N 108, a neuroblastoma cell line originating from M. Nierenberg's laboratory, National Institutes of Health, Bethesda, Maryland.

For fibroblasts and KHT, Eagle's Minimum Essential Medium plus 10% FCS were used as nutrient. For N 108 the nutrient was otherwise the same, but contained twice the amount of amino acids. Cells were cultured in the wells of the plastic microtiter plates (Nunc AB, Denmark) at +35° ± 1 °C in humidified 6% $CO_2$ atmosphere in an incubator (Assab, Medicin AB, Stockholm). They were examined under living conditions for growth and possible pathological changes daily for 5 days with an inverted microscope.

Into each culture chamber, 50 $\mu$l of growing cell suspension was added and the culture was checked the following day to verify a well-established growth. In the presence of good growth, 150 $\mu$l of nutrient containing contrast agent was added to make given contrast concentrations. At the end of the culture period the cells were fixed and stained with May-Grünwald-Giemsa stain for further microscopic examination.

Each cell type and contrast concentration was studied in four separate cultures with duplicate untreated cultures and with equimolar NaCl series on each plate.

## Contrast Media

All contrast media were administered to produce final iodine concentrations of 2.5, 5.0, 15.5, 25, and 50 mg I/ml, except for biliary contrast media, which were applied only up to the maximum concentration of 25 mg I/ml for reasons of solubility and toxicity. Untreated cells and NaCl corresponding to the molar concentrations of metrizamide in the experiment were used as controls. If significant retardation of growth or death of the cultures was observed in untreated cultures, the whole plate was discarded.

The following vascular contrast media were studied: metrizamide, iopamidol, iohexol, ioxaglate, P 297 (nonionic monomer, Guerbet), and ZK 38005 (nonionic dimer, Schering). Among biliary contrast media the following were studied: ioglycamate, iotroxinate, and iodoxamate.

The following criteria were used in the evaluation of cytotoxic changes:
Grade 0: no difference as compared to control experiments
Grade 1: retardation of growth, with or without abnormalities in the cells or fibers
Grade 2: partial death of the culture in addition to eventual changes seen in Grade 1
Grade 3: total death of the whole culture

## Results

Fibroblasts fromed a continuous layer on the chamber floor in 2–3 days. Glioma cells grew more slowly and a continuous layer was attained in 3–5 days in control experiments. Neuroblastoma formed only a scattered layer within the culture period. Progressive

**Table 1.** The effect of various contrast media on cultured fibroblasts during 5 days of cell culture

| Contrast medium | Concentration | Day of culture | | | | |
|---|---|---|---|---|---|---|
| | mg I/ml | 1. | 2. | 3. | 4. | 5. |
| Metrizamide<br>Iopamidol<br>Ioxaglate<br>Iohexol<br>ZK 38005 | | No effect in any concentration up to 50 mg I/ml | | | | |
| P 297 | 50 | 0000 | 0000 | 0000 | 1100 | 1111 |
| Ioglycamate | 12.5 | 0000 | 3222 | 3222 | 3222 | 3333 |
| | 25 | 2222 | 3322 | 3333 | 3333 | 3333 |
| Iotroxinate | 12.5 | 0000 | 2222 | 2222 | 2233 | 3333 |
| | 25 | 0000 | 3322 | 3333 | 3333 | 3333 |
| Iodoxamate | 12.5 | 0000 | 2222 | 3322 | 3322 | 3333 |
| | 25 | 0000 | 3322 | 3333 | 3333 | 3333 |

Grading: 0, no effect; 1, retarded growth and/or eventual abnormalities; 2, partial death of culture; 3, total death of culture.
Four cultures in each group

**Table 2.** The effect of various contrast media on cultured glioma cells during 5 days of cell culture

| Contrast medium | Concentration | Day of culture | | | | |
|---|---|---|---|---|---|---|
| | mg I/ml | 1. | 2. | 3. | 4. | 5. |
| ZK 38005<br>Iopamidol<br>Iohexol<br>P 297<br>Ioxaglate | | No effect in any concentration group up to 50 mg I/ml | | | | |
| Metrizamide | 50 | 0000 | 0000 | 0000 | 1111 | 1133 |
| Ioglycamate | 12.5 | 0000 | 0000 | 0000 | 1111 | 1111 |
| | 25 | 1111 | 2222 | 3333 | 3333 | 3333 |
| Iotroxinate | 25 | 0000 | 1111 | 3333 | 3333 | 3333 |
| Iodoxamate | 25 | 0000 | 1122 | 3333 | 3333 | 3333 |

Grading: 0, no effect; 1, retarded growth and/or eventual abnormalities; 2, partial death of culture; 3, total death of culture.
Four cultures in each group

**Table 3.** The effect of various contrast media on cultured neuroblasts during 5 days of cell culture

| Contrast medium | Concentration | Day of culture | | | | |
|---|---|---|---|---|---|---|
| | mg I/ml | 1. | 2. | 3. | 4. | 5. |
| Iopamidol<br>Iohexol<br>ZK 38005 | | No effect in any concentration up to 50 mg I/ml | | | | |
| Ioxaglate<br>Metrizamide | 50 | 0000 | 0000 | 0000 | 2222 | 2222 |
| P 297 | 25 | 0000 | 0000 | 0000 | 2222 | 2222 |
| | 50 | 0000 | 0000 | 2222 | 2222 | 2233 |
| Ioglycamate | 5 | 0000 | 0000 | 0000 | 2222 | 2222 |
| | 12.5 | 0000 | 2222 | 2222 | 2222 | 2222 |
| | 25 | 0000 | 2222 | 3333 | 3333 | 3333 |
| Iotrixinate | 12.5 | 0000 | 2222 | 2222 | 2233 | 2233 |
| | 25 | 0000 | 2222 | 2233 | 3333 | 3333 |
| Iodoxamte | 12.5 | 0000 | 2222 | 2233 | 3333 | 3333 |
| | 25 | 0000 | 2222 | 2233 | 3333 | 3333 |

Grading: 0, no effect; 1, retarded growth and/or eventual abnormalities; 2, partial death of culture; 3, total death of culture.
Four cultures in each group

fiber growth indicated good vitality of the neuroblastoma cells, but it was more difficult to assess minor changes in neuroblast than in the other two cell lines.

The results with fibroblasts, glioma cells, and neuroblasts are summarized in Tables 1, 2, and 3, respectively.

## Discussion

Established cell culture lines provide an economical and rapid screening method for the evaluation of direct cellular toxicity of contrast media. Among the cell lines used here, the neuroblasts pose some problem of evaluation due to slow and scattered growth and frequent failures of thrive. However, the general order of toxicity attained in the present series of experiments, is in good agreement with the results obtained with other methods [3]. Variation in the response of different cell lines points out the complexity of the problem of toxicity, which cannot be definitely evaluated with any single screening test.

Cell culture screening systems like ours and those used by others [3] are unable to give absolute values as far as the toxicity of the given contrast medium is concerned, but in the presence of known media, it will reliably indicate the ranking of the compound to be tested, in a semiquantitative fashion. If other factors than growth or death are taken into account, cell cultures can be used to study the effect of contrast media on specialized cell functions, like leukocyte locomotion [4] or myocardial function [5] as well, but such experiments may not be feasible in the early phase of testing new compounds.

All the stabile nonionic agents showed remarkably low toxicity even in high-dose long-term application. It should be pointed out that since the test was run with an equal amount of iodine, the nonionic dimer was applied in relatively much lower molar concentrations. The two unstable nonionic compounds, metrizamide and P 297 were equally well tolerated initially, but after several days both interfered with the growth of neuroblasts in the concentration of 50 mg I/ml. In addition, some interference with the growth of fibroblasts and deaths of glioma cells with the highest concentrations of P 297 and metrizamide, respectively, were observed. This may not reflect the toxicity of the compound itself but may be due to compounds formed by decomposition of the molecule [6] during incubation. Free iodide or other metabolites of contrast media are formed in the living tissue [7], and could also appear in cell cultures.

Although somewhat less toxic than ioglycamide, the newer biliary contrast media iotroxinate and iodoxomate are an order of magnitude more toxic than any of the urographic media.

*Acknowledgment.* This investigation has received financial support from the Sigrid Juselius Foundation, Helsinki, Finland.

## References


1. Kormano M, Hervonen H (1976) Use of tissue culture to examine neurotoxicity of contrast media. Radiology 120:727–729
2. Kormano M, Frey H (1980) Toxicity of X-ray contrast media in cell cultures. Invest Radiol 15:68–71
3. Sovak M, Siefert HM, Ranganathan R (1980) Combined methods for assessment of neurotoxicity: Testing of new nonionic radiographic media. Invest Radiol 15:S248–S253
4. Carr DH, Walker AC, White RG (1981) Effects of radiographic contrast media on leucocyte locomotion. Invest Radiol 16:133–140
5. Scott JA, Lader CD, Miller SW, Koloduy GM (1981) Effects of radiographic contrast material on cultured myocardial cells. Invest Radiol 16:141–151
6. Sovak M, Ranganathan R (1980) Stability of nonionic watersoluble contrast media: Implications for their design. Invest Radiol 15:S323–S328
7. Kelly M, Golman K (1981) Metabolism of urographic contrast media. Invest Radiol 16:159–164

# Effects of Contrast Media on Cell Cultures

D. Christmann and A. Wackenheim

We studied the effects of contrast media used in radiology, in particular metrizamide (Amipaque). This new water-soluble, nonionic contrast medium is used in neuroradiology for opacifying the subarachnoid spaces; it may, in some cases, be responsible for side effects. We thought it would be interesting to study the cell reactions to this contrast medium in order to determine its direct toxicity.

We utilized cell cultures of chinese hamster's ovary in permanent suspension, put on agitator and kept up in a warm chamber. Increasing concentrations of metrizamide were studied in comparison with a control culture. The concentrations were all below those reached in clinical practice. At day 1 each culture contained 30 000 cells/ml in 500 ml nutrient alpha. A cell count after vital stain was made daily, as well as a spectrophotometric dosage of the proteins. The experimentation was conducted over 4 days.

Our results show a marked decrease of the cell growth in proportion with the augmentation of the metrizamide concentration (Fig. 1). With a low concentration of contrast medium (1.71 mmol/liter ▲) the number of living cells was from the very first day inferior to the number of living cells in the control culture (Δ).

We studied the evolution of the protein amount in each culture by measuring daily the optic density of the various cultures (Fig. 2). We noted a 75% decrease of the protein amount in the cultures with a metrizamide concentration of 8.55 mmol/liter (■) or above, with regard to the control culture and to a culture with a metrizamide concentration of 1.71 mmol/liter (Δ and ▲ respectively).

After making more objective measurements, our data confirm the toxicity of metrizamide in cell cultures which had already been reported in 1980 by Kormano et al. [4]. These authors had made a morphologic study of the effects of several contrast media in cell cultures [3]. They reported retardation of growth of glioma cells to occur from the 3rd to the 5th day of culture with a metrizamide concentration of 10 mmol/liter or above. Our experiments showed a more marked toxic effect characterized by cell death occuring as soon as the 1st day of culture. The same authors also noted a marked cytotoxicity in cell cultures with a metrizamide solution which had been refrigerated for 2 weeks. We intend to confirm these data with cell cultures of chinese hamster ovary in suspension. This technique provides an approach to the evaluation of the direct cytotoxicity of contrast media and also allows one to compare their effects. It is simple, easy, and economical. Some cell lines grow particularly well in suspension, which allows one to avoid trypsinization and thus errors in the cell count.

Our experiments did not, however, allow us to make a statement on the mechanism of the cytotoxicity of contrast media, in particular of metrizamide.

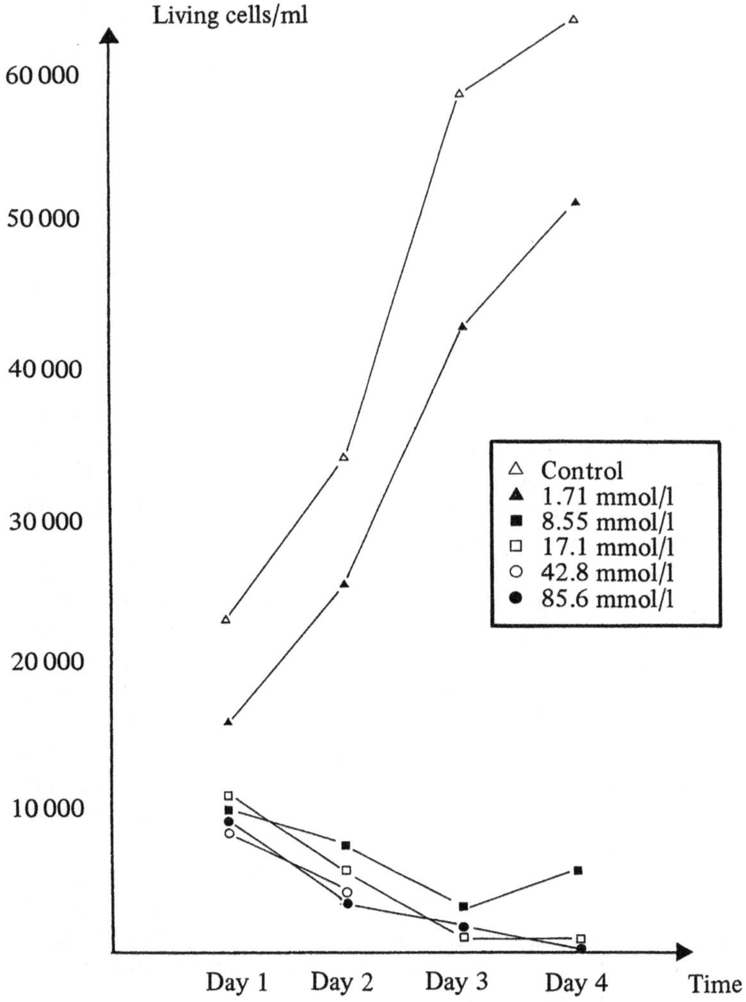


**Fig. 1.** Cell growth at different concentrations of metrizamide

According to Ambrose et al. [1] there is no intracellular penetration of the contrast media in vivo. Besides, Kormano et al. [2] have shown that the rapid extracellular distribution of the contrast medium avoids prolonged contact of the cells with the high concentrated medium which could be responsible for cytotoxic effects. It is also very likely that the hypertonicity of the contrast media, which damages the blood-brain barrier, plays an important part, which would account for the lesser cytotoxicity of metrizamide [5].

The problem of the mechanism of the cytotoxicity of metrizamide is still unsolved. A study with electron microscopy should enable this to be approached. Studies on this subject being are undertaken.

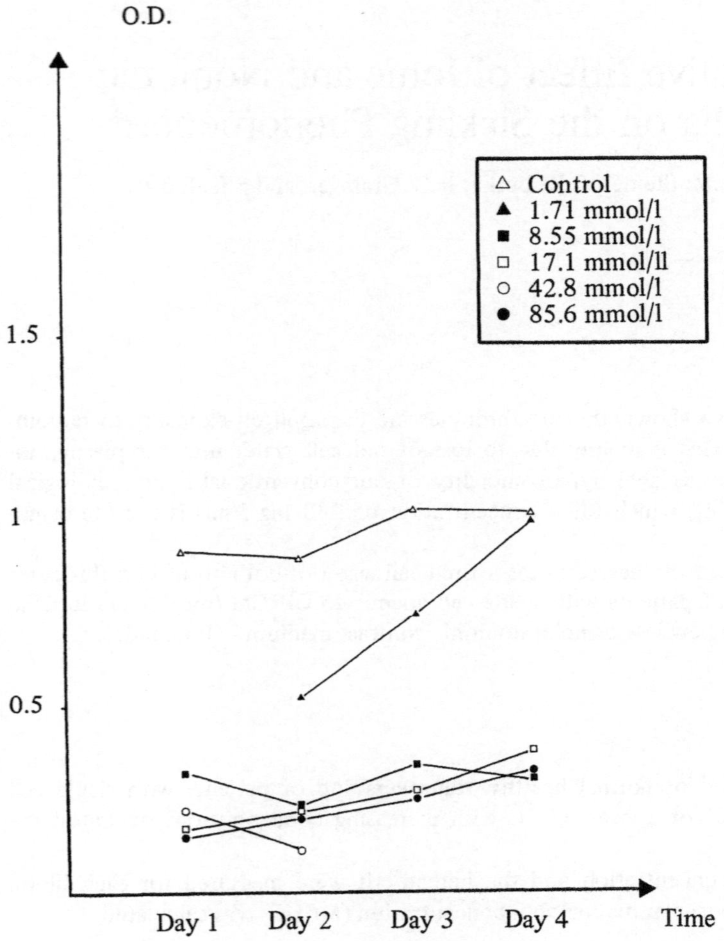


**Fig. 2.** Optic density of cell cultures at different concentrations of metrizamide

## References


1. Ambrose J, Joseph A, Taylor DM (1977) The uptake of 125 I-labelled contrast media in human intracranial neoplasms. Clin Radiol 28:529
2. Dean PB, Kormano M (1977) Intra-arterial bolus of 125 I-labelled meglumine diatrizoate-early extravascular distribution. Acta Radiol [Diagn] (Stockh) 18:425–432
3. Kormano M, Hervonen H (1976) Use of tissue culture to examine neurotoxicity of contrast media. Radiology 120:727–729
4. Kormano M, Frey H (1980) Toxicity of X-Ray contrast media in cell cultures. Invest Radiol 15:68–71
5. Raininko R (1978) Role of hypertonicity in the endothelial injury caused by angiographic contrast media. Acta Radiol [Diagn] (Stockh) 20:410–416

# The Comparative Effect of Ionic and Nonionic Contrast Media on the Sickling Phenomenon*

V.M. Rao, A.K. Rao, R.M. Steiner, E.R. Burka, R.G. Grainger, and S.K. Ballas

Aspelin and others have shown that erythrocytes are damaged on exposure to radiological contrast agents. This is mainly due to loss of red cell water into the plasma, induced by the very considerable hyperosmolality of our conventional ionic radiological contrast media (CIRCM), which (at a concentration of 280 mg I/ml) is 5 x the osmolality of plasma.

We have investigated the degree of loss of red cell water of both normal erythrocytes and the erythrocytes of patients with sickle cell anemia to CIRCM (meglumine iothalamate, Conray) and to a new low osmolar nonionic contrast medium – Iopamidol.

## Method

Aliquots of 1 ml blood of normal healthy volunteers and of patients with sickle cell anemia were incubated for 1 h at 37 °C with increasing concentrations of one of the two contrast media.

The hemoglobin concentration and the hematocrit were measured for each blood sample. The mean corpuscular hemoglobin concentration (MCHC) was calculated.

$$\text{MCHC} = \frac{\text{hemoglobin (g/100 ml)} \times 100}{\text{hematocrit \%}}$$

It is well established that MCHC correlates well with the number of irreversibly sickled cells.

The number of irreversibly sickled cells was also counted directly from each of the blood samples.

*This study was supported in part by the Pennsylvania State Regional Sickle Cell Center and the Squibb Research Foundation

## Results

### Effect of Meglumine Iothalamate on Normal Red Blood Cells

MCHC rose as the concentration of the iothalamate was increased until the red cell membrane became damaged at the higher concentrations.

No sickle cells were seen at any concentration.

### Effect of Meglumine Iothalamate on Red Cells From Sickle Patients

MCHC rose as the concentration of the iothalamate was increased. MCHC of sickle blood was significantly higher than that of normal blood at all blood contrast medium levels above 7.2 g/100 ml.

Considerable sickling was observed at the higher concentrations of contrast medium.

### Effect of Iopamidol on Normal Red Blood Cells

Iopamidol caused no increase in MCHC throughout the range of contrast medium concentration.

### Effect of Iopamidol on Red Cells From Sickle Patients

Iopamidol caused significantly less increase than iothalamate in MCHC at all comparable levels of blood contrast medium ($P > 0.001$).

Peripheral smears revealed much lesser numbers of irreversible sickle cells than with equivalent concentrations of iothalamate.

## Conclusion

Patients with sickle cell anemia or the trait are at risk of dangerous sickling after injection of radiological contrast media.

This risk is very much reduced when one of the new low osmolar contrast media is used. The present study illustrates the increased safety in sickle patients when Iopamidol is injected. Other low osmolar media such as Hexabrix, Iohexol, and Amipaque may well have the same beneficial effect.

The detailed results are presented in [1].

## Reference


1. Rao VM, Rao AK, Steiner RM, Burka ER, Grainger RG, Ballas SK (1982) The comparative effect of ionic and non-ionic contrast media on the sickling phenomenon. Radiology

# Summary of the Discussion

J. F. Moreau

Dr. Lasser thought that it is appropriate to give heparin in patients submitted for angiographies. His essay was carried out at 0 °C, in order to move all inhibitor influences and he showed a rate of conversion prekallikrein-kallikrein free of inhibitor. The influence of inhibitor is present at 37 °C. In that situation heparin is expected to potentiate the inhibitor as it does in "in vitro" studies and also to excite a second inhibitor. The overall effect will be inhibitory rather than the opposite. Dr. Revillard asked if there is any evidence that in humans the plasma component which binds to the CM molecule is indeed an antibody and, if such evidence exists, whether it is an IgG or an IgA class. Dr. Brasch recalled that the binding of CM to the body fraction of the serum proteins is demonstrated in humans by three European reports. One patient had a Prausnitz-Kuestner reaction related to an IgA antibody. The two other patients had an IgM antibody demonstrated by radio-immunological assay. The IgA antibody against CM seems to be the most informative field of research. However, IgA assay is rather difficult. Dr. Specht agreed with Dr. Brasch that cross-reactions between CM and antibodies raised against any other group of chemicals may occur in patients. However, animals experiments, as presented by Dr. Brasch, but using any other kind of drugs (steroids, antiinflammatory drugs . . .) can give the same results. The immunological binding, he reported, should be different from the CM binding to enzymes and plasma proteins described by Dr. Lasser. On the other hand, if dimers seem to be more effective as regard to these reactions than monomers, this could result from the immunologically demonstrated fact that the two benzene rings react differently with the proteins.

Dr. Louisot considered that, probably because of the transient life of the CM molecule inside the body, there is no evidence than the changes in CPK and LDH enzymatic systems (which do not result from a full inhibition) play any significant role in the clinical approach of the adverse reactions. The effects of CM in enzymes indicate that these molecules may react at a subcellular level and that CM may compete with enzymatic proteins. Dr. Touraine wondered whether CM molecules may have an effect on membranaceous enzymes, for instance on methyltransferase, which would play a prominent role in mastocytes degranulation. Dr. Louisot thought that CM might react in a B-B enzymatic system and then induce significant troubles. Dr. Kormano did not think that cell culture can yet bring a big contribution to the understanding of the effects of CM on the membranaceous enzymes, because of numerous artifacts induced by contamination. Dr. Brasch pointed out the gap existing between the clinical doses and the very high doses used for cells culture. Dr. Kormano confirmed that the phenomena described from cell culture are dose related. A long discussion followed based on the accuracy of the cells culture techniques applied to the CM toxicity study.

Is this possible to study the plasmic membrane and its enzymes? Does osmolality induce by itself difficulties in interpreting the cellular damage? Is it possible to study less severe lesions than cellular mortality by cell culture? Do the degradation products of CM molecules resulting from the very long exposure (several days) induce their own lesions? How to appraise the effects related to an possible remainder of CM? Dr. Louisot and Dr. Revillard pointed out the gap existing between the very long cellular exposure to CM requested for cell culture experiments and the transient cellular exposure observed in clinical conditions. They suggested cellular studies with smaller doses and focusing the interest on the nuclear and mitochondrial effects.

Dr. Moreau reported some cases of acute thrombosis of arteriovenous fistulae in patients treated by chronic hemodialysis and submitted for angiographies, without associated hemodynamic complications. Anuric patients belong to the small group of humans involved in possible effects from CM remainder.

A long discussion followed dealing with the opportunity for including aminocaproic acid in the pretreatment of adverse reactions. Dr. Belleville thought that caproic acid is dangerous because of its disastrous effects in patients developing disseminated intravascular coagulation. Dr. Shultz suggested giving up the acid because of its property for activating the complement system. Dr. Moreau recalled that the pretreatment associating steriods and caproic acid had been promoted by Dr. Michel in the mid-sixties because of a French report of three cases of acute fibrinolysis coexisting with anaphylactic shock. His first concept had been based on three main clinical data: steroids alone were known to be inconsistently effective as preventive agents for shocks; caproic acid was known to be an antifibrinolytic agent; preliminary trials showed that in several patients who had previously developed shocks in spite of a steroid pretreatment, no shocks occurred during further IVUS under both drugs premedication. The lack of mortal accidents in high-risk patients premedicated by Dr. Michel contributed to decreasing the often dramatic anxiety of many French radiologists having to perform IVU. Dr. Moreau agreed with Dr. Revillard and Dr. Louisot that the effectiveness of caproic acid as a preventive drug is presented more like an empirical statement than like scientifically proven data. As the specialists of coagulation attending the discussion did not share the clinical views of Dr. Michel, more and more support appeared for the idea of a randomized prospective clinical study of the effectiveness of premedications with and without caproic acid. Dr. Lasser pointed out that the antifibrinolytic effects of caproic acid have probably been overemphasized, except on the urinary tract, where the concentrations can rise to high levels. The prophylactic effects of caproic acid are probably based on other properties (effect on heparin?).

# Section B: Effect on the Heart

# Considerations of Pathogenicity and Clinical Aspects of Contrast Media Toxicity on the Heart in 1981

Ch. B. Higgins[1]

The toxicity of water soluble iodinated contrast media has been gradually reduced over the years since the introduction of these agents. Although the iodinated contrast media, used clinically during the 1970s has been considered relatively safe and associated with few important deleterious effects, the effects of contrast media on the heart still remain the most important proximate factor causing mortality and morbidity during coronary arteriography. A nationwide survey during 1970–1971, which included 46 904 coronary arteriograms, revealed an overall complication rate of 4.66% of which 1.42% were likely related to the effects of contrast media. A similar survey during 1973 which included 89 079 coronary ateriograms revealed a decline in complication rate to 2.99% but actually a slight rise to 1.84% for those complications for which contrast media could be implicated. During the time covered by these surveys most cardiovascular studies were performed with monomeric ionic contrast media at a concentration of 370 mg iodine per milliliter of contrast medium.

Contrast media cause numerous electrophysiologic and hemodynamic alterations. The most important effects on the cardiovascular system are asystole, ventricular fibrillation, myocardial depression, and vasodilatation. The timing and severity of these changes varies considerably depending upon the site of injection of contrast medium [3] and to some extent upon the preexisting circulatory status of the organism. For instance, the hemodynamic changes caused by intra-aortic and direct intracoronary injection of contrast medium are substantially different. The predominant hemodynamic effect of intravenous, ventricular, or intra-aortic injection of contrast media is hypotension as a consequence of vasodilatation. Under these circumstances, the decline in LV pressure and peak dP/dt are due to peripheral vasodilatation. On the other hand, the predominant effect of intracoronary injection of ionic contrast media is transient direct depression in myocardial contractile state causing left ventricular pressure to decline prior to the time of onset of peripheral vasodilatation.

The cardiovascular effects of contrast media can be conveniently grouped in the following manner:

I. Central circulatory effects (cardiac)
   - A. Heart rate, conduction, rhythm, excitability (electrophysiological)
   - B. Ventricular pressures, dimensions, myocardial contractile state (mechanical)

---

1 Recipient of US Public Health Service Career Development Grant Award no. 1K04HL2001 from the National Heart, Lung, and Blood Institute

II. Peripheral circulatory effects
    A. Vasoactivity
    B. Reflex activation
    C. Rheologic

As a consequence of hyperosmolality, cation content, and chemical configuration, ionic contrast media have primary or direct inhibitory actions on specialized cells of the cardiac conduction systems, on myocardial cells, and on vascular smooth muscle cells. During the past decade attempts have been made to reduce the cardiovascular toxicity of contrast media by altering the cation content of ionic contrast media through substitution of meglumine for sodium ions and by the addition of calcium ions. In this same regard a series of nonionic contrast media have been developed. The availability of these new contrast media has stimulated studies in our own and other laboratories aimed at comparing the electrophysiologic and contractile effects of these newer contrast materials with the standard monomeric ionic agents.

## Electrophysiologic Effects

### Impulse Generation and Conduction

The direct inhibitory effects of contrast media on the sinoatrial and atrioventricular nodes have been studied in an experimental model in which tiny catheters were inserted into the isolated sinoatrial nodal (SA) artery and the atrioventricular nodal (AV) artery [4]. Infusion of ionic contrast media [meglumine sodium diatrizoate, 370 mg iodine/ml (MSD)] into the SA node artery causes a dose rate dependent decrease in heart rate (Fig. 1). Solutions of saline or meglumine hydrochloride, which were equiosmolar to the contrast media, caused similar decreases in heart rate. On the other hand the nonionic contrast media, metrizamide, with the same iodine content caused substantially less decrease in heart rate.

Likewise, infusion of MSD into the AV nodal artery caused a dose-dependent increase in the PR interval (Fig. 2). Metrizamide causes substantially less increase in PR interval at the same dose rates.

### Ventricular Irritability

An important deleterious effect of contrast media in coronary ateriography is the production of ventricular fibrillation. The propensity of contrast media to induce fibrillation has been crudely assessed by injecting incremental doses of contrast media into the canine right coronary artery. These studies have suggested that the tendency to cause ventricular fibrillation is intensified by lowering of the ambient ionic calcium levels by contrast media containing chelating agents, and that this effect is alleviated by addition of an optimal amount of calcium ions [5].

A quantitative technique for evaluation of the arrhythmogenic potential of contrast media and other factors is to determine their effect on the ventricular fibrillation threshold (VFT). Wolf [6] has used VFT in the intact canine heart to demonstrate that ionic contrast media lower the threshold current needed to induce ventricular fibrillation during the vulnerable period of the cardiac cycle. The VFT was determined by finding

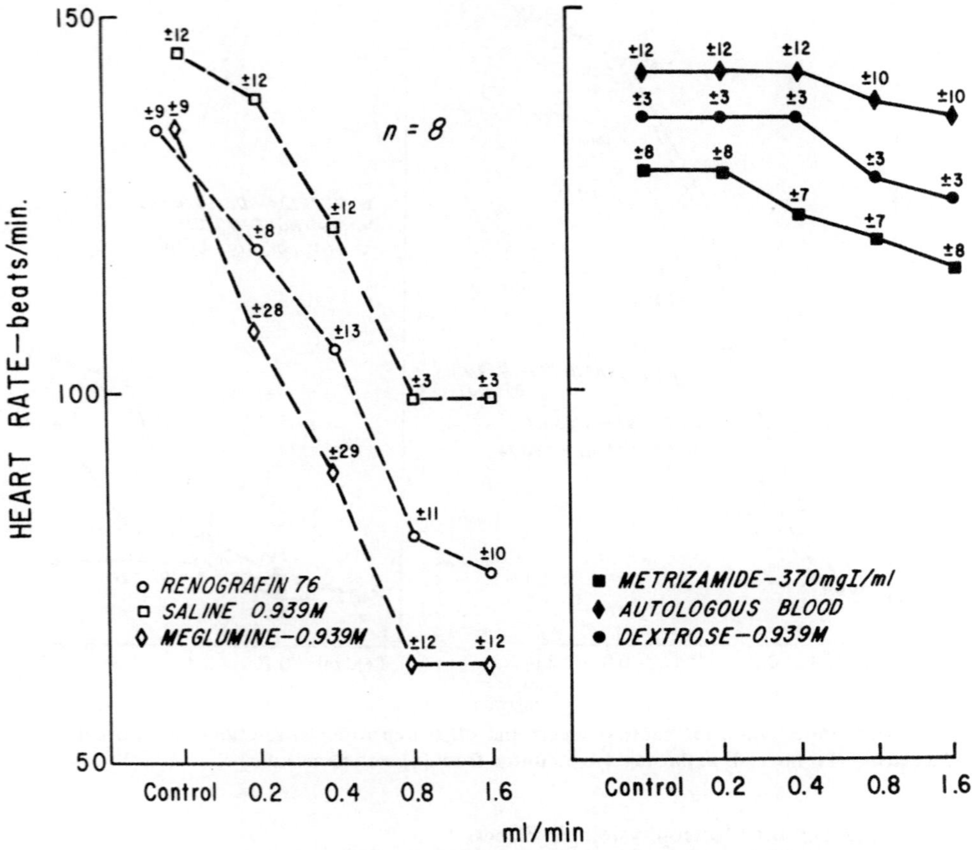


**Fig. 1.** Dose rate response for contrast media and other hyperosmolal solutions on sinoatrial node activity (heart rate) in the dog. [Reproduced from [4] with permission]

the lowest milliamperage (MA) current applied over a 2 ms period during the vulnerable period of the paced heart that induced ventricular fibrillation.

Immediately and for 60 s after the intracoronary injection of monomeric ionic contrast media (meglumine sodium diatrizoate) VFT decreases considerably (Fig. 3). There was a dose-related decrease in VFT; 2 ml contrast media decreased VFT to nearly 80% of control and 4 ml decreased it to 50% of control. For the same dose of contrast media, VFT was lowered to a greater degree by a prolonged injection and in the presence of ischemia and nonphysiologic levels of ionized calcium.

The addition of calcium ions to ionic contrast media has a salutory effect on VFT. With meglumine sodium iothalamate, the concentration of calcium ions that caused the greatest improvement in VFT is 5–10 mEq/liter [6].

Among the monomeric ionic media pure sodium salts (sodium iothalamate) causes a greater reduction in VFT than mixed meglumine sodium salts (meglumine sodium diatrizoate). Nonionic contrast media (metrizamide and iohexol) and low osmolality ionic media (Hexabrix) cause significantly less reduction in VFT than ionic media [6, 7].

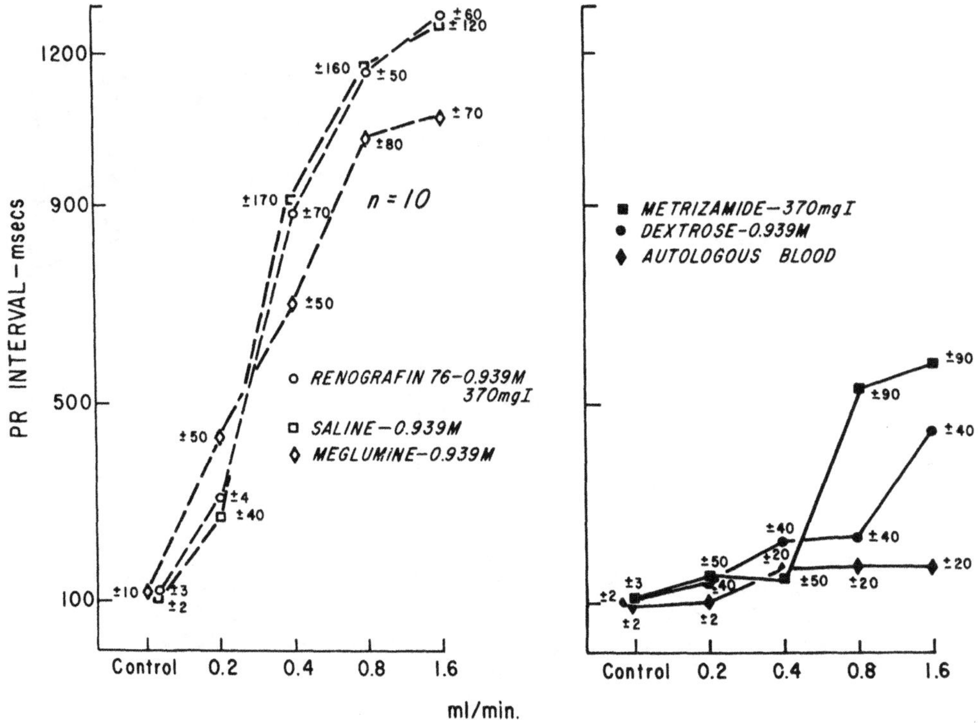


**Fig. 2.** Dose rate response for contrast media and other hyperosmolal solutions on atrioventricular nodal activity (PR interval) in the dog. [Reproduced from [4] with permission]

## Toxic Mechanism for Electrophysiologic Effects

Most of the adverse electrophysiologic effects seem to be closely related to the degree of hyperosmolality of the contrast media. Inhibition of sinoatrial nodal automaticity shows a dose-response relationship to the osmolality of the solution injected into the coronary artery [8]. Infusion of hyperosmolar ionic solutions into the sinoatrial or

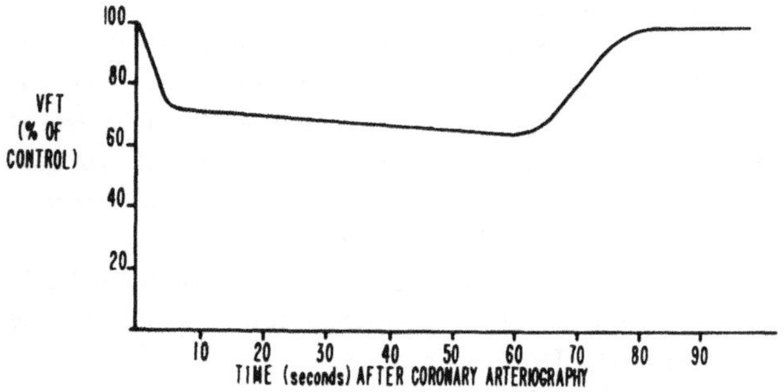


**Fig. 3.** Temporal changes in ventricular fibrillation threshold (VFT) after intracoronary injection of meglumine sodium diatrizoate (Renografin 76). Within seconds there is an abrupt decrease in VFT. This is followed by a further gradual decline. This is a smoothed curve derived from more than 200 fibrillations in 80 animals. [Reproduced from [6] with permission]

atrioventricular nodal arteries causes a dose-related response similar to that caused by ionic contrast media (Fig. 1, 2). Likewise, Popio et al. [9] showed that each of the electrophysiologic effects of ionic contrast media could be reproduced by injections of hyperosmolar solutions of dextrose (equiosmolar with MSD, 370 mg/iodine/ml (Renografin 76) but were not elicited by the injection of a saline solution containing sodium ions at a concentration equivalent with the sodium ions in MSD (Renografin 76). Finally, the nonionic media with lower osmolality induce smaller electrophysiologic alterations.

Although hyperosmolality may be the major factor responsible for electrophysiologic toxicity, a deficiency in ambient calcium ions must exert some influence. Ionic contrast media containing chelating agents cause a greater propensity for ventricular fibrillation compared to media without chelating agents [5]. Moreover, addition of calcium ions to ionic contrast media reduces the propensity for ventricular fibrillation. Older studies indicate that the frequency of ventricular fibrillation is also increased with ionic contrast media containing less than an emperically determined optimal concentration of sodium ions.

## Hemodynamic Effects

### Global Left Ventricular (LV) Function

Dogs were prepared with high fidelity solid state pressure gauges or fluid filled catheters in the LV apex and a pair of ultrasonic dimension crystals on opposing endocardial surfaces of the LV. The LV pressure and dimension signals were differentiated to give LV dp/dt and dD/dt (rate of change of dimension). The latter parameter reflects the velocity of contraction and is an ejection phase index of LV contractile state.

MSD (Renografin 76) caused a biphasic response in the normal dog consisting of initial depression in LV function characterized by decreases in arterial pressure, LV peak systolic pressure (LVP), peak dp/dt, $dtp/dt_{50}$, and slight increase in LV end diastolic pressure (LVEDP) [10]. After 10 s from the start of the injection, AP, LVP, peak dp/dt and $dp/dt_{50}$ increased above control, indicating an augmentation of LV contractile function. Responses were qualitatively similar in open chest anesthetized dogs and conscious dogs.

In this same preparation and under identical experimental conditions the nonionic contrast medium, metrizamide, caused no myocardial depression but produced a monophasic response consisting of increases in LVP, peak dp/dt, and $dp/dt_{50}$. Likewise, an ionic contrast medium with calcium ions, meglumine sodium calcium metrizoate, caused only increases in parameters of LV contractile state.

In another series of experiments the effects on LV dynamics of monomeric ionic contrast media were compared with ionic and nonionic contrast media with lower osmolality [11]. The contrast media compared were sodium iothalamate, P-286 (ioxyglate, Guerbet), metrizamide (Sterling-Winthrop), P297 (Guerbet), and iopamidol (Bracco). The latter three media are nonionic. All media were prepared in solutions with identical iodine concentrations.

The average values for each variable of LV function during the control period and during the peak of the response are displayed in Fig. 4. The maximum depression in LV function occurred within the first 10 s from the start of the intracoronary injection.

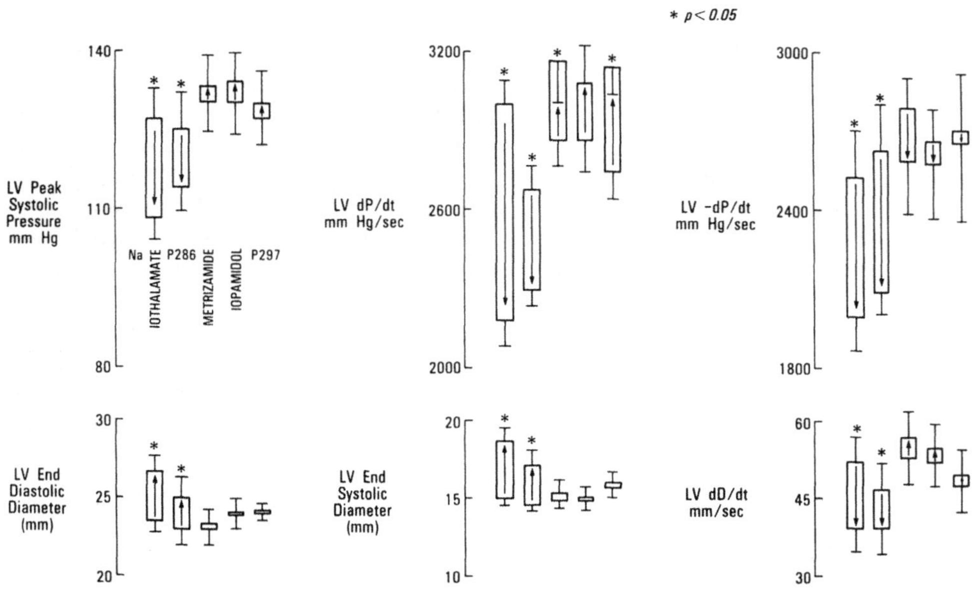


**Fig. 4.** Block diagrams depict the maximum changes in parameters of LV function during the first 10 s after intracoronary injection of two ionic [sodium iothalamate and P-286 (ioxyglate)] and three nonionic media (metrizamide, P-297, and iopamidol). For each parameter, one end of each block represents the control value and the other end the value at the peak of the response. The direction of the changes is indicated by the arrow in each block. [Reproduced from [11] with permission]

Sodium iothalamate caused the most severe decreases in LVP, peak dp/dt and dD/dt and produced significant increases in LV end diastolic and end systolic diameters. The monacid dimer P-286 (ioxyglate) also caused significant decreases in LVP, peak dp/dt, and dD/dt and increases in LV dimensions. The three nonionic contrast media caused no drepression in LV function. The actions of these three agents were similar to each other.

## Segmental Left Ventricular Function. Influence of Regional Myocardial Ischemia

Coronary ateriography is generally performed in patients with segmental myocardial ischemia. However, most studies evaluating the myocardial toxicity of contrast media have used preparations with normal coronary blood flow. In order to compare the effects of contrast media on myocardial function in the normal state and in the presence of segmental myocardial ischemia, the experimental preparation shown in Fig. 5 was employed [13]. Global parameters of LV contractile function were assessed by the catheter in the LV apex which provides LVP and dp/dt. Segmental myocardial function was monitored by a pair of ultrasonic dimension crystals implanted facing each other 1 cm apart in a subendocardial position in the region destined to become ischemic during coronary arterial stenosis. This experimental preparation has been described in detail previously [13]. The signals form the crystals provided a continuous measure of myocardial segment length and this signal was electronically differentiated to obtain rate of segment contraction (dL/dt). The effects of intracoronary injection of contrast media

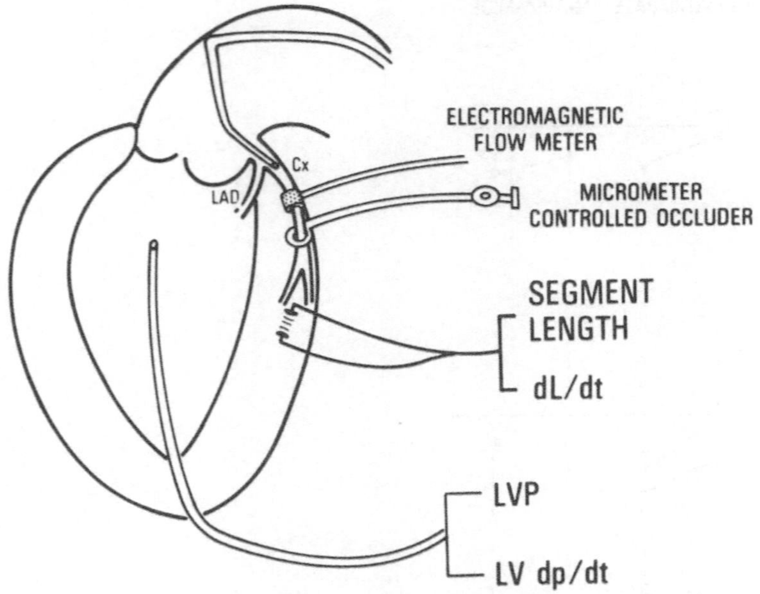


**Fig. 5.** Experimental model used for the study of the effects of contrast media on global and regional contractile function in the normal state and in the presence of regional myocardial ischemia. Ultrasonic crystals were placed 1 cm apart in the subendocardial layer of the LV wall in the area supplied by the circumflex (Cx) coronary artery. Critical coronary arterial stenosis was produced by a micrometer-controlled occluder on the Cx artery. [Reproduced from [16] with permission]

were evaluated in the normal state and after a micrometer-controlled occluder had caused a slight reduction in resting coronary blood flow (critical coronary arterial stenosis, CAS).

In the normal state the ionic contrast media, MSD (Renografin 76) caused a biphasic response consisting of an initial depression in regional contractile function characterized by increases in end diastolic segment length (EDL) and end systolic segment length (ESL) and decreases in dL/dt (Fig. 6). This was followed by an augmentation in segmental contractile state characterized by decreases in segment lengths and increases in extent of contraction and dL/dt.

In the presence of regional myocardial ischemia (CAS), MSD caused a more profound initial depression in regional contractile function. This effect persisted and replaced the secondary positive inotropic effect observed in the normal state (Fig. 6).

A monomeric ionic media with calcium ions (meglumine sodium calcium metrizoate) and a nonionic media (metrizamide) caused no myocardial depression in either the normal or ischemic state (Fig. 6). These contrast media produced only positive inotropic effects.

In the same experimental model the effects of ioxyglate (Hexabrix) and ioxyglate with calcium ions were compared with MSD and metrizamide in the normal and regional ischemic states [14] (Fig. 7). All contrast media were prepared in solutions with identical iodine concentrations. In the normal state MSD produced an early (0–10 s) decrease in regional contractile state followed by a late (10–20 s) rebound augmentation in contractile state. In the presence of regional ischemia the depression of regional contractile function in response to MSD was prolonged (Fig. 7). Ioxyglate induced a similar biphasic

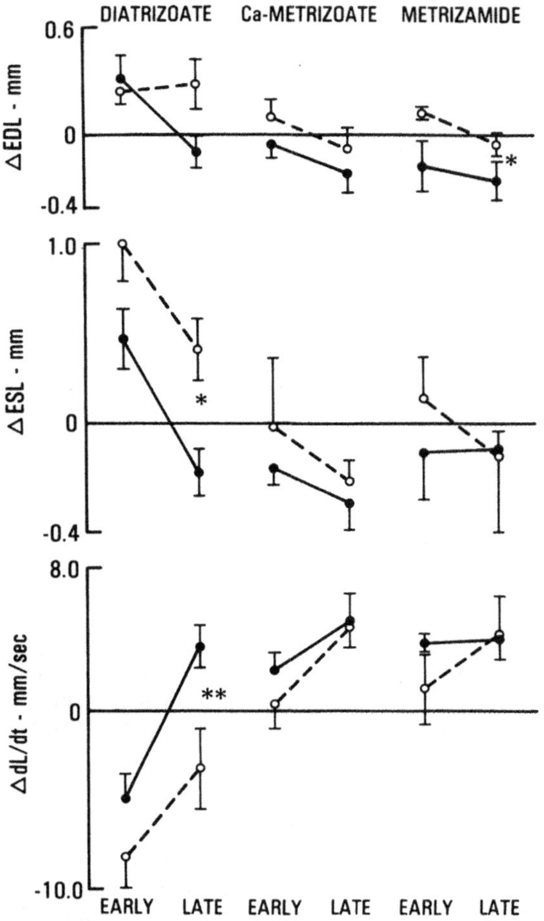


**Fig. 6.** Graph compares the effects of three contrast media on segmental LV function in the normal state and in the presence of regional myocardial ischemia. [Reproduced from [13] with permission]

response in the normal state although the initial depression of myocardial contractility was significantly less than that observed with MSD. The negative effects of ioxyglate were *not* intensified in the presence of segmental ischemia. Ioxyglate with added calcium ions and metrizamide produced only augmentation in parameters of regional LV contractile function in the normal state. Ioxyglate with calcium caused a slight transient initial decrease in dL/dt in the ischemic state while metrizamide caused only increases in dL/dt. In both the normal and ischemic states, ioxylate and ioxyglate with calcium ions caused less myocardial depression than MSD.

The above studies have consistently shown that nonionic contrast media cause no myocardial depression but actually induce a slight positive inotropic effect. However, the prototype nonionic media, metrizamide, is hydrolytically unstable. This and its expense have rendered the media less than ideal for cardiovascular angiographic studies. In recent years newer nonionic media have been developed which are hydrolytically

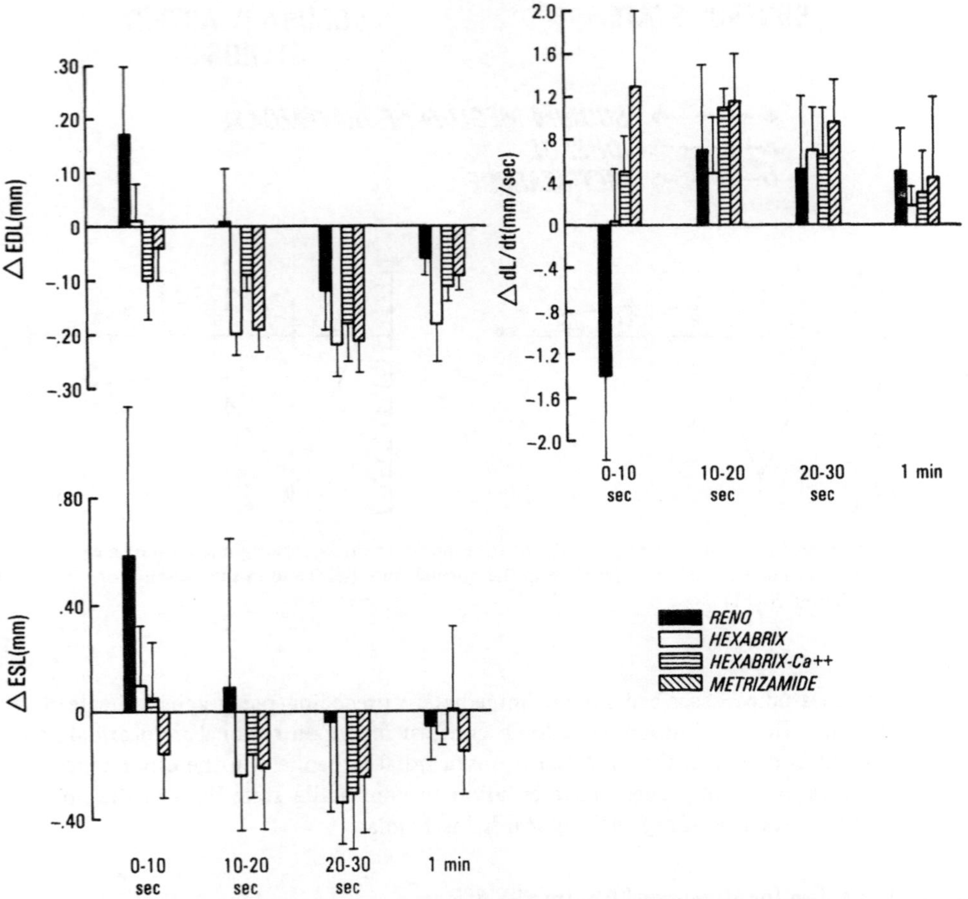


**Fig. 7.** Graph shows the effects of four contrast media on dL/dt in the normal (left) and ischemic states (right). The absolute changes are indicated at various time intervals during the first minute after the start of the intracoronary injection [reproduced from [14] with the permission of author and Invest. Radiol.]

stable and may be financially realistic for use in angiographic procedures requiring large volumes of contrast media. The effects of one of these new hydrolytically stable non-ionic media, iohexol, was compared with MSD and metrizamide in the experimental model of segmental myocardial ischemia. The effects of each agent on regional contractility were compared in the normal state and in the presence of regional ischemia (critical coronary arterial stenosis).

In the normal state, MSD caused an initial transient decrease in rate of segment contraction (dL/dt), which subsided in less than 10 s (Fig. 8). With CAS, this ionic contrast media caused a more severe and prolonged decrease in dL/dt, which did not return to control within the 2-min observation period. In contradistinction, iohexol caused a mild increase in dL/dt, which returned to control within 1 min. With CAS the changes caused by iohexol were not significantly different from those in the normal state. The responses to metrizamide were similar to those of iohexol.

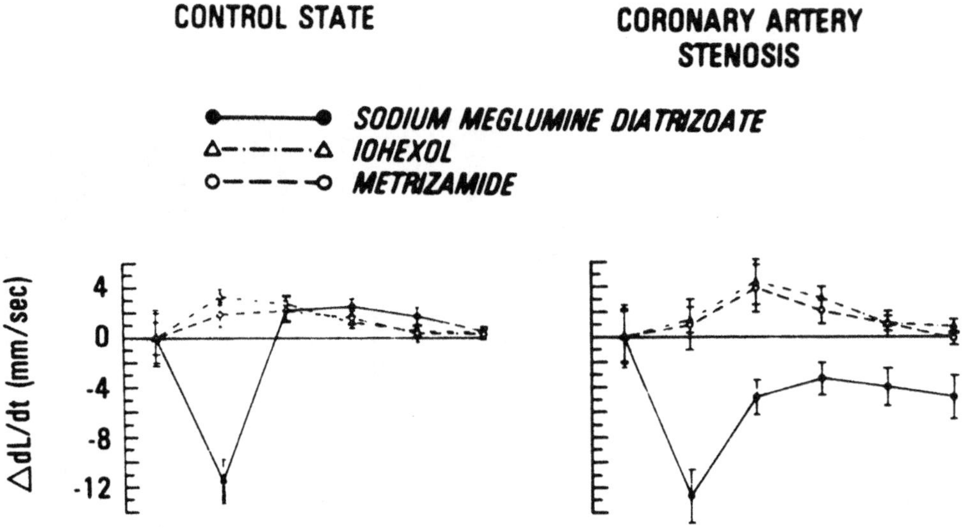


**Fig. 8.** Graph shows the absolute changes in dL/dt in response to intracoronary injection of meglumine sodium diatrizoate, iohexol, and metrizamide in the normal state (left) and in the presence of regional myocardial ischemia (right)

The three studies described in the immediately preceding paragraphs indicate that the deleterious effects of monomeric ionic contrast media on regional myocaridal contraction are accentuated in the presence of myocardial ischemia. On the other hand, the nonionic media cause only slight augmentation in contractile state both in the normal state and in the presence of regional myocardial ischemia.

### Toxic Mechanism for Myocardial Contractile Effects

The lack of any myocardial depressant effect of nonionic contrast materials, in spite of an osmolality more than twofold that of normal serum, prompted us to reexamine the notion that hyperosmolality per se is at least partially responsible for the myocardial depression caused by contrast media. In a recent series of experiments [15] the effects of intracoronary injection of hyperosmolal solutions of glucose and mannitol on LV dynamics were assessed. Surprisingly, there was a progressive increase in parameters of LV contractile state with increasing osmolality of these two nonionic or molecular solutions. On the other hand, intracoronary injection of hyperosmolal ionic solutions (saline) cause severe myocardial depression. These results suggest that hyperosmolality alone has a positive, rather than a negative, inotropic influence. However, an imbalance of single valence cations, particularly sodium, exerts an important negative inotropic effect.

A study in our laboratory [12] and early work by Salvesen, et al. showed that an imbalance in sodium and calcium ions in ionic contrast media is an important mechanistic factor for myocardial depression. In our study a close temporal relationship was observed between decrease in ionic calcium levels after intracoronary injection of MSD and depression in myocardial contractility. The decline in the levels of ionic calcium was not merely a dilution effect since the ratio of ionic to total calcium also fell, suggesting that the contrast material caused chelation. Moreover, addition of MSD (Renografin 76) to blood in vitro produces a dose-related decline in ionized calcium; this implies that some component of this contrast media binds calcium ions or at least causes a decrease in bioactivity of calcium ions [16]. This effect has been implicated as the cause of rare instances of electromechanical dissociation occurring during clinical coronary arteriography [16].

## References


1. Adams DF, Fraser DB, Abrams HL (1973) The complications of coronary arteriography. Circulation 48:609–618
2. Adams DF, Abrams HL (1979) Complications of coronary arteriography: A follow-up report. Cardiovasc Radiol 2:89–96
3. Higgins CB (1980) Overview and methods used for the study of cardiovascular actions of contrast materials. Invest Radiol [Suppl] 15:S188–S193
4. Higgins CB (1977) Effects of contrast media on the conducting system of the heart. Radiology 124:599–606
5. Thomson KR, Violante MR, Kenyon T, et al. (1978) Reduction of ventricular fibrillation using calcium-enriched Renografin 76. Invest Radiol 13:238–240
6. Wolf GL (1980) The fibrillatory propensities of contrast agents. Invest Radiol [Suppl] 15: S208–S214
7. Wolf GL, Mulry CS, Kilzer L, et al. (1980) New angiographic agents with less fibrillatory propensity. Invest Radiol 16:320–323
8. White CW, Eckberg DL, Ihaska T, et al. (1976) Effects of angiographic contrast media on sinoatrial nodal function. Cardiovasc Res 10:214–223
9. Popio KA, Ross AM, Oravec JM, et al. (1978) Identification and description of separate mechanisms for two components of Renografin cardiotoxicity. Circulation 58:520–528
10. Higgins CB, Schmidt W (1978) Direct and reflex myocaridal effects of intracoronary contrast materials in the anesthetized and conscious dog. Invest Radiol 13:205–216
11. Higgins CB, Sovak M, Schmidth WS, Kelley MJ, Newell JD (1980) Direct myocardial effects of intracoronary administration of new contrast materials with low osmolality. Invest Radiol 15:39–46
12. Higgins CB, Schmidt W (1978) Alterations in calcium levels of coronary sinus blood during coronary arteriography in the dog. Circulation 58:512–519
13. Green CE, Higgins CB, Kelley MJ, et al. (1981) Effects of intracoronary administration of contrast materials on left ventricular function in the presence of critical coronary artery stenosis: Advantages of newer contrast materials over standard materials. Cardiovasc Radiol 4:110–116
14. Deutsch AL, Gerber KH, Haigler FH, Higgins CB (to be published) Effects of low osmolality contrast materials on coronary hemodynamics, myocardial function and coronary sinus osmolality in normal and ischemic states. Invest Radiol
15. Newell JD, Higgins CB, Kelley MJ, et al. (1980) The influence of hyperosmolality on left ventricular contractile state. Disparate effects of nonionic and ionic solutions. Invest Radiol 15:363–370
16. Caulfield JB, Zir L, Harthorne JW (1975) Blood calcium levels in the presence of arteriographic contrast material. Circulation 52:119–123

# Effects on Cardiac Function of Contrast Media Used in Angiography: An Experimental Study

P. Besse, M. Sicart, S. Bonoron-Adele, L. Tariosse, Ph. D'Agatha, and G. Delorme

## Introduction

Angiocardiographists are daily confronted with the problem of toxicity of the contrast media used. Most often it results in ECG changes and blood pressure decrease or fall. Fortunately, few accidents occur. They must be feared all the more as cardiac function is altered: myocardial failure, variant angina. Many workers have tried to determine precisely the advantages and the disadvantages of the various media used.

We chose to study the specific muscular function on the preparation of the papillary muscle isolated from the cat heart and to study its variations when in touch with the contrast media.

## Methodology

The preparation of the cat's papillary muscle has been studied by several authors and answers to a precise protocol [2, 3]. We consider here three parameters: V max (maximum velocity of shortening), PF (peak of developed force), TPF (time to peak force). The variations of these parameters were measured on series of five muscles, each series being in touch with a contrast medium added at increasing dose to the preparation bath. These parameters were measured a second time during a hypoxia-reoxygenation test. The tested media were Telebrix 38 (Na ioxitalamate, Guerbet), Radioselectan (Na amidotrizoate, Schering), Hexabrix (Na ioxaglate, Guerbet), Iopamidol 370 and Iopamidol 300 (triiodoisophtaldiamide, Schering).

## Results and Comments

When we compare the effect of contrast media on cardiac contraction parameters, i.e., V max and PF (Fig. 1), we notice that all of them have more or less a cardiodepressive action. As long as the concentration is low, V max and PF are high, showing a positive inotropic effect. But, as soon as the concentration increases, a quick fall of V max and PF appears. The most depressive medium is Telebrix, followed by Radioselectan. Iopamidol 370 is clearly less cardiotoxic than these, but more however, than Iopamidol 300 and Hexabrix. This depression cannot be considered due to the variations of the calcic charge of the bath, which steadily decreases as dilution increases, whatever the medium used.

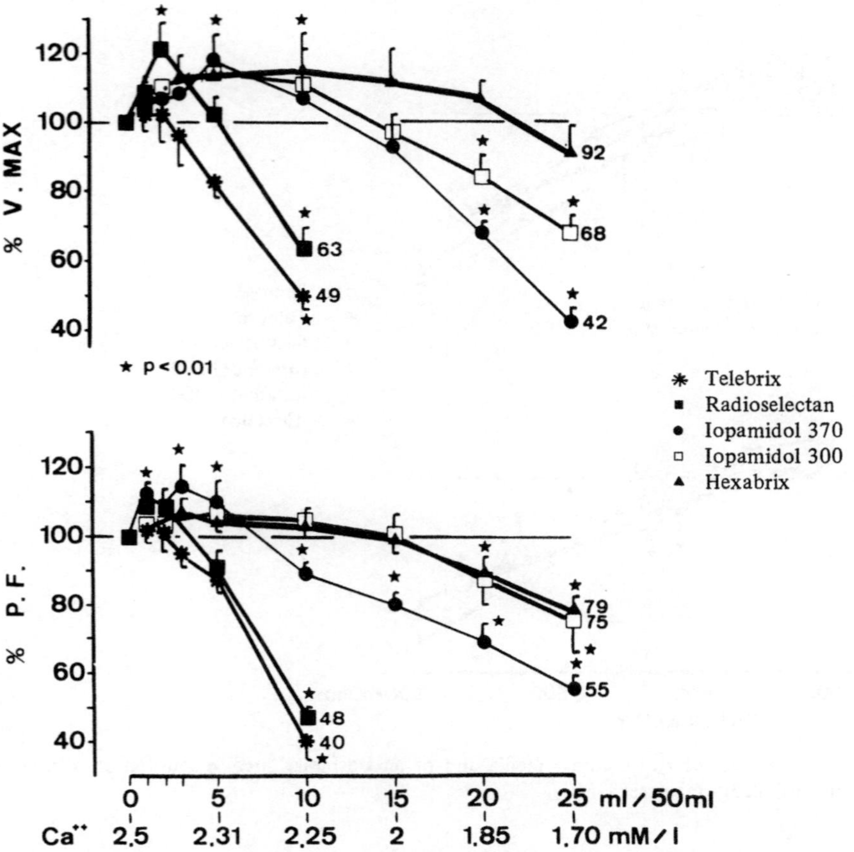


**Fig. 1.** Comparative effects of five contrast media at increasing doses on V max and PF. The calcic concentration of the solution is notified for each dilution

For a same calcic dilution, the effect depends upon the media. So, other factors interfere with the depressive mechanism induced by contrast media. The variations of TPF, which measures the activation time, do not seem involved. While the calcic charge of the bath decreases, TPF quickly falls to a minimum, then becomes normal, and then increases except for Hexabrix, which makes it fall gradually. Moreover, whereas TPF decreases at low concentrations, the inotropism is kept or increased.

When the concentration increases, the reverse phenomenon appears (except for Hexabrix), TPF increases, and the contractility falls. If the modifications of TPF and of the calcic rate do not seem involved in the effect on inotropism, we must notice that the effect of the media is all the more obvious as their osmolality is more important. The osmolality of pure Telebrix is 2060 mOsm, 1750 mOsm for Radioselectan, 1075 mOsm for Iopamidol 370, 770 mOsm for Iopamidol 300, and 680 mOsm for Hexabrix.

When we compare the effects of the various media at isosmolar concentrations to the effect observed with a sucrose dilution at the same osmolality (Fig. 2), we can see that V max and PF graphs are practically superimposable. Up to concentrations of 400 mOsm,

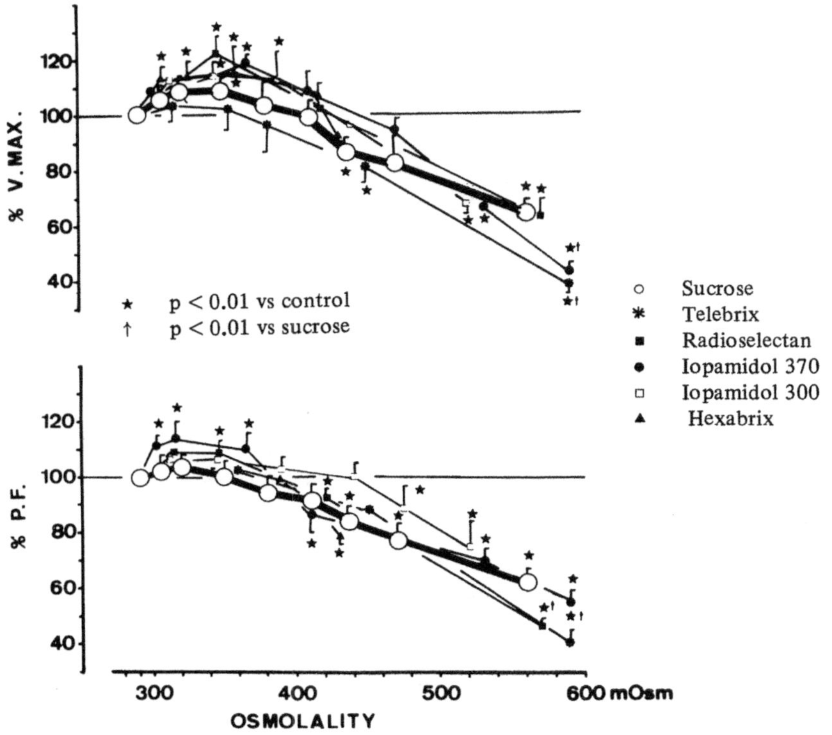


**Fig. 2.** Comparative effects of five contrast media and of an isosmolar sucrose solution on V max and PF, when the osmolality increases

V max and PF are slightly increased, showing a positive inotropic effect independent of the molecule used. Beyond 400 mOsm, PF and V max fall. Differences are not significant from one medium to another, so that the Na differences induced in the bath by the various media do not seem involved (Iopamidol) has no Na, Telebrix has 25.5 g/100 cc, Hexabrix 19.67, and Radioselectan 10). Thus, the contrast media seem to have a cardiodepressive effect correlated with the osmolality they induce. At low concentrations this effect is counterbalanced by a positive inotropic effect since V max and PF are all over control up to 400 mOsm.

The positive inotropic effect at a low concentration was well shown during the study under hypoxia-reoxygenation condition. Iopamidol 300 at 5 ml (340 mOsm) is compared with the test solution and with an isomolar sucrose solution (Fig. 3). We can see that V max and PF fall during hypoxia and are quickly restored by reoxygenation. There is no significant difference between Iopamidol and sucrose whereas these two graphs are higher ($P < 0.01$) than that obtained with the test solution. Thus it seems that the moderate hyperosmolality protects the muscle from hypoxia.

On the contrary, if Telebrix is used at the same dose, the osmolality of the mixture is higher (440 mOsm) and we fall into the cardiodepressive effect zone. But, the isosmolar sucrose solution always has a significant protective effect ($P < 0.01$) (Fig. 4) on V max as well as on PF. Telebrix induces a more important fall than the test and a longer reco-

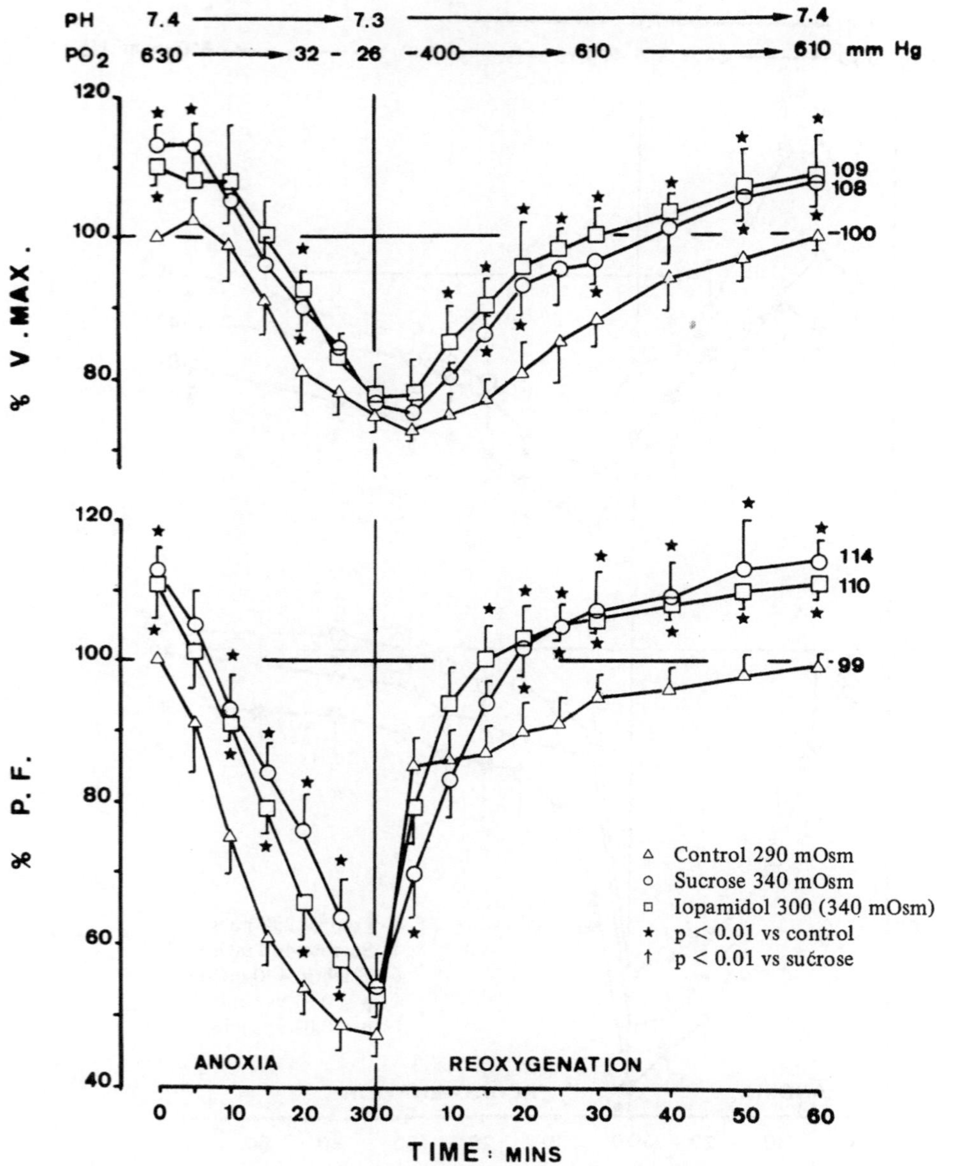


**Fig. 3.** Comparative effects of Iopamidol 300, of an isosmolar sucrose solution, and of a control solution on V max and PF, during the hypoxia-reoxygenation test

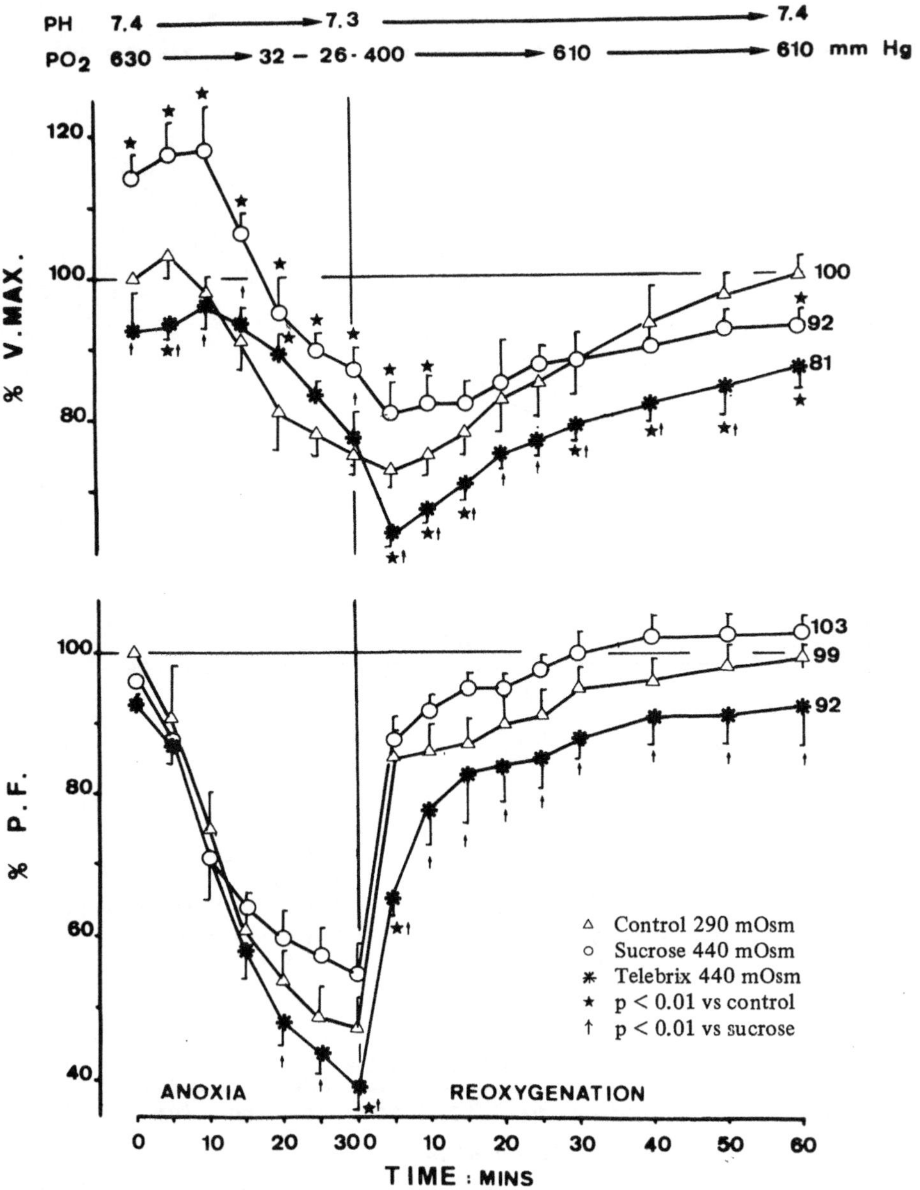


**Fig. 4.** Comparative effects of Telebrix, of an isosmolar sucrose solution and of a control solution on V max and PF during the hypoxia-reoxygenation test

very, thus showing a specific toxicity of the medium; this toxicity appears as significant ($P < 0.01$) compared with the isosmolar solution. Hypoxia shows there an effect which was not appreciable on normal muscles at that same concentration (Fig. 2).

## Conclusion

Therefore, the contrast media exert a complex action on cardiac function. They depend essentially upon the solution osmolality. The role of calcium seems to be unimportant since the concentration of this ion gradually decreases, whereas the inotropic effect is positive at first, then gradually decreases, and finylla becomes negative. Perhaps the Ca effect is hidden by the osmolality of the bath. This effect was shown by Goethals et al. [4] in a dual calcium-osmolality study.

The explanation could be a relative cellular dehydration that would give a calcic cellular hyperconcentration at low osmolalities [1].

Moreover, the study under hypoxia-reoxygenation condition shows that the medium used has to be taken into account: if the contractility graphs are parallel for normal muscles and whatever the medium used at the same osmolality, the hypoxia test affects the muscle: Iopamidol has the same effect as sucrose, i.e., a protective effect at a low osmolality (340 mOsm). On the contrary, Telebrix at the same dose (5 ml) is hyperosmolar (440 mOsm). It has a very clear cardiodepressive action whereas the isoosmolar sucrose solution still protects the muscle. This is due to the Telebrix molecule, which is a Na "rich" acid (25.5 g/100 cc) and which clearly changes the Na concentration of the bath. We must emphasize the fact that Iopamidol is not ionized and does not contain Na. A similar effect was noticed by Goethals et al. [4], correlated with the Na increase in the bath.

From this experimental work it would be hazardous to draw conclusions extrapolated to humans.

The role of calcium seems passive in our study. The effect of adding calcium to the preparation might be beneficial [4], especially at high sodium concentrations.

## References


1. April E, Brandt P (1973) Myofilament lattice studies on isolated fibers. J Gen Physiol 61:490–508
2. Bonoron-Adele S, Besse P, Tariosse L, Bricaud H (1974) Effets des derives nitres sur la contractilite et la relaxation du muscle papillaire en hypoxie et en reoxygenation. Arch Mal Coeur 4:414
3. Brutsaert D, Claes V (1974) Onset of mechanical of mammalian heart muscle in calcium and strontium containing solutions. Circ Res 35: 345–357
4. Goethals M, Adele S, Brutsaert D (1975) Contractility in mammalian heart muscle calcium and osmolality. Circ Res 36:27–33

# Comparison of Iopamidol, Ioxaglate, and Diatrizoate During Coronary Angiography in Dogs

C. A. Evill, G. T. Benness, and R. Hassam

## Introduction

The influence of contrast medium osmolality, and ionic composition on the toxic effects seen during coronary angiography, has received considerable attention. In this laboratory studies were undertaken to examine the influence of contrast medium composition on the blood in the coronary venous sinus, following intracoronary injections [1]. At the same time, changes in ECG and blood pressure parameters were examined. Diatrozoate (as Urografin 76), iopamidol, and sodium/meglumine ioxaglate were compared. In general it was found that iopamidol was the most benign, but the ioxaglate preparation used had a sodium concentration of 205 mEq/liter, which is considerably above physiological.

In view of the possible detrimental effects [2] of the high sodium level in the ioxaglate it was decided to carry out further studies comparing iopamidol with ioxaglate preparations having lower sodium concentrations.

## Methods

Coroary angiography was carried out on six greyhound dogs of either sex, weighing from 28 to 35 kg. The dogs were anesthetized with 10 g intravenous sodium thiopentone. Anesthesia was maintained by a nitrous oxide, oxygen, and halothane mixture, with respiration being controlled by an Oxford ventilator.

Catheters were placed in the left ventricle, and the left coronary artery, via the femoral artery. The left ventricular pressure was differentiated electronically to give a recording of LV dP/dt.

Peak LV dP/dt and depression of the ST segment of the ECG were measured before injection and at 7-s intervals up to 1 min post injection.

Two ioxaglate solutions were prepared, one with a sodium concentration of 140 mEq/liter (physiological), and one with sodium ioxaglate and meglumine ioxaglate in the ratio 10 : 66 by weight (ratio). These solutions were compared with iopamidol, and sodium/meglumine diatrizoate (Urografin 76). All contrast media had an iodine concentration of 370 mgI/ml.

Each dog received two injections of each contrast agent in random order. The injection volume was 10 ml, delivered at 1 ml/s by hand injection. All injections were monitored fluoroscopically to ensure delivery of the test volume to the coronary artery.

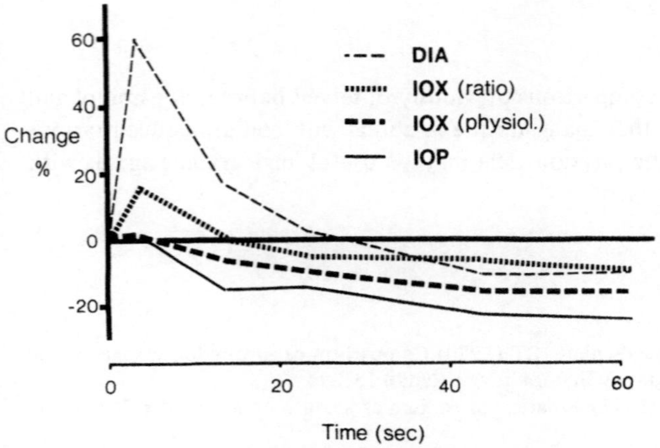


**Fig. 1.** Mean ST segment depression expressed as percent of control values, following contrast medium injection

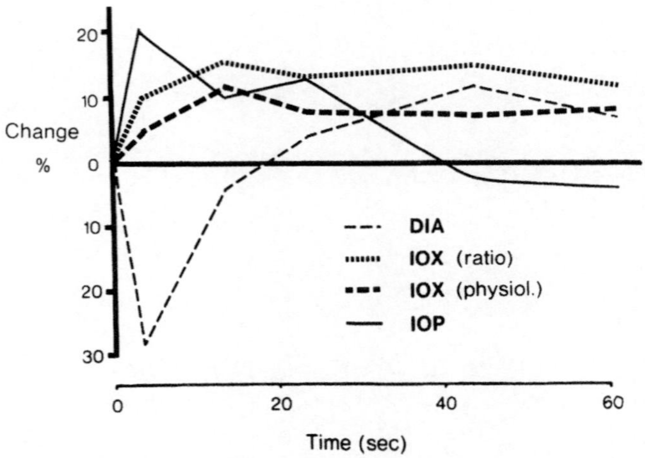


**Fig. 2.** Mean change in peak LV dP/dt following contrast medium injection, expressed as percent of control value

## Results

The results for ST segment depression are shown in Fig. 1. Diatrizoate caused the most marked depression immediately after injection while the changes with the low osmolality agents were relatively minor. Figure 2 shows the changes observed in peak dP/dt. Diatrizoate provoked a marked decrease in cardiac contractility immediately after injection, followed by a rebound after about 20 s. The other three agents, on the other hand, all showed a degree of positive inotropy. This was most rapid with iopamidol but was more prolonged with the ioxaglate preparations.

## Discussion

This limited study confirms the comparisons previously observed between iopamidol and diatrizoate. In addition it shows that ioxaglate preparations with sodium concentrations that more closely approximate the physiological may be useful angiographic agents with a toxicity similar to the nonionic agents.

## References


1. Thomson KR, Evill CA, Fritzche J, Benness GT (1980) Comparison of iopamidol, ioxaglate, and diatrizoate during coronary angiography in dogs. Invest Radiol 15:234
2. Snyder C, Cramer R, Amplatz K (1971) Isolation of sodium as a cause of ventricular fibrillation. Invest Radiol 6:245

# Effects of Iohexol on Heart Functions During Coronary Arteriography in Dogs

B. Trägårdh and P. Lynch

Iohexol is a new nonionic contrast medium with low toxicity, suitable for cardiovascular use. During coronary arteriography in dogs we compared diatrizoate (Urografin 76%), metrizoate with added calcium ions (Isopaque Coronar), metrizamide (Amipaque), 711 (a nonionic compound), and iohexol regarding their effects on electrical and mechanical heart functions. ECG was recorded during right and left coronary injections in intact dogs. Contractile force, left ventricular pressure, aortic pressure, and aortic blood flow were recorded during left coronary injections.

The nonionic media prolonged the PQ, QRS, and QT intervals significantly less than diatrizoate. This smaller effect of the nonionic media on cardiac conduction may decrease the frequency of AV blocks and of ventricular fibrillation, which occur during coronary arteriography.

The nonionic media and metrizoate with calcium ions reduced contractile force, LVP, LV dp/dt, stroke volume, and stroke work significantly less than diatrizoate. No significant differences were observed between the various contrast media regarding the increased heart work, which follows the initially reduced pumping efficiency.

No significant differences were found between the nonionic contrast media in regard to the recorded parameters.

We conclude that in comparison to diatrizoate the new nonionic medium iohexol like metrizamide produces less alterations of the electrical and mechanical functions of the heart during coronary arteriography in dogs.

# The Importance of Electrolyte Shifts and Calcium Binding on Cardiotoxicity of Contrast Media*

G. Hellige, D. Baller, A. Hoeft, H. Korb, H. G. Wolpers, and J. Zipfel

The summary of our experimental and clinical examinations on cardiac side effects of coronary angiography is that the acute phenomena are mainly caused by physicochemical properties of the contrast media [1, 2]. This seems to be true in case of the well-known hemodynamic side effects: acute cardiodepression followed by a delayed positive inotropic effect and long-lasting increase of coronary blood flow combined with reduction of coronary vascular resistance and increase of coronary venous $O_2$-saturation. The same properties seem to be responsible for the typical electrocardiographic effects: hypervoltage combined with shift of the electrical axis of the heart, disturbance of electrical activation- and repolarization waves and dysrhythmias.

These side effects are accompanied by electrolyte shifts in the coronary venous blood, dependent on the physicochemical properties and ion composition of the used contrast media. Common ionic contrast media cause an increase of osmolality, decreases of calcium and potassium content, and, dependent on their sodium content, changes of plasma sodium levels. The electrolyte shifts results from dilution of plasma ions by the contrast media themselves, from watershift caused by hyperosmolality, and, as discussed later on, from calcium-binding properties of the angiographic media. First of all the consequence of this electrolyte constellation is an imbalance of the sodium to calcium ratio of plasma particularly in the case of high sodium content of contrast medium or strong calcium binding [2, 3]. In accordance with the basic knowledge of exitation-contraction coupling of the heart muscle, the degree of increase of this ratio correlates well with the negative inotropic effect of the contrast medium. E.g., the mentioned high sodium preparations are more cardiodepressive than commonly used sodium meglumine diatrizoates with physiologic sodium concentration. Resulting from this theory are two possiblities for prevention of cardiodepression. First the compensation of an increase of this ratio by addition of calcium to the contrast medium [4] and second the use of substances without influence on the sodium to calcium ratio like the nonionic metrizamide or iopamidol. Both approaches prevent severe cardiodepression as is well known in practical use [4, 5]. The addition of calcium reduces the negative inotropic effect markedly but not completely. This incomplete reduction is in our opinion due to the ineffectiveness of added calcium on the sinus slowing, which may additionally cause a negative frequency inotropism. Metrizamide and iopamidol cause no cardiodepression but indeed a positive inotropic effect, which will be discussed later on.

---

* Supported by the Deutsche Forschungsgemeinschaft, SFB 89 – Kardiologie Göttingen

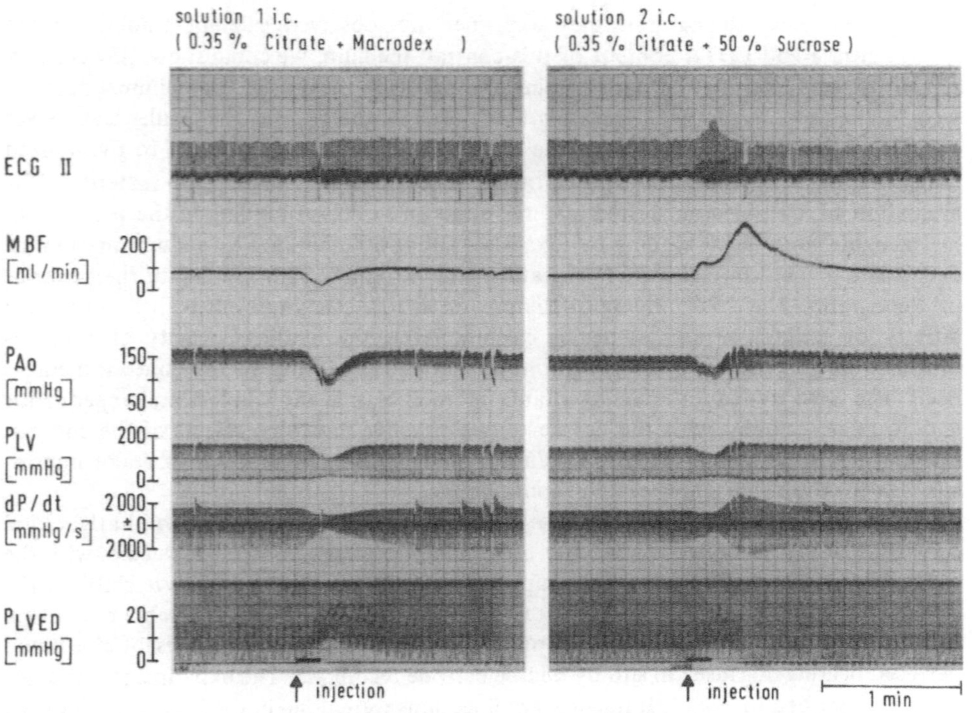


**Fig. 1.** Effects of an isoosmotic (*left*) and a hyperosmotic (*right*) sodium citrate solution on ECG, myocardial blood flow, aortic and left ventricular pressure, dP/dt, and left ventricular diastolic pressure

The validity of this theory of the importance of the sodium to calcium ratio for cardiac side effects of contrast media is easily examined by use of different test solutions with model compounds [2]. Figure 1 demonstrates one example of a lot of tested solutions. A hyperviscous sodium citrate-saline solution which causes an increase of the sodium to calcium ratio as described above leads to a marked cardiodepression. Compared to the corresponding contrast medium, however, no secondary positive inotropic effect, no increase of coronary blood flow, and no hypervoltage in ECG is achieved. The complete picture of coronarographic side effects requires additionally, as demonstrated in the right part of the figure, hyperosmolality of the injected solution, obtained by addition of highly concentrated sucrose. The secondary positive inotropic effect of common ionic contrast media and the primary positive inotropic effect of nonionic media should, in our opinion, be interpreted on the basis of the hyperosmolality of contrast media. A simple explanation without postulation of baroreflectory counterregulation can be given based on systematic examinations of Koch-Weser in 1963 on the influence of osmolality on myocardial contractility. These results indicate that hypertonic solutions improve contractility by increase of intracellular calcium levels due to a dehydration of the myocardial cells, which is in our opinion also to be expected during the presence of contrast media in the coronary vascular bed [2]. The above-mentioned overproportional decrease of ionic calcium concentration in coronary venous blood was first described by investigators using Renografin; they explained the observed calcium binding by the sodium citrate and EDTA content of this contrast medium. We could show, however, by in vitro experiments that calcium binding also occurs in the presence of minimal doses or even in the absence of added chelating agents due to the contrast molecules themselves [6]. This effect is demonstrable by the relation of total calcium content to the ionized calcium level in a saline solution in the presence of different contrast materials. The evaluation of the different tested material shows no calcium binding in the presence of metrizamide, only 15% binding by ioxaglate, about 40% binding by sodium meglumine diatrizoate as used in Germany (Urografin), and extremely high binding in the presence of Renografin. The 73% binding of Renografin at low calcium levels is due to the high affinity of sodium citrate; at higher calcium levels the binding capacity of citrate is saturated and the slope equals Urografin, indicating the affinity of the contrast medium itself. The same graduation is demonstrable in blood plasma and whole blood experiments and correlates closely with the degree of the negative inotropic effects of the contrast materials. This indicates that the calcium binding within the blood is of major importance for the influence on myocardial contractility.

All acute side effects may be caused indirectly by electrolyte shifts within the blood contrast material mixture without any direct contact of the contrast molecules with the cardiac muscle cells. This theory presupposes that the observed electrolyte shifts in the coronary venous blood reach and affect the cardiac cells. We believe to be able to confirm this by recent experiments with recordings of transmembrane potentials of the blood perfused beating dog heart in situ by microelectrode technique. The experimental arrangement is described in Fig. 2. Intracoronary injections were done in the LAD branch of the left coronary artery; venous blood samples were taken from the great cardiac vein; the membrane potential was recorded in the supply area of the LAD. Stable positions of the microelectrodes were achieved by a special technique of support of the heart and soft coupling of the micro glass electrodes [7]. The right part of Fig. 2 shows parallel recordings

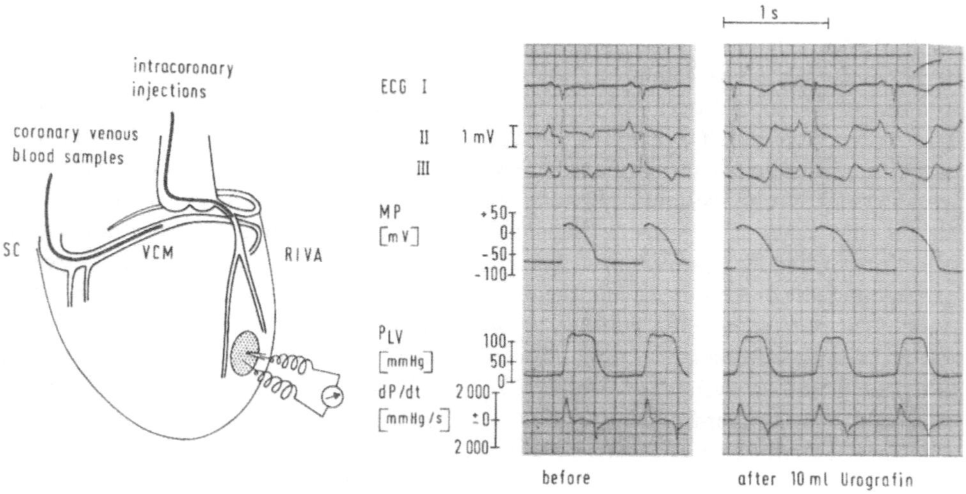


**Fig. 2.** Arrangement of microelectrode experiments (*left*) and affects of coronary angiography on ECG, transmembrane potential, ventricular pressure, and dP/dt (*right*) compared to control conditions

of ECG, transmembrane potential, and ventricular pressure before and under coronary angiography, indicating a hyperpolarization of resting potentials and prolongation of action potentials by contrast materials. Comparative experiments show that these effects are dependent on the injected contrast medium and correspond to the isolated effects of the accompaning electrolyte shifts. Low sodium diatrizoates, e.g., Urografin, show, as described in the figure, hyperpolaization and prolongation due to combined low potassium and hypocalcemia; high sodium diatrizoates show, corresponding to the increase of sodium content, an excessive prolongation of action potential. Metrizamide affects membrane potential less due to the reduced shifts in electrolyte concentrations [7]. The close correlation of plasma electrolyte shifts with effects on membrane potential proves the efficacy of these plasma ion alterations on the cardiac cell and supports thereby the assumption that acute cardiac side effects are mainly caused by physicochemical properties of the contrast materials. On the other hand these electrophysiological side effects of angiography may be helpful in explaining not only disturbance in cardiac exitation but also disturbances in function of other cells with electrical activity, e.g., smooth muscle cells, receptor cells, and neurons.

## References


1. Hellige G, Baller D, Prennschütz-Schützenau H, Sigmund-Duchanova H, Zipfel J (1978) Analyse von Kontrastmittelwirkungen auf die Funktion des linken Ventrikels. Z Kardiol 67:222
2. Hellige G (1981) Elektrolytverschiebungen durch Kontrastmittel und ihre Rückwirkung auf die Funktion des Herzens. In: Lang E, Weikl A (eds) Kontrastmittel in der Kardiologie. Steinkopff, Darmstadt, pp 35–51
3. Zipfel J, Baller D, Karsch R, Rentrop P, Hellige G (1979) Cardiotoxity of contrast media used in coronary angiography. Decrease by correcting intravascular $Na^+/Ca^{++}$ – imbalance. Circulation 59, 60 [Suppl II]:162
4. Zipfel J, Baller D, Karsch R, Rentrop P, Hellige G (1980) Decrease in cardiotoxity of contrast media in coronary angiography by addition of calcium ions. Clin Cardiol 3:178–183
5. Zipfel J, Baller D, Blanke H, Ensink FBM, Karsch R, Rentrop P, Wiegand VW, Wolpers HG, Hellige G (1980) Möglichkeiten der Reduktion kardialer Nebenwirkungen der Angiokardiographie – Klinische Vergleichsstudie unter Verwendung des Kaliziumzusatzes und Einsatz eines nichtionischen Kontrastmittels. Klin Wochenschr 58:1339–1346
6. Wolpers HG, Baller D, Ensink FBM, Zipfel J, Hellige G (1981) Influence of arteriographic contrast media on the $Na^+/Ca^{++}$-ratio in blood. Cardiovasc Intervent Radiol 4:8–13
7. Wolpers HG, Baller D, Ensink FBM, Hoeft A, Korb H, Hellige G (1982) Einfluß von Röntgenkontrastmitteln auf das Membranpotential am schlagenden Herzen. Z Kardiol 71:82–86

# Regional Myocardial Hemodynamic and Metabolic Effects of Ionic and Nonionic Contrast Media in the Normal and Ischemic State*

Ch. B. Higgins[1] and K. H. Gerber[2]

## Introduction

Intracoronary injection of ionic contrast media produces myocardial depression [1, 2] which is apparently related to the induction of an imbalance in the ratio of sodium to calcium ions in the myocardium [2]. An approach to alleviating the myocardial toxicity of contrast media has been the development of nonionic contrast media which have a lower osmolality and are essentially devoid of sodium and other single valence cations. The nonionic contrast media, metrizamide, which was the initial nonionic contrast agent introduced, has no sodium and has approximately one-third of the osmolality of the standard ionic contrast media. It has been shown to cause no negative inotropic effects [1]. Unfortunately, this medium is hydrolytically unstable and must be reconstituted from the lypholized form just prior to use. Iohexol is a new nonionic contrast agent which is hydrolytically stable and has a shelf life similar to diatrizoate preparations.

The purposes of the current study were: (1) to compare the myocardial contractile effects of nonionic contrast materials (metrizamide and iohexol) with the ionic contrast medium, sodium meglumine diatrizoate, which is currently used for coronary arteriography in the United States; (2) to determine the alterations in chemical composition of coronary sinus blood after intracoronary injection of these three contrast media; and (3) to compare the effects on myocardial contractility of each of the three agents when injected into a coronary artery without coronary stenosis and with a critical coronary artery stenosis (CAS). The latter goal was important since most previous studies on the myocardial effects of contrast media have utilized models with normal coronary blood flow. These models are not closely germane to clinical coronary arteriography, which is frequently performed on patients with obstructive coronary disease and regional myocardial ischemia.

---

* This research project was supported in part by a research grant from the Sterling Winthrop Research Institute

1 Recipient of US Public Health Service Career Development Grant Award no. K04HL2001 from the National Heart, Lung, and Blood Institute

2 Recipient of the NIH Training Grant Program Award no. NIHPHSHL07447-01

## Materials and Methods

The study was conducted on a total of 14 mongrel dogs, weighing 20–32 kg. All animals were premedicated with morphine sulfate, 1.5 mg/kg subcutaneously, and anesthetized with pentobarbital sodium, 25 mg/kg intravenously. Respiration was mechanically controlled with a Harvard respiratory at 12 cycles/min.

The contrast materials studied in each dog were sodium meglumine diatrizoate (R76) (Renografin 76, Squibb Co.), iohexol (C545, Sterlin-Winthrop Co.), and metrizamide (Amipaque, Sterling-Winthrop Co.). Each material was prepared in a solution of 370 mg iodine/ml.

Two experimental models were used in this study. One was used to study the effects on chemical composition of coronary sinus blood (experimental model 1) and the other to study the effects on contractile state (experimental model 2). In six dogs, the experimental protocol was designed to study the effects of the contrast media on left ventricular contractile function in the normal state and in the presence of critical coronary arterial stenosis. In these animals the proximal portion of the circumflex coronary artery was dissected free to accept a micrometer controlled snare-type coronary artery occluder. A catheter was positioned in the outflow tract of the left ventricle (LV) through a small apical stab wound. A stable position in the LV outflow tract was confirmed fluoroscopically in order to avoid catheter entrapment in the LV apex. Left ventricular pressure (LVP) was measured with a Statham P23 strain gauge manometer, and this signal was also differentiated using an operational amplifier differentiator to yield LV dp/dt. A modified Judkins catheter was introduced into the femoral artery and advanced into the circumflex coronary artery under fluoroscopic guidance. A pair of ultrasonic dimension crystals were positioned through small myocardial stab wounds in a subendocardial position in the region destined to become ischemic during the coronary stenosis.

The ultrasonic dimension system continuously measures transit time between the piezoelectric crystals and thereby monitors instantaneous myocardial segment length. Segment length (L) was also electronically differentiated to provide a measure of the velocity of contraction of the myocardial segment (dL/dt). Left ventricular pressure (LVP), LV dp/dt, segment length (L), and dL/dt were recorded on a multichannel recorder during the control period prior to each intracoronary contrast injection and at 10 s, 20 s, 30 s, 1 min, and 2 min after each injection. Following injection of contrast media in the normal state, the occluder was gradually tightened until an initial increase in end diastolic segment length (EDL) or end systolic segment length (ESL), or a decrease in contraction velocity (dL/dt) was observed.

In eight additional animals, a polyethylene catheter with a flared tip was inserted through a small incision into the coronary sinus and held in place with a purse string suture. The incision in the coronary sinus was located approximately 2 cm proximal to its ostium. The position of the catheter tip in the coronary sinus was confirmed by a small injection of contrast material under fluoroscopic observation. A modified Judkins left coronary artery catheter was introduced into the right femoral artery and advanced into the left coronary artery under fluoroscopic guidance.

After injection of 3 ml of contrast media, fluoroscopic visualization was used to time the peak opacification and clearance of contrast material from the coronary sinus after coronary arterial injection. The time of peak opacification (Tp) averaged 6.6 s, and the time of clearance of contrast from the sinus (Tc) averaged 13.9 s after the start of each injection. The duration of each injection was 3 s. After the injection of 3 ml of each of the three contrast media, blood samples were withdrawn from the coronary sinus for the determination of ionized calcium ($Ca^{++}$), sodium ($Na^{+}$), potassium ($K^{+}$), hematocrit (Hct), and osmolality (Osm). These samples were obtained at Tp, Tc, and 10 s after clearance (Tc + 10 s). It required approximately 3 s to withdraw the requisite 8 ml blood from the coronary sinus. Hematocrits were determined in duplicate on each sample immediately after withdrawal. When a suitable clot had formed in the blood specimen tubes, the samples were centrifuged and the serum was decanted. Potassium, sodium, and ionized calcium were determined on the fresh serum samples using ion selective electrode techniques (Clin-ion, Model AI-3, Applied Medical Technology, Inc., Palo Alto, Calif.). Commercially available reagent standards were used to calibrate the instrument before analysis of each set of serum samples.

## Statistical Analysis

The data were analyzed to determine the overall differences between effects of the three contrast media in each experimental state and for the same contrast media in the normal vs CAS state. The methodology utilized included a repeated measurements mixed model univariate analysis of variance, and a multivariate analysis of variance (ANOVA) procedure specifically applicable to growth curve analyses. In addition, pairwise t tests were used to compare matched variables for a particular contrast medium at individual time points.

## Results

The contractile effects on the left ventricle in response to intracoronary injection of each of the three contrast media are displayed in Fig. 1, both in the normal state, i.e., no coronary stenosis (left column), and in the presence of a critical coronary artery stenosis (right column). With the exception of EDL in the normal state, R76 caused a significantly

**Table 1.** P values from the repeated measurements analysis of variance for each parameter of LV function [Reproduced from [10] with the permission of the author and the American Heart Association]

| | LVP | dp/dt | $dp/dt_{50}$ | EDL | ESL | dL/dt |
|---|---|---|---|---|---|---|
| Normal state | | | | | | |
| R76 vs iohexol | 0.0045 | 0.0077 | 0.0106 | 0.2340 | 0.0064 | 0.0002 |
| R76 vs metrizamide | 0.0107 | 0.0080 | 0.0165 | 0.4260 | 0.0205 | 0.0063 |
| Iohexol vs metrizamide | 0.9323 | 0.6710 | 0.6167 | 0.6870 | 0.7971 | 0.5400 |
| Ischemic state | | | | | | |
| R76 vs iohexol | 0.0077 | 0.0010 | 0.0016 | 0.0216 | 0.0066 | 0.0003 |
| R76 vs metrizamide | 0.0122 | 0.0011 | 0.0018 | 0.0225 | 0.0073 | 0.0010 |
| Iohexol vs metrizamide | 0.6427 | 0.5807 | 0.6291 | 0.5850 | 0.4082 | 0.6657 |

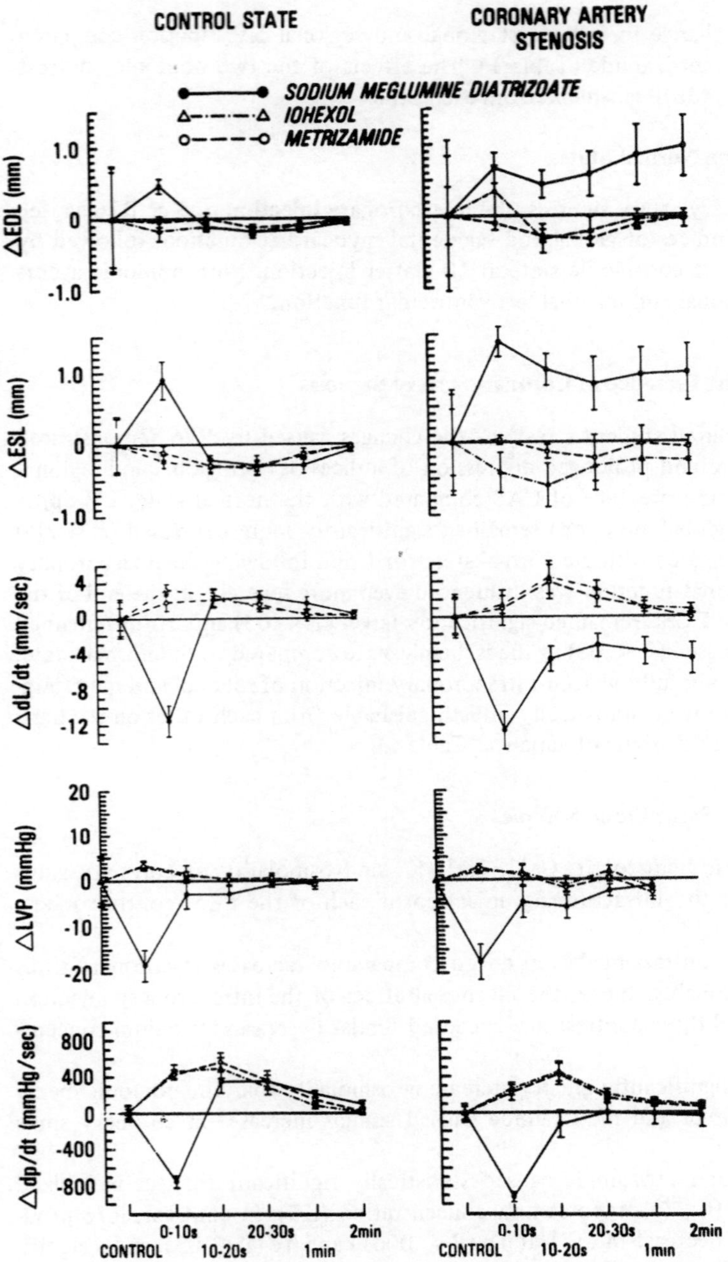


**Fig. 1.** Time sequence of the alterations in indices of global and regional myocardial function after injection of each of the three contrast media. The alterations in the normal state (left column) are contrasted with those in the presence of a critical coronary artery stenosis (CAS) (*right column*). Δ *LVP*, change in left ventricular peak systolic pressure; Δ *EDL*, change in end diastolic segment length; Δ *ESL*, change in end systolic length; Δ *dL/dt*, change in velocity of contraction of the myocardial segment length; Δ $LVP_{50}$, change of rate of rise of LV pressure at LVP of 50 mmHg [Reproduced from [10] with the permission of the author and the American Heart Association]

different (Anova test) change in indices of global and regional LV function compared with either iohexol or metrizamide (Table 1). The effects of the two nonionic contrast media were statistically indistinguishable from each other.

### Contractile Effects in the Normal State

In the absence of coronary artery stenosis, the intracoronary injection of 3 cc R76 caused transient decreases in indices of global and segmental myocardial function, followed by increases in parameters of contractile state at 10 s after injection. Both nonionic agents augmented indices of global and regional left ventricular function.

### Contractile Effects in the Presence of Coronary Artery Stenosis

Pairwise comparison (paired student *t* test) of the changes caused by R76 demonstrated significantly more severe and prolonged depression of indices of both global and regional myocardial function in the presence of CAS compared with the normal state. LV dp/dt and LV $dp/dt_{50}$ (i.e., global function) remained significantly more depressed ($P < .05$) in the ischemic state compared with the normal state for 1 min following the intracoronary injection of R76. Regional function was influenced even more severely; at the end of the 2-min observation period ESL remained significantly larger ($P < .05$) and dL/dt remained significantly more depressed ($P < .02$) in the ischemic state compared to the normal state.

Overall, the changes resulting from intracoronary injection of iohexol and metrizamide in the ischemic state were statistically indistinguishable from each other on the basis of repeated measurements analysis of variance (Table 1).

### Alterations in Coronary Sinus Blood Samples

The absolute values for hematocrit, $Ca^{++}$, $Na^+$, $K^+$ and osmolality of coronary sinus blood before and after the intracoronary injection of each of the three contrast media are displayed in Fig. 2.

Each of the three contrast media produced comparable decreases in coronary sinus hematocrit at Tp, presumably due to the dilutional effect of the intracoronary injection of contrast material. All three contrast media caused similar decreases in sodium concentration.

The R76 caused a significantly greater increase in osmolality than the nonionic media at Tp ($P < .03$). Iohexol and metrizamide caused similar increases in coronary sinus osmolaity.

Neither iohexol nor metrizamide caused statistically significant changes in ionized calcium concentration ($Ca^{++}$) or potassium concentration ($K^+$). In contrast, R76 produced both a significant decrease in $Ca^{++}$ at Tp ($P < .0001$) and Tc ($P < .03$), and a significant drop in $K^+$ at Tp ($P < .0001$).

## Discussion

Intracoronary administration of ionic contrast media is known to induce a number of alterations in myocardial function [1, 2]. The current study and previous studies show

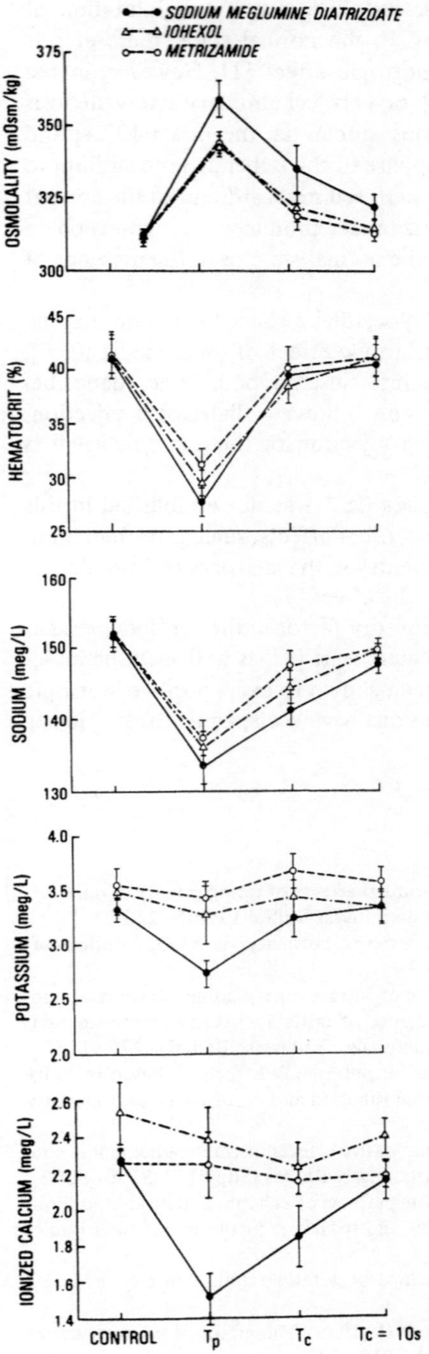


**Fig. 2.** Time sequence of the alterations in coronary sinus blood osmolality, hematocrit, sodium, potassium, and ionized calcium in response to intracoronary injection of each of the three contrast materials [Reproduced from [10] with the permission of the author and the American Heart Association]

that the initial effect includes decline in LV peak systolic pressure and inhibition of global and regional myocardial contractile function. In the normal state, these effects are transient and followed by a reflex positive inotropic effect [1]. However, in the presence of acute heart failure [2], hypocalcemia [2], or a critical coronary artery stenosis [3] these deleterious effects are prolonged. Previous studies in the intact [3, 4] and isolated heart [5] have shown differences in the response of the ischemic myocardium to intracoronary contrast media compared to normally perfused myocardium. In the current study, the two nonionic media, iohexol and metrizamide, produced no depression in either global or regional left ventricular function in the normal state or in the presence of a critical coronary artery stenosis.

An imbalance in sodium and calcium ions in myocardial extracellular fluid may be the important factor responsible for the negative inotropic effect of ionic media [2, 6]. The present study and a previous study [2] demonstrate close temporal concordance between coronary sinus $Ca^{++}$ and ventricular depression following diatrizoate injection. The absence of a significant drop in $Ca^{++}$ following injection of the nonionic agent is consistent with their lack of cardiodepressant effects.

The exact mechanism by which the R76 depresses $Ca^{++}$ was not established in this study. While dilutional effects may play a minor role, other effects, such as protein binding of free $Ca^{++}$ or chelation of $Ca^{++}$ by constituents of the diatrizoate formulation (specificially, citrate and EDTA) likely contribute to the effect [7].

Hyperosmolality has been suggested as a contributory factor in the cardiodepressant effects of contrast media. However, both in the isolated heart [8], as well as in the intact animal [9], nonionic hyperosmolal solutions have been shown to exert positive inotropic effects. On the other hand, ionic hyperosmolal solutions have a disparate effect, causing a decrease in myocardial contractile state [9].

## References


1. Higgins CB, Schmidt W (1978) Direct and reflex myocardial effects of intracoronary administered contrast materials in the anesthetized and conscious dog. Invest Radiol 13:205–216
2. Higgins CB, Schmidt W (1978) Alterations in calcium levels of coronary sinus blood during coronary arteriography in the dog. Circulation 58:512–519
3. Green CE, Higgins CB, Kelley MJ, et al. (1981) Effects of intracoronary administration of contrast materials on left ventricular function in the presence of critical coronary artery stenosis: Advantages of newer contrast materials over standard materials. Cardiovasc Radiol 4:110–116
4. Deutsch AL, Gerber KH, Haigler FH, Higgins CB (to be published) Effects of low osmolality contrast materials on coronary hemodynamic, myocardial function and coronary sinus osmolality in normal and ischemic states. Invest Radiol
5. Serur JR, Als AV, Miner Green N, Paulin S (1981) Comparative effects of three radiographic contrast agents in isolated normal and ischemic canine hearts. Invest Radiol [Suppl] 15:S196–S202
6. Salvesen S, Nilsen PL, Holterman H (1967) Amerliorating effects of calcium and magnesium ions on the toxicity of Isopaque sodium. I. Acute toxicities and toxicities in the brain. Acta Radiol [Diagn] (Stockh) [Suppl] 270:17–29
7. Wolpers HG, Baller D, Ensink W, et al. (1981) Influence of arteriographic contrast media on $Na^{+}/Ca^{++}$ ratio in blood. Cardiovasc Radiol 4:8–13
8. Lipton MJ, Higgins CB, Wiley AA, Angell WW, Barry WH (1978) The effect of contrast media upon the isolated perfused canine heart. Invest Radiol 13:519–522
9. Newell JD, Higgins CB, Kelley MJ, et al. (1980) The influence of hyperosmolality on left ventricular contractile state. Disparate effects of nonionic and ionic solutions. Invest Radiol 15:363–370
10. Gerber KH (1982) Circulation (in press)

# Modifications in Coronary Flow After Injection of Contrast Media

M. E. Bertrand, M. R. Delforge, J. M. Lablanche, P. Y. Tilmant, and F. A. Thieuleux

The modifications in coronary flow induced by a contrast agent (methylglucamine amidotrizoate) were studied in 15 patients undergoing coronary arteriography. Ten patients (group A) had normal coronary arteries. Five patients (group B) displayed significant (> 50%) atherosclerotic lesions of the left coronary artery.

A special 8F catheter bearing two thermistors was introduced into the coronary sinus to measure the coronary flow using Ganz's continuous thermodilution method. The patients' cardiac rhythm was kept stable by supraventricular electrical stimulation at a rate ten beats per minute above the control rate. Selective injection of 5 ml methylglucamine amidotrizoate into the left coronary artery was carried out, and coronary flow and aortic pressure were measured every 10 s for 1 min, then again at 3 min and 5 min after coronary opacification. From aortic pressure and coronary flow was calculated coronary resistance.

Ten seconds after injection of contrast material both groups showed an increase in coronary flow. In group A the increase was significant ($P < 0.001$), reaching an average of 47% and lasting for 50 s after injection. Coronary flow was back to normal at 1, 3, and 5 min. In group B the flow rose very quickly (10 s), but in the increase, of 28%, was significantly ($P < 0.05$) less than in group A and was not observed to last longer than 30 s before returning to normal.

In conclusion, the usual hyperemic effect of contrast material is less marked and less durable in coronary patients than in those free from coronary lesions.

# Changes in Left Ventricular Preload and Afterload Induced by Coronary Angiography: Influence of Contrast Medium Osmolality

H. Petitier, D. Crochet, P. Wanlin, J. de Laguerenne, and D. Krause

Coronary angiography using conventional contrast media with high osmolality induces an immediate and brief deterioration of myocardial contractility which, in animals, is less severe when contrast media with low osmolality are used [2, 4]. Studies in humans [2] have not confirmed these results although contractility has been assessed by a different method only 10 min after the last coronary injection. We have found, however, that diatrizoate (Radioselectan 76%, Schering) with high osmolality enhances the ejection fraction whereas ioxaglate (Hexabrix, Guerbet) depresses it; moreover the two products have opposite effects on left ventricular end diastolic volume and aortic pressure. As this suggests different effects on left ventricular loading conditions, the purpose of our study was to compare modifications of preload and afterload observed during the first 10 min after coronary angiography using the same contrast media as in our previous studies.

## Population

Our study concerned 34 patients (32 males and 2 females, mean age 47.8 ± 7.6 years) with coronary artery disease, but no associated cardiac disease. Fourteen presented an unstable angina, 13 a stable angina, and 7 were asymptomatic with a previous history of myocardial infarction. Coronary artery disease was localized in one vessel in 13 cases two vessels in 12 cases, and three vessels in 9 cases. Left ventricular contraction was normal in 15 cases, presented hypokinetic segments in 16 cases, and akinetic segments in 3 cases.

## Methods

Hemodynamic data were recorded during a right and left heart catheterization. Before coronary angiography, left cineventriculography was performed with ioxitalamate (Telebrix 30, Guerbet) in all patients. Coronary angiography performed either with diatrizoate (osmolality 1800 mosm/kg $H_2O$) or ioxaglate (osmolality 580 mosm/kg $H_2O$) lasted an average of 19 ± 7 min with 68.5 ± 20.5 ml contrast medium for 7.6 ± 1.5 manual intracoronary injections. The following parameters were recorded or calculated before and 1, 2, 4, 6, 8, and 10 min after coronary angiography: heart rate, aortic and pulmonary pressures, cardiac output, stroke volume, left ventricular total stroke work per minute and per beat, and systemic and pulmonary resistances. Student's $t$ test was used for statistical comparisons between the two groups when different contrast media were employed. Within each group, basal and post coronary angiographic data were compared using Student's paired $t$ test.

## Results

Our population was divided into two groups of 17 patients according to the contrast medium used for coronary angiography, diatrizoate in group I and ioxaglate in group II. The two groups were not differentiated as to sex, clinical status, severity of coronary artery disease, basal hemodynamic parameters, or technical data of coronary angiography. Patients of group I (51.7 ± 8.5 years) were older ($P < 0.05$) than those of group II (45.1 ± 6.6 years).

Within each group basal parameters were compared to post coronary angiographic ones in order to assess modifications induced by coronary angiography.
Modifications of general cardiac performance are summarized in Figs. 1 and 2.
Modifications of left ventricular afterload are summarized in Fig. 3.
Modifications of left ventricular preload are summarized in Fig. 4.

### Modifications of Left Ventricular Function

These modifications were assessed according to a methodology developed by Ross [6], simultaneous variations in left ventricular total stroke work per beat and diastolic pulmonary artery pressure being noted during the first 10 minutes following coronary angiography. The results are summarized in Fig. 5.

## Discussion

Contrast media used for coronary angiography induce direct, deleterious myocardial effects, with no clinical disturbance. In animals [6] those effects are briefer and slighter when new products with low osmolality are used, but the results have not been confirmed

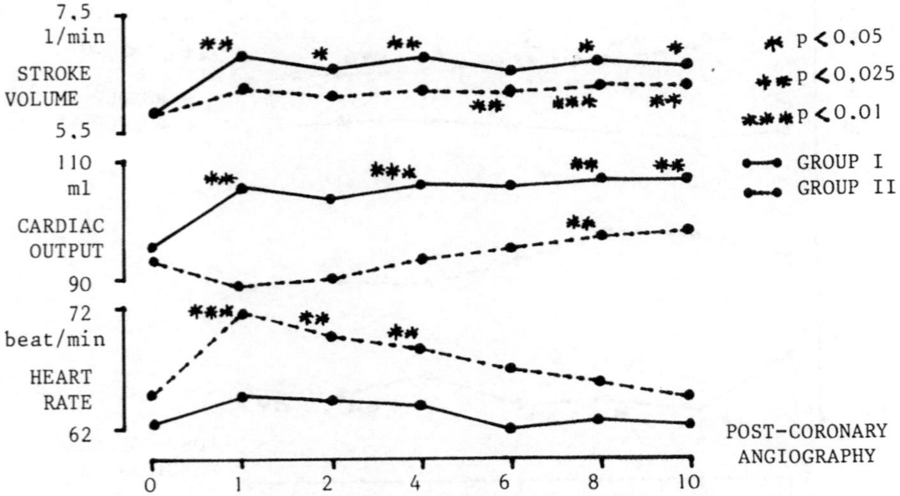


**Fig. 1.** Modifications of cardiac output, stroke volume, and heart rate induced by coronary angiography

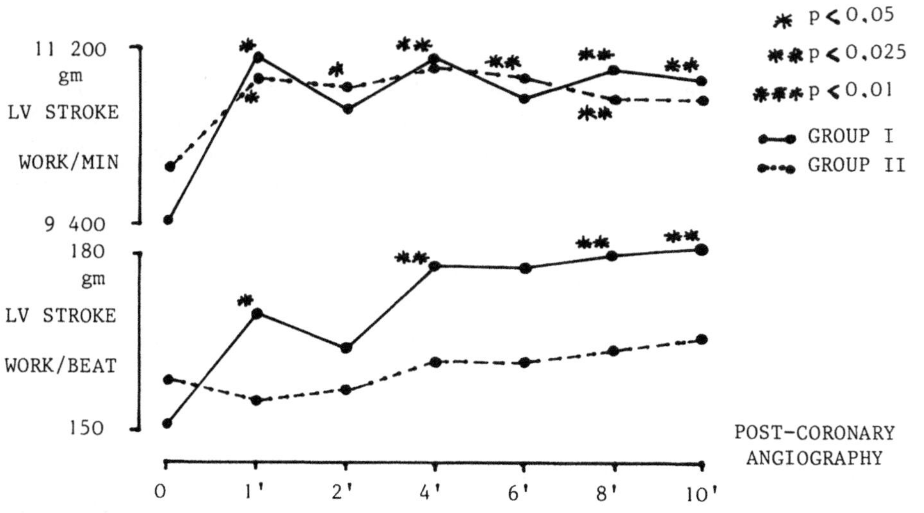


**Fig. 2.** Variations of left ventricular (LV) stroke work per minute and per beat observed after coronary angiography

in human experiments [3]. For the present study we observed modifications of left ventricular function, preload, and afterload during the first 10 min following coronary angiography. Our results show that coronary angiography using a conventional product with high osmolality (group I) induces and increase of stroke volume and stroke work per beat ($P < 0.05$) which are not observed when a new product with low osmolality is

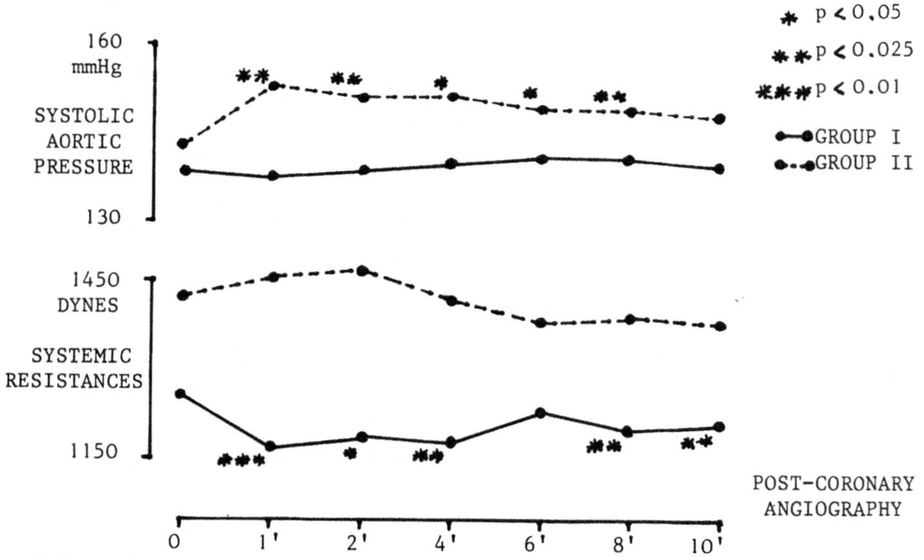


**Fig. 3.** Changes of afterload induced by coronary angiography

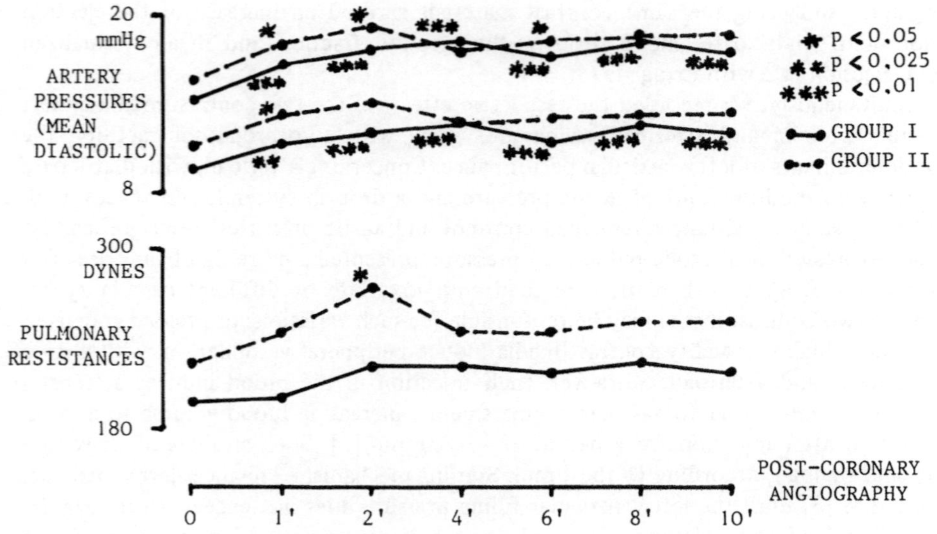


**Fig. 4.** Modifications of pulmonary pressures and resistances observed after coronary angiography

used (group II). Coronary angiography, considered as a stress test and employed to build left ventricular function curves as with Ross' method [6] induces an abnormal response with diatrizoate. With ioxaglate, during a short period of 2 min, there was an increase of preload and a simultaneous insignificant drop in stroke work. If these changes are confirmed in a larger series, they will indicate a more severe depression of left ventricular function with a low osmolality product. This finding is in agreement with our previous work [1], in which a left cineventriculographic study performed 10 min after coronary

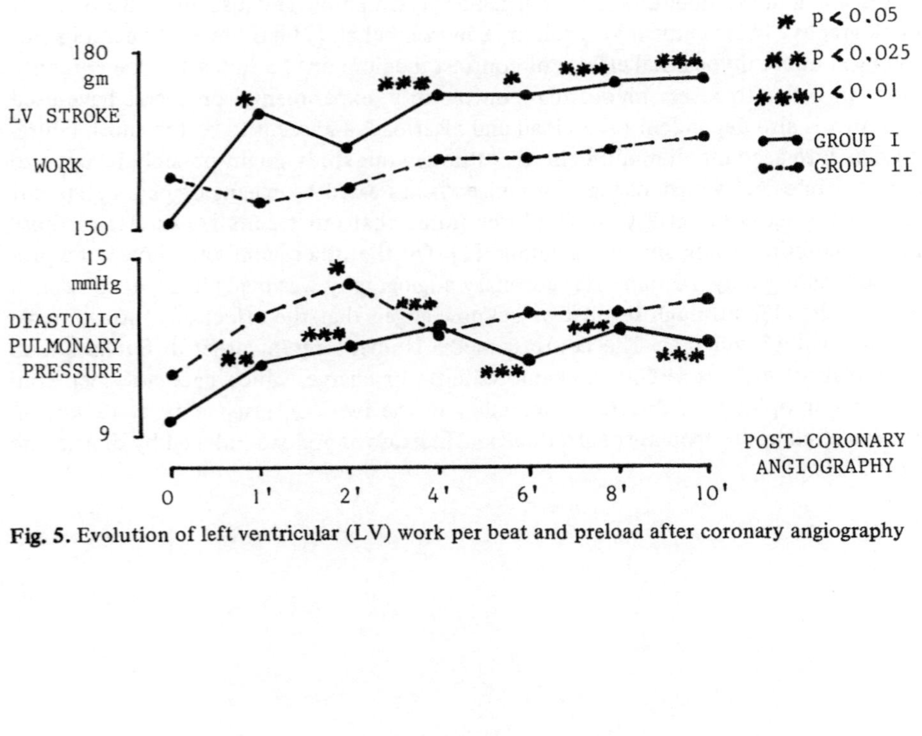


**Fig. 5.** Evolution of left ventricular (LV) work per beat and preload after coronary angiography

angiography and using the same contrast materials showed an increase of the ejection fraction with diatrizoate and a drop in the ejection fraction and mean normalized systolic ejection rate with ioxaglate.

Simultaneously, we recorded the respective effects of the two contrast media on left ventricular preload and afterload which are, along with myocardial contractility, the major determinants of left ventricular performance. Concerning afterload, with diatrizoate there were no modifications of aortic pressure and a drop in systemic resistances; with ioxaglate, systemic resistances remained constant and aortic pressures rose significantly. Preload, expressed in diastolic pulmonary pressure, presented a more significant rise after coronary angiography with diatrizoate than with ioxaglate. A different osmolality between the two contrast media may be responsible for such variations of preload and afterload because high osmolality contrast media induce peripheral vasodilation, with a drop in resistances and afterload. Moreover, their injection in the blood induces a transfer of fluid from interstitial to vascular compartments, increasing blood volume to a maximum 1 min after injection for a period of 15–20 min [3]. Such an increase of venous return and preload, according to the Frank Starling mechanism, enhances left ventricular performance [5] until the left ventricular filling pressure does not exceed 18 mmHg. Increase of preload was deleterious for only two patients in group I who had pressures above that optimal level. For others, late change in the conditions of left ventricular loading after coronary angiography with high osmolality contrast medium had beneficial effects, although in experimental studies it has been claimed that early direct myocardial effects [2, 4] are more deleterious than those induced by low osmolality products.

The apparent discrepancy between our results and those of experimental studies may be explained by several factors concerning the model, protocol and parameters recorded. In experimental works [2, 4], effects of coronary angiography were studied by means of one intracoronary injection of contrast material, generally in normal dogs or pigs, with recording of various hemodynamic parameters during 2 min after injection. In clinical practice, the conditions are quite different because coronary angiography requires seven to ten injections of a total amount of 70 cc contrast medium in patients with coronary artery disease and, frequently, left ventricular dysfunction and usually follows a left ventriculography. In ischemic myocardium, Yamazaki et al. [7] have recently demonstrated prolonged direct myocardial effects of contrast medium until 3 min after one coronary injection. In order to assess myocardial contractility, experimental protocols have used dP/dt, which is also dependent on preload and afterload, and seem to be too short a duration to take into account all modifications. Although our study might possibly be open to criticism because left ventricular performance was assessed by means of parameters not directly measuring contractility, it should be noted that our results are similar to those previously published using such parameters [1]. On the other hand, our choice of a protocol study lasting only 10 min after coronary angiography was made in order to explain previous results [1], although it must be acknowledged that the effect of contrast media lasts more than 15 min [3]. The contrast media studied present other differences than their osmolality, such as viscosity, chemotoxicity, or charge, which have not been considered. In our opinion, a different osmolality in the two contrast media by its known effects, can explain the decrease of afterload and increase of preload induced by diatrizoate (high osmolality).

Such late modifications of left ventricular loading conditions should be beneficial to left ventricular performance, even if early direct myocardial effects [2, 4] are more deleterious than those induced by low osmolality products.

In conclusion, it should be said that more extensive work, in the form of experimental and clinical studies according to the type of contrast medium employed, is needed to confirm all the modifications and their final results on left ventricular function as induced by coronary angiography.

## References


1. Crochet D, Petitier H, De Laguerenne J, Wanlin P (1979) Modifications de la performance ventriculaire gauche induites par la coronarographie avec un nouvel opacifiant à faible osmolarité. Ann Radiol 22:313–314
2. Higgins CB, Schmidt W (1978) Direct and reflex myocardial effects of intracoronary administered contrast materials in the anesthetized and conscious dog: comparison of standard and newer contrast materials. Invest Radiol 13:205–216
3. Iseri LT, Kaplan MA, Evans MJ (1965) Effect of concentrated contrast media during angiography on plasma volume and plasma osmolarity. Am Heart J 69:154
4. Lautrou J, Bergin M, Cardinal A (1978) Action des solutions des produits de contraste sur l'hémodynamique cardiaque au cours de la coronarographie chez le porc. Ann Radiol 21:261
5. Ross J jr (1976) Désadaptation de la post charge et réserve de précharge: un concept utile à l'analyse de la fonction ventriculaire. Acquis Nouvelles Pathol Cardiovasc 18:473
6. Ross J jr, Gault JH, Mason DT, Linhart JW, Braunwald E (1966) Left ventricular performance during muscular exercise in patients with and without cardiac dysfunction. Circulation 34:597
7. Yamazaki H, Banka VS, Bodenheimer MM, Hattori S, Agarwall JB, Helfant RH (1981) Differerential effects of Renografin 76 on the ischemic and non ischemic myocardium. Am J Cardiol 47:597

# Influence of Ioxaglic Acid on Hemoglobin Affinity During Selective Coronarography

M. Seurot, F. Volter, M. Paris, B. Teissere, A. Raynaud, V. Bismuth, and J. C. Gaux

## Introduction

The principal modifications induced by intracoronary artery contrast media injection has been extensively published in the past and consist in myocardial contractility status and cellular electrophysiologic changes [1].

These modifications are in part due to direct action of osmolality and ionic composition of compounds used. In addition, toxicity induced by these compounds could also be due to a change in oxyhemoglobin affinity in relation to the level of osmolality. Very few studies emphasize this point [2].

The aim of the present study was to appreciate modifications of oxyhemoglobin affinity parameter (P 50) induced by a new contrast medium agent, ioxaglic acid.[1]

## Methodology

Studies were performed in 34 patients during coronary angiography in some for ischemic heart disease evaluation (n = 24) and in others for cardiac disease (n = 10). All coronary heart disease patients had the left anterior descending artery significantly involved. The following protocol was performed before (group B: n = 27) or after (group A: n = 7) left ventricular angiography with Ioxaglate (7 ml/kg).

Simultaneous blood samples were performed in aorta and in venous coronary sinus before (0) and 1 mn (1), 3 mn (T3) and 10 mn (T10) after left main intra coronary injection of 8 ml of Ioxaglate. These following parameters were measured in blood samples:

- osmolality (mOsm/kg $H_2O$)
- P 50 (Torr)
- red blood cell 2–3 DPG ($\mu$mol/gHb)

Average results are given in mean ± SEM. ANOVA was used for statistical analysis.

## Results

*Role of total amount of contrast media agent on different parameter modifications.* No particular different trend and magnitude (NS) were observed due to starting the left ventricular angiography study (before $n$ = 27, after $n$ = 7).

---

1 Laboratoires Guerbet, Aulnay sous Bois, France

*Changes in osmolality of venous coronary sinus blood.* Maximal modifications were observed in both groups, 1 min after intracoronary injection.
Gr A TO: 296.5 ± 2.9 mOsm/kg $H_2O$ vs T1: 299.8 ± 2.7 mOsm/kg $H_2O$ (NS)
Gr B TO: 296.3 ± 2.8 mOsm/kg $H_2O$ vs T1: 299.7 ± 2.7 mOsm/kg $H_2O$ (NS)

*Changes in P 50 of venous coronary sinus blood.* No changes of this parameter were observed when protocol was performed after left ventriculography (Gr A) TO: 25.63 ± 0.51 torr; T1: 25.84 ± 0.48; T3: 26.08 ± 0.59; T10: 26.10 ± 0.58 (NS).

A slight P 50 decrease was observed in group B, 3 min after injection. TO: 27.48 ± 0.3 torr vs T3: 26.47 ± 0.8 torr (NS). None of these modifications reached the significant level ($P < 0.05$).

*Changes in red blood cell 2.3 DPG.* No change was observed.

*Difference between atherosclerotic coronary artery and normal artery.* Even if modifications were more pronounced in patients with coronary artery disease, we did not find any significant difference in these cases from the control value or from the value observed in the normal coronary artery group.

## Discussion

In a previous study with exactly the same protocol performed in another group of 13 patients, we observed with diatrizoate, a significant decrease of P 50 at T1 and T3, a significant increase of osmolality at T1, and a significant decrease in red blood cell 2.3 DPG at T1. [3].

Comparison in main modification patterns with both compounds are shown in Fig. 1. No clear hypothesis can explain the difference in the effect of compounds in oxyhemoglobin affinity (4). Nevertheless composition of both compounds are different with a lesser osmolality in ioxaglate than diatrizoate (ioxaglate 580 mOsm/kg $H_2O$, diatrizoate 1900 mOsm/kg $H_2O$).

Changes in oxyhemoglobin affinity cannot be explained by secondary increase in coronary blood flow after injection of ioxaglate or diatrizoate. From a safety point of view, changes of oxyhemoglobin affinity (or myocardial oxygen avaibility) are certainly important during coronary angiogram particularly in ischemic disease. So with equal imaging quality it seems better to use a compound which does not increase oxygen affinity.

## Conclusion

Among cases of myocardial toxicity of contrast media during coronary angiography in ischemic patients, increase of red blood cell oxygen affinity probably plays a role.

Ioxaglic acid was studied from this point of view in 34 patients during coronary angiography and no significant change of P 50 was observed with this compound as opposed to a previous study of a group using diatrizoate.

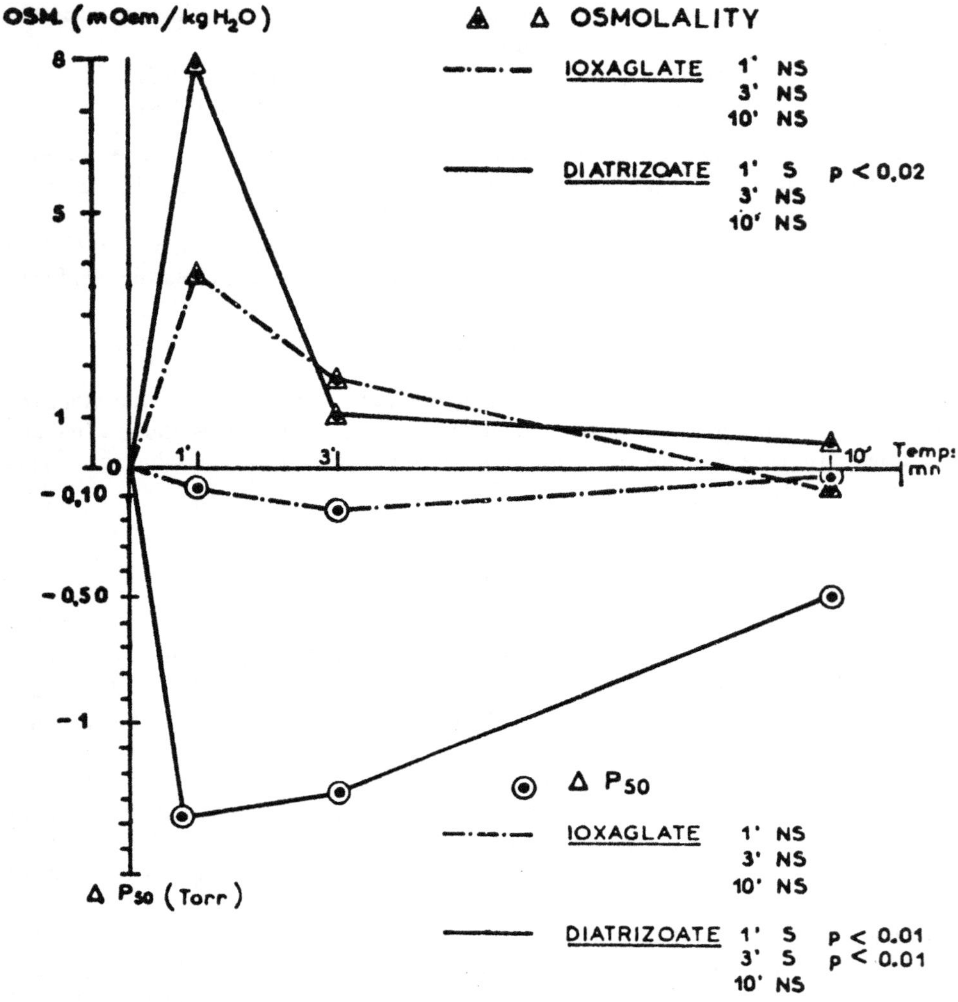


**Fig. 1.** Comparative study between ioxaglate ($n$ = 34) and diatrizoate ($n$ = 13): variations of osmolality and P 50 after left intracoronary injection of 8 ml contrast medium

## References


1. Fischer HW, Thomson KR (1978) Contrast media in coronary arteriography: a review. Invest Radiol 13:450
2. Sheps DS, Cameron BF, Mallon SM, Sommer LS, Lo WC, Harkness DR, Myerburg RJ (1980) Depression of intramyocardial oxyhemoglobin dissociation by angiographic contrast media. Am Heart J 99:193
3. Gaux JC, Blanchet F, Bismuth V, Bourdarias JP, Lesseng G, Rocha P, Duchatelle C, Eveleigh MC, Bardet J, Frija G (to be published) Effects of diatrizoate on hemoglobin affinity for oxygen during coronary arteriography. Ann Radiol
4. Rosenthal A, Mesrobian A (1975) The relationship between angiography, intraerythrocytic pH and hemoglobin equilibrium. Invest Radiol 10:140

# The Use of Amipaque in Pediatric Angiocardiography

H. A. Baltaxe, P. Mooring, P. Hofschire, J. Kugler, W. Pinsky, and W. Chu

The outlining of abnormal cardiac structures in cases of congenital heart disease requires angiocardiography with multiple views of the heart during the intracardiac injection of iodinated contrast materials. The administration of large volumes of contrast material during such examinations can result in serious complications and in death. Particularly in small infants the physician is limited by the total amount of contrast material that he can inject with impunity. The deleterious effects resulting from these injections is caused to a large extent by the hyperosmolarity of the contrast material. The contrast materials currently used in angiocardiography are hyperosmolar monomeric agents. Previously obtained experimental data seem to indicate that nonionic contrast materials have less deleterious effects upon the myocardium when injected either directly into the coronary arteries or into the left ventricle. The purpose of our study was to compare Renografin 76, a hyperosmolar monomeric agent, with metrizamide, a nonionic agent, in a group of patients studied by angiocardiography to diagnose congenital heart disease.

## Method

Sixteen patients under the age of 2 years suspected of complicated congenital heart disease were submitted alternately to either Renografin 76 or metrizamide during the investigation of their condition. The protocol consisted in obtaining baseline parameters and follow-up studies after the injection of contrast material into the left ventricle. The following parameters were obtained.

Heart rate 1, 2, 3, 4, 5, 10, 15, 30 min
Left ventricular pressure 1, 2, 3, 4, 5, 10, 15[1] min
Echocardiogram (end systolic and end diastolic) immediately post, 5, 15 min
Hematocrit 15 min
Serum osmolality 15 min
Serum electrolytes 15 min

Renografin 76 or Amipaque at a concentration of 370 mg I/ml were injected at a dose of 1.5 ml/kg.

---

[1] Measurement will be repeated at 30 min if the value at 15 min has not returned to control level

## Results

*Heart Rate.* An inital rise at 1 min after the injection of contrast material was noted with both contrast media. At 3 min the heart rate in the Renografin group seemed to fall below baseline. The Amipaque group seemed to experience less rise at 1 min and only a slight fall below baseline at 10 min. Being that the number of patients was small and the standard deviation high, the differences between mean values of the two data groups were normalized by their pooled variance. A set of normalized mean differences, as defined below, were obtained as a result of evaluating difference for each time interval of interest.

Normalized Mean Difference $= M_1 - M_2/S\sqrt{1/n_1 + 1/n_2}$

1, Renografin
2, Amipaque
$M$, mean value
$n$, sample number
$S$, pooled standard deviation

These differences confirm that Renografin 76 produces a higher initial rise in heart rate at 1 min and a significant drop at 3–4–5 min in comparison to metrizamide.

## Peak Systolic Left Ventricular Pressure

An initial rise of peak systolic pressure up to 12% from baseline was noted with both contrast media with maximum rise at approximately 2 min after the injection. Analysis by mean normalized differences showed a greater rise of peak systolic LV pressure with Renografin 76 which lasted until 5 min after the injection.

## Peak End Diastolic Pressure

This rose up to 40% from baseline with both contrast media, with maximum rise at 2–3 minutes. Large standard deviations were noted but normalized mean difference analysis showed that the end diastolic pressure rose more significantly with Renografin 76.

## Echocardiographic Findings

No significant left ventricular functional changes were noted by echocardiography either during systole or diastole after injection of either contrast medium as assessed by echocardiography.

## Other Findings

Serum osmolality rose by an average of 2% with either contrast medium. Hematrocrit fell by an average of 8% with either contrast medium. Serum sodium fell by an average of 1.6% with either contrast medium. Serum potassium fell by an average of 11% with either contrast medium. No difference in the amount of changes was noted with Renografin 76 and Amipaque in the analysis of blood.

## Conclusion

Although the number of patients studied was small, statistical analysis of our data seems to indicate that the use of metrizamide in the angiocardiography of patients under the age of 2 with congenital heart disease produces less initial rise and subsequent drop in heart rate, less rise in peak systolic and end diastolic pressures. Contrary to what one might expect changes in serum osmolality, hematocrit, serum sodium, and serum potassium are the same for both contrast media.

# Comparative Study in Small Infants of the Hemodynamic Effects of Ioxaglate and Diatrizoate Contrast Media in Left Ventriculography

V.H. de Villeneuve, M. Meradji, A. Penning, and A. van de Wiel

## Introduction

Rapid intravascular injection of a fairly large volume of radiopaque material induces an acute increase in blood volume. A hyperosmotic contrast agent gives an additional influx of extravascular fluid into the circulation, thus resulting in hypervolemia.

In the normal heart this triggers the Frank-Starling mechanism and hemodynamic adaptation will ensue.

Infants with congenital heart defects often are referred in heart failure. In this situation acute volume overload is less well tolerated and a low-osmolarity contrast agent could be advantageous to avoid the aforementioned undesirable secondary effects of angiocardiography [1].

This study was intended to compare the hemodynamic effects produced by two contrast media: ioxaglate and diatrizoate.

## Material and Methods

In 21 infants with various forms of congenital heart disease, below 5 kg in weight, ioxaglate or diatrizoate was injected into the left ventricle. Ioxaglate (Hexabrix) has a low osmolarity of 580 mosmol/kg and contains 32% iodine.

Diatrizoate 76% has a high osmolarity of 1800 mosmol/kg and contains 37% iodine. The injected volume of contrast agent was 2 ml/kg body weight and the flow rate was also kept constant at 7 ml/s. Preceding contrast injection, and 1 and 10 min after injection samples were taken to obtain biochemical as well as physiological data.

**Table 1.** Patient material

| | Ioxaglate | Diatrizoate |
|---|---|---|
| Number of patients | 11 | 10 |
| Age (days) | 46 | 52 |
| Weight (g) | 3465 | 3586 |
| Length (cm) | 52.6 | 55.1 |
| Body surface area ($m^2$) | 0.21 | 0.22 |
| Ejection fraction | 52% | 60% |

A complete cardiac catheterization with percutaneous catheter insertion in the femoral vein and an arterial line in the femoral artery was performed. Cardiac output measurements (including sampling in the pulmonary artery) were performed shortly before and approximately 10 min after left ventriculography. Calculations of pressures, flows, and pressure-derived conceptions (dp/dt and Vmax) were performed with the aid of the Philips Automated Catheterization System.

A steady state for the infants examined was obtained by diazepam 1 mg/kg rectally and ketamine 3 mg/kg intramuscularly as premedication, if necessary supplied by ketamine 1 mg/kg intravenously.

The infants in the ioxaglate group were slightly younger and lighter than those in the diatrizoate group.

In view of the ejection fraction, calculated from the left ventricular angio, the ioxaglate group presents itself less favorably condition than the diatrizoate group. The data are presented in Table 1.

## Results

The biochemical findings are presented in Table 2. Arterial pH showed a slight and transient decrease following ioxaglate administration, whereas diatrizoate caused a somewhat deeper drop and slower return to its preinjection level. Arterial $O_2$ saturation was not significantly affected by both contrast media.

Hemoglobin showed a transient drop in the same order of magnitude for both media (0.5–0.6 mmol/liter), apparently caused by hemodilution, followed by diuresis.

Osmolality increased sharply 1 min after injection of diatrizoate and was still somewhat above its preinjection level 10 min later. Ioxaglate on the contrary showed a minimal decrease, apparently caused by renal contrast excretion. As far as pressures and pressure-derived data are concerned, they have been summarized as mean values in Table 3.

Peak systolic and end diastolic pressures in the left ventricle were hardly influenced by both media let alone a small temporary increase in the end diastolic pressures. Peak systolic femoral artery pressure follows the same trend.

In an attempt to assess myocardial function peak left ventricular dp/dt (using a differentiator) has been calculated before and after contrast injection. Its increase parallels enhanced contractility, and diminution is found in conditions associated with depressed myocardial activity. Although augmented preload, which is achieved by contrast injec-

**Table 2.** Biochemical dates

| | Ioxaglate | | | Diatrizoate | | |
|---|---|---|---|---|---|---|
| | Before | After 1min | After 10min | Before | After 1 min | After 10min |
| pH | 7.38 | 7.37 | 7.38 | 7.38 | 7.35 | 7.36 |
| $O_2$ (%) | 91 | 91 | 91 | 93 | 92 | 92 |
| Hb (mmol) | 7.0 | 6.5 | 6.7 | 6.2 | 5.6 | 6.2 |
| Osmol | 291 | 290 | 289 | 292 | 304 | 296 |

**Table 3.** Functional analysis

| | Ioxaglate | | | Diatrizoate | | |
|---|---|---|---|---|---|---|
| | Before | After 1min | After 10min | Before | After 1min | After 10min |
| LV peak syst. (mmHg) | 86 | 88 | 86 | 84 | 83 | 82 |
| Lv end diast. (mmHg) | 11 | 12 | 10 | 13 | 15 | 13 |
| DP/DT | 1433 | 1145 | 1406 | 1586 | 1418 | 1531 |
| Vmax | 66 | 64 | 68 | 71 | 58 | 82 |
| Heart rate | 141 | 141 | 141 | 138 | 144 | 138 |

tion, tends to increase the peak dp/dt, a transitory decrease, caused by both agents was noted. This forms some evidence for a transitory depressive effect.

Another parameter for myocardial contractility based on the force-velocity relation of the left ventricle is Vmax [2] (maximal velocity of shortening at zero load). As distinct from dp/dt, Vmax is independent from preload and afterload, while positive inotropic interventions produce an increase of Vmax. As is shown in Table 3 ioxaglate hardly influences Vmax, while diatrizoate produces an initial dip followed by a boost 10 min later.

The heart rate was not affected by ioxaglate, while diatrizoate injection resulted in a transient rise in heart rate.

Systemic and pulmonary vascular resistances (Table 4) in the two groups are far from comparable, owing to the fact that more shunts were to be found in the trizoate group and some coarctations in the ioxaglate group.

However, pulmonary vascular resistance tends to decrease slightly after ioxaglate and increases somewhat after diatrizoate.

Finally the contrast qualities of ioxaglate and diatrizoate were assessed by a pediatric radiologist and a pediatric cardiologist independent of each other and without advance knowledge of the contrast media used. A striking consensus of opinion was present.

Contrast density as well as detailed structural information were considered to be superior after ioxaglate injection. The low viscosity of ioxaglate undoubtedly enhances

**Table 4.** Vascular resistances (in dynes s $cm^{-5}/m^2$)

| | Ioxaglate | | Diatrizoate | |
|---|---|---|---|---|
| | Before | After | Before | After |
| Pulmonary | 671 | 644 | 249 | 290 |
| Systemic | 1530 | 1330 | 1019 | 958 |

Preceding and 10 min after ventriculography

bolus formation during contrast injection, and this could contribute to the opacifying properties of ioxaglate.

## Conclusion

From the data presented we conclude that ioxaglate is to be recommended for angiocardiography in the small infant because it hardly affects the hemodynamic state and thus seems to be better tolerated than diatrizoate. In addition its opacifying qualities are excellent.

## References


1. Petitier H, Crochet D, Bizais Y, Dehumeau J, Laguererme J, Le Donarin L (1978) Etude des effects hémodynamiques d'un nouveau produit de contraste à structure dimère mono-acide. Ann Radiol 21:297–300
2. Hugenholtz P, Mirsky I, Urschel CW, Sandler H, Kaplan E, Sonnenblick EH (1968) Vmax and myocardial force-velocity relations: A useful and sensitive measure of contractility in man. Circulation [Suppl II] 37:186

# A Comparison Between the New Low Osmolality Contrast Agent, Hexabrix, and a Conventional One

F.D.M. Haagen, M.L.F. Landsman, L.E.J.M. Schrijvers, and J.H. Pasteuning

## Effects on Left Ventricular Function During Selective Coronary Angiography. A Clinical Trial

The purpose of this paper is to present the results of a clinical trial in which a new, low osmolality contrast agent was compared with a conventional compound.

Investigated were, among others, changes in the left ventricular function during selective coronary angiography. This is the first time that left ventricular pressure was recorded continually during this procedure.

Coronary angiography still carries a small but distinctive morbidity and mortality [1]. In the last decade the great importance of the osmolality of the contrast media has become increasingly appreciated as a toxic effect, responsible for a certain part of the complications. Erythrocytes lose intracellular fluid and because of their increased rigidity will obstruct the capillaries, which may lead to local tissue anoxia [2].

Platelet aggregation and thrombosis may occur on places where endothelial cells are disrupted and plasma elements are exposed to underlying collagen [3].

These effects can be dangerous in the discrete coronary or cerebral circulation, in particular when exposure time is long, as is often the case where flow is restricted by obstructive lesions.

High osmolality may furthermore increase circulating volume after ventriculography [4] and this overloading can lead to deterioration of an already poor left ventricular function.

The appreciation that the high osmolality of current contrast agents can lead to major adverse reactions has encouraged the synthesis of low osmolality compounds.

One of these is Hexabrix, a solution of salts of ioxaglic acid. It contains six iodine atoms in each molecule with only one acid group. This modification lowers the number of dissociated particles in comparison with the conventional triiodinated organic acids like metrizoic acid.

This new agent has none or only slight subjective adverse reactions in angiography [5] as is our experience. But the effect on left ventricular function *during* selective coronary angiography initiated our interest.

A clinical trial was therefore instituted, comparing Hexabrix with sodium, calcium, meglumine metrizoate (Isopaque, Coronar). The osmolality of the agents is 600 and 2150 mmol/kg water respectively.

In a double blind cross-over study in 24 patients, referred for evaluation of angina pectoris, left ventricular pressure was continually recorded during 4 min, four times, by means of a catheter-tip pressure transducer. After the first minute selective coronary angiography was performed. Changes in the first derivative, dp/dt, were analyzed.

The order in which the left or right coronary artery were injected was selected randomly as was the sequence of the compounds.

To avoid Valsalva maneuvers, the patients were not asked to hold their breath.

The films were assessed for quality of contrast. We could not determine a clear difference in opacification of the arteries and the small branches; neither could we observe any difference in clearance time.

We noted a striking difference in subjective reactions: 30% of the patients complaining of anginal pain or dyspnea when Isopaque was injected in the left coronary artery and no patients complaining when Hexabrix was used. In the right coronary artery the numbers were 10% and 15% respectively.

## Data

Over the 1st min the mean value was calculated of heart frequency, diastolic, end diastolic and systolic pressure and dp/dt of left ventricle. These data were considered as reference.

During selective coronary angiography maximal and minimal values of these hemodynamic parameters were determined. The same was done for the 3 min after injection. Calculated were maximal and minimal disturbances expressed in percentages of the reference value.

Statistical analysis was carried out according to paired Student's t text.

## Results

### Heart Frequency

Hexabrix (H) produces significantly less bradycardia compared to Isopaque (I). (H:5.6% in LCA and I:17.1% in LCA; H:3.8% in RCA and I:21.2% in RCA). Difference in acceleration was less striking (H:11.8% in LCA and I:8.4% in LCA; for RCA the difference between H and I was not significant).

### Left Ventricular Diastolic Pressure

The difference between the two contrast agents was hardly or not significant.

### Left Ventricular End Diastolic Pressure

No significant difference between Hexabrix and Isopaque.

### Left Ventricular Systolic Pressure

Hypertensive effect of Hexabrix is significantly less than that of Isopaque when injected in the left coronary artery (H:5%, I:9%). Hypotensive effect not significantly divergent. In RCA the hypotensive effect is now significantly more for Isopaque (H:8.8, I:15.5).

**First Derivative of Left Ventricular Pressure**

Difference between the agents not significant for the RCA, but in the LCA more positive inotropic influence by Isopaque (H:16.6%, I:34.0%) and less negative inotropic effect (H:7.8, I:4.1).

## Conclusions

Hexabrix is a new low osmolar contrast medium with good radiographic qualities. The subjective adverse effects are clearly less compared to conventional contrast agents. Hemodynamic disturbances are significantly less during selective coronary angiography, which means a great advantage. Hexabrix may be the contrast agent of choice for coronary angiography particularly in critically ill patients.

*Acknowledgement.* Thanks are due to Mrs. J. Reinders Folmer-Spaans for her assistance.

## References

1. Davis K, Kennedy JW, Kemp HG jr et al. (1979) Complications of C.A.G. from the collaborative study of coronary artery surgery CASS. Circulation 59:1105
2. Aspelin (1978) Effect of ionic and nonionic contrast media on morphology of human erythrocytes. Acta Radiol 19:675
3. Almen T, Hartel M, Nylander G et al. (1973) Effect of metrizamide on silber staining of aortic endothelium. Acta Radiol [Suppl] 335:233
4. Izeri I, Kaplan MA, Evans MJ, et al. (1965) Effect of concentrated contrast media during angiography on plasma volume and plasma osmolality. Am Heart J 69:154
5. Holm M, Praestholm J (1979) Ioxaglate, a new low osmolar contrast medium used in femoral angiography. Br J Radiol 52:169

# Summary of the Discussion

Dr. Petitier: We are offered a limited time for discussion. In order to facilitate this discussion perhaps we could retain two main subjects: the myocardial toxicity of contrast media (CM) used in coronary angiography, and the hemodynamic tolerance following angiocardiography, especially in neonates and infants. In theory, according to the experimental and clinical hemodynamic studies, everyone here seems to agree with the fact that we have to prefer low osmolality CM (LOCM) rather than high osmolality CM (HOCM) for our patients. Nevertheless, in practice, I think we are all daily using HOCM and occasionnally LOCM. Have we to make up our mind about this point?

Dr. Baltaxe: We have to look at the better care of our patients. If we consider large series of coronary angiographies, collecting up to 50 000 patients during the last 2 years, we find a 1%–1.5% mortality. This mortality means that our patients have no adverse effects when receiving sodium meglumine diatrizoate. Some years ago I compared this last CM with another one containing calcium. As we know calcium protects the myocardium. This new compound was better. However, even in patients with bad left ventricles, the effects of the two CM were not significantly different. So there is no doubt that the nonionic CM are better than the ionic CM, but when considering the cost of the products, I think that we have no true reason for abandoning the ionic CM in coronary angiography. We only expect that the manufacturers will offer a nonionic product as cheap and as easily usable. On the other hand I think that nonionic CM have to be used in the special group of critically ill neonates and infants where the anatomy must be precisely defined.

Dr. Crochet: When comparing the experimental and the clinical studies of the hemodynamic effects of CM we find some discrepancies. They could be explained by the fact that some experimental conditions are quite different from the clinical conditions. So we are not allowed to compare the effects of only one intracoronary injection in animals with the effects of 5–10 injections in human patients. Let us not forget that the preload and afterload status is highly and proportionally influenced by the amount of CM introduced in the intravascular bed. Similarly the effects of CM on the normal heart of an animal cannot be compared with those of CM on a human heart with altered left ventricular function and 1, 2, or 3 coronary vessels disease.

Dr. Haagen: Some years ago we studied the hemodynamic and ECG effects of repeated CM intracoronary injections. We have found no significant difference between the effects of the first and the fourth injection. The consequences of each injection were analyzed during a limited period of 60 s following the end of injection.

Dr. Bertrand: Some pitfalls have to be avoided in the methodology of CM hemodynamic studies. Heart rate, contractility, preload, afterload and coronary flow are the main parameters influenced by CM. I think that dP/dt is not a good index because it is too much dependant on heart rate. The best index could be Vmax, which was used by Dr. de Villeneuve. But when we use Vmax we have to reject the patients suffering from a valvular insufficiency.

Dr. X.: Indeed, the control of the exact status of the patient is not easy. The effect of a Valsalva maneuver during the coronary angiography can obscure a lot of potential differences between the CM. We have seen that there are no significant differences between ioxaglate solution and calcium metrizoate. It would be preferable to compare ioxaglate compound with products without calcium because the addition of calcium to metrizoate tends to remove some negative inotropic effects.

Dr. Petitier: Our opinion is that the nonionic LOCM and the ioxaglic acid, which is a ionic but low osmolar CM, have very similar myocardial and hemodynamic effects. We currently use the ioxaglic acid for angiocardiography in our pediatric patients.

Dr. Baltaxe: In the United States we have a very limited choice, due to the FDA rules. We have no experience with ioxaglic acid. We have analyzed metrizamide, which is an expensive but very interesting contrast material. However, it has some drawbacks: it is presented as a powder which has to be mixed; it does not stay in solution.

Dr. Pinet: I am sorry but we are obliged to stop this discussion. Many thanks to all speakers for their excellent contributions in this afternoon devoted to the heart.

# Section C:
# Effects on the Nervous System

# The Neurotoxicity of Water-soluble Contrast Media: Actual Concepts and Future

R.E. Gonsette

## Introduction

Neurotoxicity of water-soluble contrast media (CM) is involved when radiopaque compounds come into contact with the brain tissue.

This was observed from the outset of neuroradiology, during cerebral angiographies, when lesions of the blood-brain barrier (BBB), either provoked by CM itself or associated to a preexisting pathology (tumor, infarction), permitted access of the radiopaque substance to brain cells. Impaired permeability of the BBB provoked by CM after intracarotid injection has been recently confirmed in man by cerebral computed tomography. In these cases, leakage of iodine through altered brain capillaries provoked abnormal gray matter enhancement for as long as for 1 h.

On the other hand, there is an increasing development of new neuroradiological techniques bringing the CM directly into contact with the central nervous system (CNS), in order to visualize ventricular, cisternal, and perimedullary spaces. Neurotoxicity of CM has been therefore gaining more and more interest during recent years.

## Vascular Toxicity

Since neurological reactions were first observed after cerebral angiographies, prime attention has been paid to the toxicity of CM for the brain capillaries. Using the Blue Trypan test, Broman and Olsson observed 33 years ago that CM injected into the carotid arteries in rabbits increased the permeability of cerebral capillaries, provoking a subsequent blue staining of the brain.

Since then, increasingly sensitive techniques have been developed, detecting the penetration of radioisotopes (NaI, 32 P, 197 Hg) by the degree of blackening they produce on macro- or microautoradiographies, or by measuring the brain tissue radioactivity in a gamma counter. BBB lesions can also be detected by direct observation of the passage of fluorescent markers (Evan's Blue) in optic microscopy, and of electron opaque substances (ferritin, horse radish peroxydase) in ultramicroscopy.

There are sometimes disparities between the results of different laboratories, due to variations of experimental techniques or to animal species specificity. Discrepancies are also observed due to differences between the markers in protein binding, passage through the altered BBB, or elimination from the brain parenchyma. It is therefore of the utmost importance when comparing the toxicity of different CM to carry out exactly the same experimental procedure for each.

In a first series of experiments, the BBB toxicity of different CM was studied in our laboratory using both radioisotopes (P 32) and fluorescent markers (Evan's Blue). We observed BBB toxicity in decreasing order for acetrizoate, diatrizoate, metrizoate, iothalamate, and iodamide. Moreover, for each CM, the sodium salt was more toxic than the meglumine salt. Addition of calcium and magnesium ions to CM solutions, as suggested by Holterman, had an ameliorating effect on the BBB damage. The most important progress during this preliminary phase was achieved by the synthesis of ioxithalamate.

The classification of actual CM according to their respective toxicity for the BBB, determined in our laboratory under the same experimental conditions, is listed in Table 1.

Even if there are minor discrepancies between different authors about the ranking of CM according to their BBB toxicity, it is generally admitted that the two major steps forward were made by the synthesis of ioxythalamate and of further slightly hypertonic (monoacid dimers and nonionic substances).

Even if new compounds with negligible adverse effects on the brain capillaries have been recently synthetized, the exact mechanism of the vascular toxicity of CM still remains unclear. It is well known that injections of CM break through the endothelial barrier by increasing pinocytotic activity and/or by opening tight junctions between the endothelial cells. But opinions are still controversial concerning the nature of factors possibly affecting each of those mechanisms.

It is generally admitted that hypertonicity causes shrinkage of the endothelial cells with subsequent opening of the tight junctions, while chemotoxicity is mainly directed toward the endothelial cell membranes. In fact there is no clear-cut distinction between respective specificity of hypertonicity versus chemical toxicity. Indeed it has been recently suggested that chemotoxicity could also affect desmosomes and influence the passage of substances between cell junctions.

When effects on the microcirculation are concerned, it has been shown that following intracarotid injection of CM, the overall cerebral blood flow increases, but most of

**Table 1.** Blood-brain barrier toxicity of contrast media

| Contrast media | Highest iodine content of 1 ml CM not incurring BBB damage (% wt/vol) |
|---|---|
| Highly hypertonic compounds (ionic monomers as Na salts) | |
| Acetrizoate | 15 |
| Diatrizoate | 23 |
| Metrizoate | 24 |
| Iothalamate | 26 |
| Iodamide | 30 |
| Ioxithalamate | 34 |
| Slightly hypertonic compounds | |
| Metrizamide (nonionic) | 38 |
| Iopamidol (nonionic) | 40 |
| Ioxaglate (ionic monoacid dimer) | 41 |

the blood is shunted from the arterioles to the venules via bypass channels, and capillary circulation is slowed down. Those effects on microcirculation probably explain why BBB lesions are preferentially localized on arterioles (60%) and venules (25%) rather than on capillaries (12%).

Finally it must be said that other factors, like acute elevation of intracarotid pressure, may provoke lesions of the BBB. On the other hand, attention has been recently drawn to foreign bodies of varying origin and ranging in size from less than 0.5 Mm to 450 Mm in CM for angiography. These particles are likely to be responsible for thromboembolic complications.

As a matter of fact, the vascular tolerance of very recent CM is exceptionally good. Indeed iodine concentrations not provoking lesions of BBB in animal experiments are now definitely higher than the optimal iodine content requested for cerebral angiography in man. Moreover, new low osmolality CM produce less peripheral vasodilatation and less discomfort for the patients.

Nevertheless there is a need for an ideal, inert CM because of new diagnostic procedures like prolonged cerebral angiography in which large amounts of CM are injected for 3 or 4 s allowing a better demonstration of cerebral neoplasms.

Moreover, recent studies have been published reporting that the BBB could be disrupted in humans without significant toxicity after intracarotid injection of hyperosmolar solutions, in order to increase drug delivery into the brain, particularly for chemotherapy. Controls of "therapeutic" lesions of the BBB are made on CT scan after i.v. injection of CM. Definite enhancement of the gray matter of the entire perfused hemisphere is observed. Several patients developed motor seizures due to the epileptogenic activity of the injected CM, and nonepileptogenic substances would be safer.

Angiography has become more frequent in patients with cerebrovascular diseases due to the increased use of surgical therapy. But patients who can benefit most from surgery are those with severe stenoses or multiple transient ischemic attacks, and are the very ones for whom angiography is the most dangerous.

## Brain Tissue Toxicity

Another aspect of the neurotoxicity of CM which has prevented their use for intrathecal opacification until recent years is their toxicity for brain neurones, causing epileptic fits and/or toxic encephalopathy. Conventional water-soluble CM are very potent epileptogenic substances, and seizures during cranial computed tomography have been reported. In these cases, BBB damage associated with brain infarction or more permeable neoplastic vessels enable CM to leak into the brain and to provoke convulsions.

A better understanding of the toxicity of CM toward the brain tissue is probably the most important contribution to the development of new CM in neuroradiology, and the first attempt to fill the cerebral ventricles with a substance that could mingle with the cerebrospinal fluid (CSF) was made by Dandy. The various CM used in pyelography (thorium, potassium iodide, collargol, argyrol, etc.) were injected into the ventricles of dogs, but always with fatal results. Macroscopic controls of the brain showed a marked edema and petechial hemorrhages.

After the synthesis of the sodium salt of iodmetanesulfone acid (Abrodil), severe complications were reported after intracisternal injections in man, and no one has used it since then.

Thorium dioxide injected into the ventricles of rabbits and dogs visualized the ventricular system to a degree which had never been achieved before. Thorotrast was used in man extensively for a few years, but further animal experiments demonstrated severe arachnoiditis and led to the abandonment of this CM.

The next step was made after comparative studies failed to show a consistent correlation between intracisternal and intravenous toxicities of watersoluble CM. This observation led to an ever increasing specific interest in the neurotoxicity of CM. Striking differences in toxicity to the brain between CM available for angiography was demonstrated, and intracisternal injections in rabbits revealed that meglumine iothalamate was at least 3 times less toxic than its diatrizoate counterpart.

The first systematic experimental study of the neurotoxicity of CM with a view to possible further clinical application was published by Campbell et al. in 1964. Iothalamate was injected into the cisterna magna in dogs. EEG and electrocorticography revealed dose-dependent seizure activities. Histological studies in optic microscopy failed to demonstrate any changes, but were performed 1 week to 1 month after injection. Studies with labeled iothalamate showed a total elimination of the CM in the urine within 24 h, and autoradiographies indicated a penetration of the substance into the brain and the spinal cord. Iothalamate was no longer visible on serial rx films 30 min after injection. The first iothalamate (Conray) ventriculography in man was performed by Heimburger almost 20 years ago, on 4 April 1962.

Since 1966, we have developed an experimental technique for the screening of CM using pericerebral injection in the guinea pig and based on clinical reactions, usual EEG recordings, and EEG frequency analysis as well as histological changes observed in optic and electronic microscopy.

The same year, Hayes et al. reported that the dimer of iothalamate proved to be less neurotoxic than the monomer, and in a first series of experiments, we compared the neurotoxicity of sodium monoiodomethanesulfonate (methiodal), meglumine iothalamate, and meglumine iocarmate.

Until then, histological examinations published by different authors had been performed several weeks after intracisternal or intracerebral injection. Since water-soluble CM are rapidly eliminated, we found it more suitable to carry out serial histological investigations during the 1st week after injection.

In those experimental conditions, we were able to observe edematous and inflammatory reactions in brain tissue as well as hemorrhagic suffusions. Vessels of the choroid plexus were frequently dilated. The better tolerance of iocarmate was confirmed since histological reactions were definitely less marked.

EEG recordings revealed that current CM used in cerebral angiography were epileptogenic even at low doses, and that iocarmate was half as epileptogenic as iothalamate. Our preliminary clinical experience with this new substance (Dimer X) was published in 1971.

In further experiments, in collaboration with the Nyegaard Laboratories, we found that the epileptogenic activity and the cellular toxicity of newly synthetized dissociable CM was but slightly improved. It was also demonstrated that injections of equimolar solutions of meglumine hydrochloride produced EEG changes and cellular alterations. This ion appeared therefore as a supplementary factor of toxicity.

According to the suggestion of Almen, nondissociable CM were investigated. We observed a striking reduction of the toxicity and of the epileptogenic activity when changing the dissociable "amine" of metrizoic acid into the nondissociable "amide." Finally, metrizamide was chosen among different nondissociable CM because of its exceptional tolerance for the CNS.

From 1969 to 1972, neurophysiological of this new CM was thoroughly tested in various laboratories and the different investigated parameters are summarized in Table 2. We must stress the fact that a considerable amount of experimental results were collected before metrizamide (Amipaque) was injected in man for the first time on 31 March, 1972 in our clinical department.

Simultaneous development of CT scan and metrizamide led to new neuroradiological techniques like CT cisternography, bringing the CM directly into contact with the brain tissue. A wide clinical use has confirmed the good tolerance of metrizamide but unexpected CNS reactions were observed. It soon appeared that metrizamide induces unusual changes of the EEG in man, different from those provoked by other CM. Indeed high voltage slow waves like in toxic encephalopathies were definitely more frequently observed than typical epileptic discharges. It was therefore our first impression that the mechanisms supporting the neurotoxicity of metrizamide were different from those of other CM.

Another unexpected and still unexplained side effect is the "psycho-organic syndrome". These "provoked" psychic disturbances, ranging from the temporary lack of concentration to the typical paranoia, raise the question of a possible organic substratum in some human mental disorders.

The fact that animal experiments failed to predict some of the complications observed after clinical use of metrizamide has stimulated and renewed interest in investigations into possible mechanisms of the neurotoxicity of CM and their site of action.

At first considerable discrepancies between results published by different authors were observed, due to variabilities in the site of injection, techniques of anesthesia, concentrations of solutions, etc.

Using hypertonic commercial solutions, an early loss of the monosynaptic H reflex is observed after peripheral stimulation of tibial nerve while cortical evoked potentials remain unchanged. In contrast, after instillation of isotonic solutions, both the amplitude of the corticoevoked potentials and the response of polysynaptic segmental reflex are increased. The monosynaptic segmental spinal reflex response remains stable. It appears therefore that the net neurotoxic effect of CM is a composite of two factors: the depressing action of hypertonicity and the irritating activity of the chemotoxicity. When the mode of action of CM is concerned, there is some evidence suggesting that they may selectively diminish synaptic inhibition. However, the type of this dysinhibition (pre- or postsynaptic) cannot be determined in the actual stage of those experiments.

Even if there is no systematic correlation between osmotic properties and neurotoxicity, the latter was reduced indeed by the synthesis of CM with a lower osmolarity (dimers and polymers).

Another factor, the electrical charge of ions, may interfere with conduction of nervous impulses or affect electrolyte balance. The dramatic reduction of the neurotoxicity of CM achieved by the synthesis of nonionic compounds probably results from a composite of two factors: absence of electrical charge and low osmolarity.

**Table 2.** Metrizamide: preliminary animal experiments (1969–1973)

| Laboratories | Animals | Way of injection | Observed parameters | Anesthesia |
|---|---|---|---|---|
| Salvesen S | Mice | Suboccipital | L.D. 50 | Ether |
| | Rats | | | Urethane |
| | Rabbits | (Chronic catheters) | Clinical reactions | No anesth. |
| | | | Histological changes (opt. micr.) | |
| Gonsette R.E. | Guinea pigs | Pericerebral | Clinical reactions | No anesth. |
| | | | EEG | |
| | | Chronic exp. | Histological changes | No anesth. |
| | | | Opt. micr. | |
| | | | Electr. micr. | |
| Grepe A., Widen L. | Dogs | Suboccipital | EEG | Neurolept. analgesia |
| | | | ECG | |
| | | | CSF pressure | |
| Oftedal S.I. | Rabbits | Cortical application | E corticogr. | Urethane |
| | Cats | | EEG | Nimbutal |
| | | Suboccipital | Evoked potentials | |
| | | Intraventric. | ECG | |
| | | Lumbar | Blood pressure | |
| | | | CSF pressure | |
| | | | Respiration | |
| | | | CSF cells | |
| | | | protein | |
| Skalpe I.O. | Cats | Lumbar | EMG | Nimbutal |
| | | | Blood pressure | |
| | | | Intravesical pressure | |
| | | | ECG | |
| | Rats | Suboccipital (chronic exp.) | Clinical reactions | Ether |
| | | | Histological changes | |

When the chemotoxicity is concerned, differences between various CM are most often set down to their liposolubility, which is determined by the nature of the substituents attached to the triiodobenzene ring. Indeed the synthesis of new nonionic CM by addition of more hydrophilic polyhydroxymoieties or hexoses seems very promising.

It must be also kept in mind that other biological factors like enzymatic or competitive mechanisms may also intervene. Recent in vitro experiments have shown that metrizamide inhibits hexokinase through competition with the substrate glucose. Penetration of metrizamide into the intercellular spaces of the brain in man is generally accepted and it is likely that, to some extent, there is an intracellular penetration as well.

It has been calculated that after intrathecal injection of 6.75 g metrizamide, the concentration in the CSF was about 57 m*M*, which is definitely higher than the CSF glucose content (3.6 m*M*). A possible competitive effect could be observed indeed in such concentrations.

Finally we know from animal experiments and from clinical observations, that "external" factors affecting the distribution and the elimination of CM may contribute to individual reactions. The site of injection, the presence or not of the CM in the basal cisterns, the position of the patient during and after the examination are mechanical factors of the utmost importance. Moreover it has been shown that dehydratation, preexisting arachnoiditis, spinal block, and neuroleptic treatments may influence the biological mechanisms involved in the resorption of CM.

## Conclusions

When the vascular toxicity is concerned, it appears that the most recent CM do not interfere with the BBB mechanism in normal conditions. But we do not know if they are still inert when there is a preexisting fragility of the BBB. Therefore better compounds should be synthetized and the criteria of the ideal vascular CM have been recently defined by Sovak et al.: osmotic pressure close to that of the body fluids, no electrical charge (nonionic), highly hydrophilic character for minimum interaction with biomacromolecules.

For what concerns the intrathecal use, recent advances in the development of CM have produced nonionic compounds much less neurotoxic than previous ionic substances. On the other hand, wide clinical experience with metrizamide has confirmed its good tolerance, but on the other hand the incidence of unusual side effects caused by this compound shows that it is far from being biologically inert.

New experimental tests for neurotoxicity assessment are continuously being developed in order to detect more subtle side effects. The more recent ones are continuous EEG frequency analysis, animals behavior tests, measurement of discomfort by aversive conditioning, and experimental arachnoiditis.

There is reasonable hope that a wider battery of neurophysiological tests will enable the criteria for the ideal CM already defined by Dandy in 1918 to be satisfied: "in addition to its radiographic properties, any substance injected into the ventricles must satisfy two very rigid exactions (1) it must be absolutely non-irritating and non-toxic; and (2) it must be readily absorbed and excreted".

## References


1. Broman T, Olsson O (1948) The tolerance of cerebral blood vessels to a contrast medium of the diodrast group. An experimental study on the effect on the blood-brain barrier. Acta Radiol 30:326–342
2. Dandy WE (1918) Ventriculography following the injection of air into the cerebral ventricles. Ann Surg 68:5–11
3. Gonsette R (1971) An experimental and clinical assessment of watersoluble contrast medium in neuroradiology. A new medium – Dimer X. Clin Radiol 22:44–56
4. Gonsette RE (1972) The neurophysiologic action of contrast media. Acta Radiol 13:889–904
5. Gonsette RE (1973) Biologic tolerance of the central nervous system to Metrizamide. Acta Radiol [Suppl] 335:25–44
6. Heimburger RF, Campbell RL, Kalsbeck JE, Mealey J, Goodell CL (1966) Positive contrast cerebral ventriculography using water soluble media. 1. Animal studies. Confin Neurol 28:97–116
7. Sovak M, Ranganathan R, Lang JH, Lasser EC (1978) Concepts in design of improved intravascular contrast agents. Ann Radiol 21:283–289

# A Nonionic, Isotonic Dimer Iotrol: A New Contrast Medium for the Intrathecal Space. A Review of Pharmacological Evaluation*

M. Sovak, R. Ranganathan, and C. Kerber

## Introduction

A completely biologically inert contrast medium (CM) for the subarachnoid space is not yet available. The goal of our research was to develop a CM which would not affect the functions of the central nervous system or the dynamics of the arachnoides and the CSF, and would accurately delineate the structures.

Ionic media are strongly epileptogenic and they often elicit late chronic arachnoiditis [1]. Although these CM are extremely economical and thus used to a considerable degree for lumbar myelography in Europe, they are not safe and their epileptogenic potential dictates limitations of both dose and technique. Metrizamide, a nonionic water-soluble contrast medium, does not induce chronic inflammatory changes, but it does produce acute side effects with severity correlating with the degree of metrizamide's ingress into the cranial intrathecal space [2]. Furthermore, metrizamide is hydrolytically unstable, which necessitates preparation of its solutions ad hoc. Nonionic iopamidol is hydrolytically stable, but a controlled clinical myelography study has shown similar incidence of adverse effects for iopamidol and metrizamide [3]. Although the potential of seizures elicited by the two nonionic media is low, the incidence of side effects ranging from nausea and headache to psychotic and depressive syndromes convinced a large number of radiologists both in Europe and in the United States to continue the use of the oily medium iophendylate (Pantopaque). Although Pantopaque has practically no acute neurotoxicity, by being immiscible with CSF, it does not provide accurate delineation of the structures. Most importantly, Pantopaque induces late chronic arachnoiditis which sometimes becomes clinically significant only after a number of years [4]. The so-called "safety" of Pantopaque is therefore an illusion afforded only by long-term periods elapsing between the procedure and the first occurrence of symptoms. Thus, it can be seen that there is a considerable need for an improved CM for the intrathecal space.

## Methods and Results

*Development of a new molecule.* A number of nonionic dimers have been prepared by Nyegaard Co., Schering AG, and Bracco Industries. None of these compounds, nevertheless, were further developed for intrathecal use, which suggested to us that substituents other than derivatives of aminopropanediol or serinol were needed. To this end, we de-

* Supported in part by PHS Grant no. GM-22911

veloped a novel synthesis which yielded D,L-amino-erythritol and D,L-amino-threitol, which are new racemic amino-alcohols. The isomeric forms, D-amino-erythritol and L-amino-threitol were not previously described. These substituents proved to be highly hydrophilic and to have a water-solubilizing capability. From a series of compounds, a nonionic dimer, DL-3-117[1], was chosen by us for further development. At the concentration of 300 mgI/ml the dimer is isotonic with the cerebrospinal fluid. At 37 °C it has an acceptably low viscosity of 9.1 cps. It is chemically stable and infinitely water soluble. The molecule contains 46.8% iodine (Fig. 1).

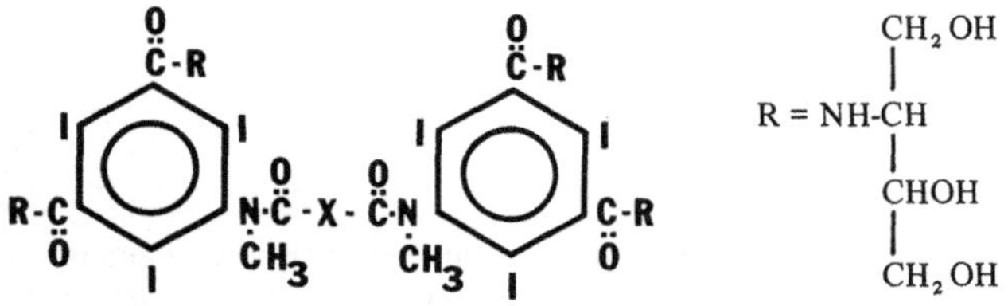

**Fig. 1.** Formula of D,L-3-117. *R* = rest of D L-amino-threitol; *X* = $CH_2$

By *octanol/water partition method*, it is about twice as hydrophilic as metrizamide and thus the most hydrophilic compound known. This observation was confirmed by serum complement-mediated hemolytic assay [5]. In this assay, which measures the effect of interference of contrast media with functional proteins, DL-3-117 proved to be about half as active as metrizamide while iopamidol was equal to metrizamide.

The *intravenous lethal dose* was determined in three groups of ten mice and five rats (330 mgI/ml, 1.1 ml/min). The majority of injected mice survived 27 gI/kg. Increase of dose was prevented by volume effect consideration. In rats, the i.v. $LD_{50}$ was found to be in the range of 12–14 gI/kg.

*Injection of contrast media into the diencephalon* of lightly anesthetized rats in 80 μl volume at doses ranging from 20 to 196 mgI/kg was conducted in groups of ten animals per dose and five dosages per compound. The animals were observed for the occurrence of neural deficits and motor coordination. Expressed in mgI/kg, iopamidol gave $ED_{50}$ 158.2 (128.2–212.4), which made it superior to metrizamide with $ED_{50}$ 60.1 (47.2–73.7). The nonionic iohexol's $ED_{50}$, reported elsewhere, was 67.9 mgI/kg (50.4–84.4) [6]. In contradistinction, the $ED_{50}$ of DL-3-117 was 219 mgI/ml (194.5–249.1), which statistically is significantly better than any other compound tested, at 98% confidence level.

*Intraventricular injections* of 400 mgI/ml DL-3-117 (300 mgI/kg) were performed on nonanesthetized rats with chronically implanted cannulas in the right lateral ventricle. Alertness, motor coordination, locomotion and responsiveness were tested during 3 hours of continuous observation following the injection. The average scores of neurofunctional deficits derived from ten animals gave 1.66 ± 2 for DL-3-117 and 22 for iopamidol. Due to high death occurrence, no scores for metrizamide were obtainable.

---

[1] Generic name: Iotrol

Using the same surgical model, we also applied a standard method of behavioral research by pairing the experience of an intraventricularly injected CM with a given flavor in an attempt to *condition the rats against contrast media*. From the change of consumption of the same flavor later on, an index of aversion was calculated [7]. We were able to produce significant aversion against both iopamidol and/or metrizamide but not against the new dimer.

*Nephrotoxicity* was tested in a pilot study by histological examination of kidneys from the mice which survived in the $LD_{50}$ group for 7 days. As a control, metrizamide and/or iopamidol were used. The animals were kept in metabolic cages and no hematuria or anuria was observed. The histological examination of the mice kidneys revealed a mild vacuolization in the proximal tubular cells similar to iopamidol and/or metrizamide and previously described as "osmotic nephrosis" [8]. It is highly improbable that the phenomenon could be induced by the small amounts of CM used in the intrathecal space. In a pilot study, we injected 150 µl DL-3-117, at a concentration of 400 mgI/ml, into the cisterna magna of lightly anesthetized rats, and studied the kidneys histologically after 3 days. No abnormalities could be found.

Encouraged by these findings, we injected 0.5 ml/kg of 300 mgI/ml DL-3-117 into the *subarachnoid space of four Cynomolgus monkeys*. The injection was carried out through a chronically implanted silastic catheter, connected to an Ommaya reservoir at the lumbar level in a nonanesthetized animal. The contrast medium was then allowed to flow into the cranial space. EEG was recorded immediately prior, during and 3 after the injection. Computer-assisted spectral analysis of the EEG revealed no frequency shifts and only a statistically insignificant decrease of the average amplitude (Figs. 2, 3). No spikes were seen. In contradistinction, metrizamide was epileptogenic in three monkeys out of three (Fig. 4); the epileptic activity made spectral analysis impossible. Iopamidol was less

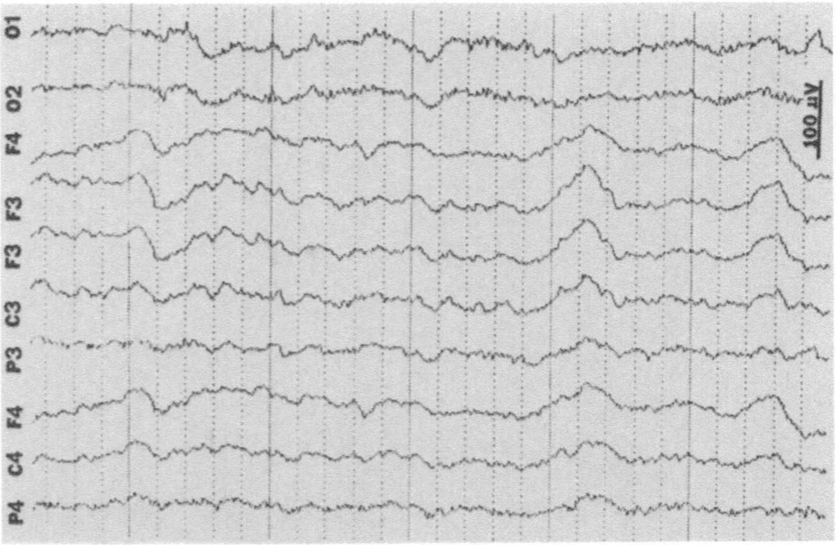


**Fig. 2.** Normal EEG of a *Cynomolgus* monkey 45 min after 0.5 mg/kg intrathecal injection of DL-3-117, 300 mgI/ml

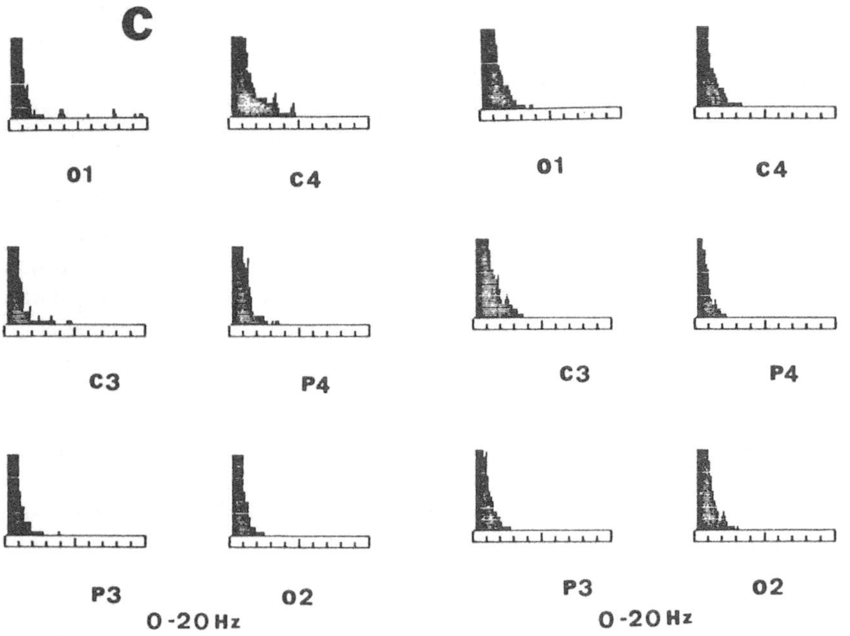


**Fig. 3.** EEG power spectrum before (*C*) and 45 min after DL-3-117 (0.5 ml/kg, 300 mgI/ml)

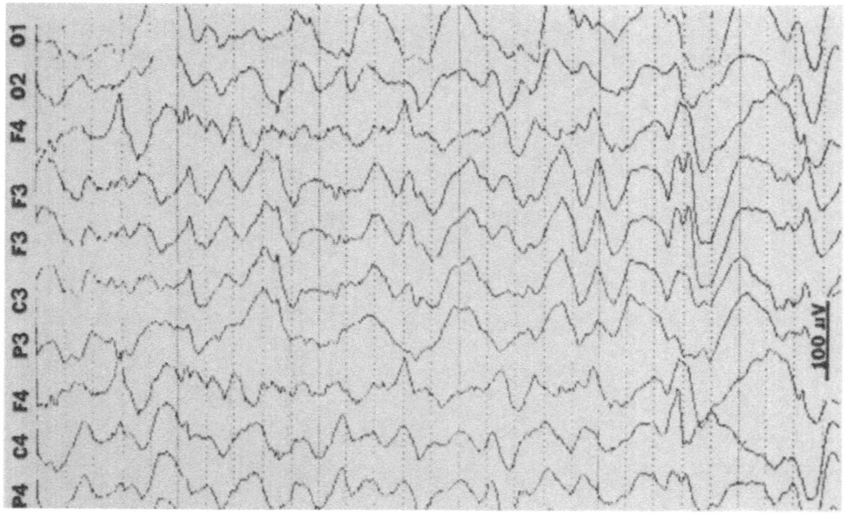


**Fig. 4.** EEG of a *Cynomolgus* monkey 45 min after 0.5 ml/kg, 300 mgI/ml intrathecal injection of metrizamide. Slow waves, spikes, and disappearance of the fast activity can be seen

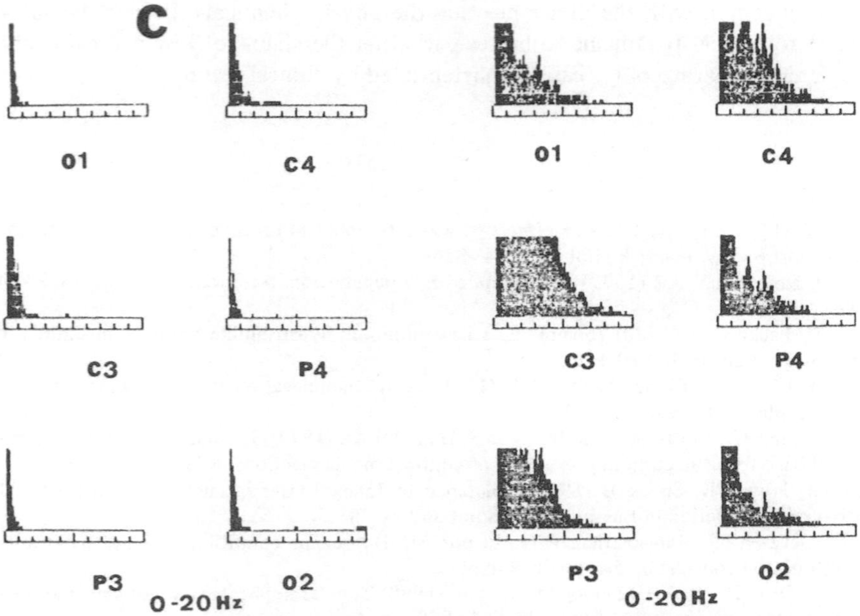


**Fig. 5.** EEG power spectrum before (*C*) and 45 min after 0.5 ml/kg, 300 mgI/ml iopamidol injected intrathecally

epileptogenic than metrizamide but it produced a shift of EEG spectral energy toward the slow frequencies (Fig. 5) [9].

In a series of five anesthetized monkeys, 0.5 ml/kg of CM was maneuvered into the cranial space following lumbar injection, and persistence of CM in the ventricles, *gray and white matter were studied by CT scans* over a period of 48 h. The density increase caused by metrizamide was about twice that of DL-3-117, iopamidol, and/or iohexol. The latter three CM were not statistically different [10].

## Conclusion

Neurotoxicity of CM in the subarachnoid space has been identified as a composite effect of chemotoxicity, including charge and hyperosmolality of solutions vis a vis the cerebrospinal fluid [11]. Charge makes the molecule act as an electrolyte and thus explains the toxicity on the basis of a disturbed electrolytical balance. Chemotoxicity is based on the compound's hydrophobicity; that is, its capability to interact with body biomacromolecules and perturb their functions. Therefore, an improved intrathecal contrast material should be highly hydrophilic, nonionic, and isosmolal with cerebrospinal fluid at the concentrations needed for intracranial radiography; i.e., at least 250 mgI/ml [12].

We realize that the isosmolality could not be achieved with nonionic monomers and that nonionic polymers would be forming hypoosmolal solutions. Therefore, the logical choice was an oligomer, with the dimer meeting the physicochemical criteria of stability and biological tolerance. It remains to be seen whether the claims of low neurotoxicity suggested by animal pharmacology can be substantiated by clinical testing.

## References


1. Ahlgren P (1980) Early and late side effects of water soluble CM for myelography and cisternography: a short review. Invest Radiol 15:S264–S266
2. Drayer BP, Rosenbaum AE (1977) Metrizamide brain penetration. Acta Radiol [Suppl] (Stockh) 355:280–293
3. Hammer B, Lackner W (1980) Iopamidol, a new nonionic hydrosoluble contrast medium for neuroradiology. Neuroradiol 19:119
4. Mayher WE III, Daniel EF Jr, Allen MB Jr (1971) Acute meningeal reaction following pantopaque myelography. J Neurosurg 34:396–404
5. Lasser EC, Lang JH, Sovak M, Kolb W, Lyon S, Hamblin AE (1977) Steroids: theoretical and experimental basis for utilization in prevention of contrast media reactions. Radiology 125:1–9
6. Siefert HM, Press WR, Speck U (1980) Tolerance to Iohexol after intracisternal, intracerebral and intra-arterial injection in the rat. Acta Radiol 362:78–81
7. Sovak M, Deutsch JA, Ranganathan R (to be published) Aversion conditioning in rats by evaluation of intrathecal contrast media. Invest Radiol
8. Moreau JF, Droz D, Noell H, Leibovitch J, et al. (1980) Tubular nephrotoxicity of water soluble iodinated contrast media. Invest Radiol 15:S54–S60
9. Sovak M, Kerber CW, Ranganathan RS (to be published) EEG spectral analysis in nonanesthetized Cynomologus: evaluation of a new nonionic, isotonic dimer. J Neuroradiol
10. Kerber CW, Sovak M (to be published) Radiography of the subarachnoid space and brain penetration of a new nonionic dimer in Cynomolgus monkeys. J Neuroradiol
11. Sovak M, Ranganathan R, Lang JH, Lasser EC (1978) Concepts in design of improved intravascular agents. Ann Radiol 21:283–289
12. Roberson GH, Ellis G, Brumar J, Taveras JM (1977) Cisternography with Metrizamide and hypocycloidal tomography. Acta Radiol [Suppl] (Stockh) 335.314–322

# Excretion of Aqueous Contrast Media From the Subarachnoid Space of Primates

V.M. Haughton, O.P. Eldevik, E.A. Sasse, and B.T. Lipman

## Introduction

Some adverse effects of aqueous myelography including nausea, vomiting, headache, and altered mental function [1, 9] may be due to contrast medium reaching the brain. Therefore, we measured the contrast medium in the serum and in the CSF after lumbar myelography in monkeys. Measurements were made in conditions simulating routine clinical practice and also in animals that were recumbent after myelography, dehydrated, or that had arachnoiditis.

## Materials and Methods

Macaque, nemestrina, or bonnet monkeys weighing 5–7 kg that had satisfactorily passed parasite testing and other health examinations were used for the study. Myelography was performed in the animals, with the technique previously described in detail [1]. The technique includes lumbar puncture at the L3–4 interspace under fluoroscopic monitoring and the injection of 1.2 ml contrast medium into the lumbar subarachnoid space. Radiographs were obtained to verify that the contrast medium is subarachnoid and to study the appearance of the arachnoid sac. The animal was then positioned sitting in a primate restraint chair to minimize gravitation of the contrast medium toward the head. Blood samples were withdrawn from a femoral vein catheter before and at selected intervals after the injection of the myelographic contrast medium. Serum was removed by centrifugation of the clotted blood. Cisternal cerebrospinal fluid was sampled by suboccipital puncture before and periodically after the myelographic contrast medium injection. Iodine was measured in the serum and in the cerebrospinal fluid with an automated catalytic technique [4].

## Results

### Normal Animals

In normal monkeys undergoing myelography, serum iodine concentrations rise rapidly while cisternal iodine concentrations rise much more slowly [6]. For example, in one animal (Fig. 1) serum iodine concentrations reached 100 mg/ml within 15 min, while CSF iodine concentrations reached only 3 mg/ml and not before 1 h after myelography.

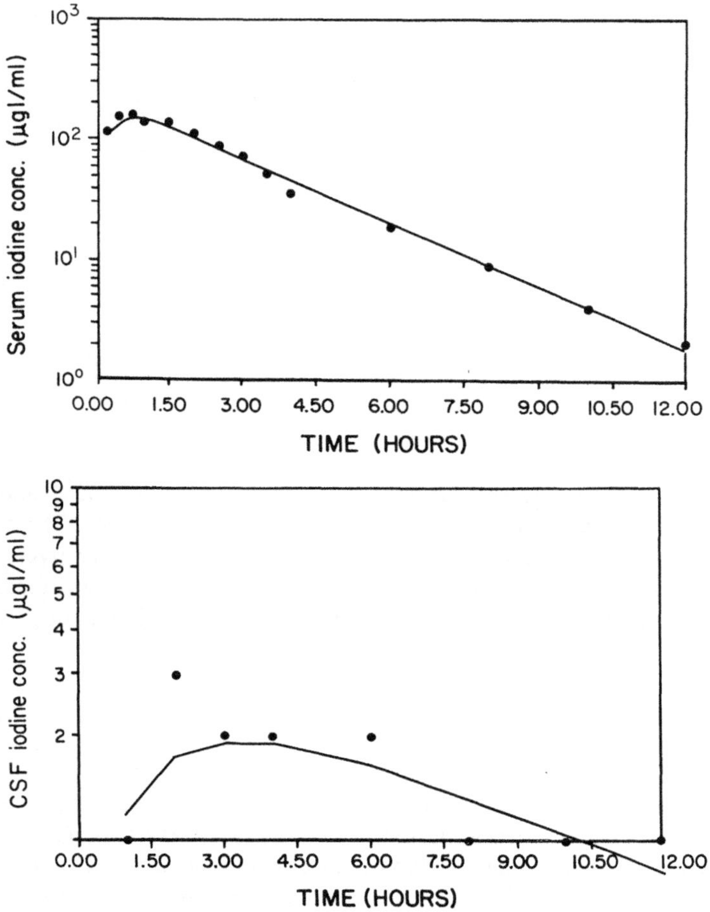


a

b

**Fig. 1a, b.** Serum (**a**) and cisterna magna (**b**) iodine concentrations in a monkey after iocarmate myelography

Minor differences were observed in serum and cisternal iodine concentrations from iocarmate, metrizamide, and iopamidol myelography. This data indicates that the aqueous myelographic contrast medium is eliminated into the primate vascular circulation predominantly across the lumbar arachnoid, presumably through the villi (Pacchionian bodies) present in the root sheaths. Only a small fraction of the contrast medium circulates with the cerebrospinal fluid into the cranial cisterns to be eliminated through the arachnoid villi there.

## Sitting Versus Decubitus Position

Cisternal and serum concentrations of iodine were compared in monkeys having myelography while in decubitus and in sitting positions. Four animals underwent metrizamide myelography twice; once sitting in a primate restraint chair for the first 16 h after the

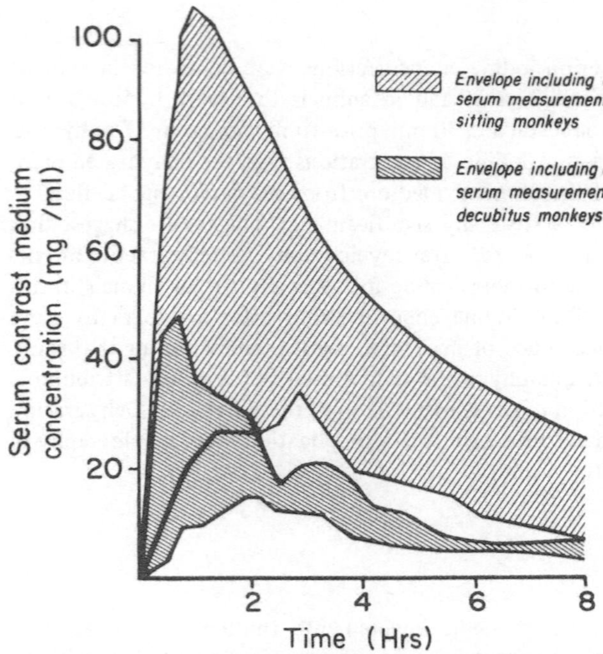


**Fig. 2.** Serum iodine concentrations in animals undergoing metrizamide myelography in sitting and in decubitus positions

procedure, once decubitus for 16 h after the procedure (Fig. 2). The myelograms were performed 7 days apart and in alternating sequence. Cisternal and serum iodine concentrations were also compared in four monkeys having iocarmate myelography followed by 16 h in a sitting position and four animals having iocarmate myelography followed by 16 h in the decubitus position. Serum iodine concentrations were significantly ($P < 0.02$), Wilcoxan Paired Rank Test) higher in animals that were sitting than in animals that were decubitus after myelography (Haughton, unpublished results). Cisternal iodine concentrations were also substantially and significantly higher, in some cases by a factor of 10 (Haughton, unpublished results).

Effect of Previous Myelogram

Iodine concentrations in cisternal cerebrospinal fluid and serum were compared in animals undergoing initial and repeat myelograms [5]. Somewhat lower and significantly later ($P < 0.05$, Wilcoxan Rank Rest) peak serum iodine concentrations were noted in the repeat than in the first myelogram. This delay of excretion was attributed to arachnoiditis, which was demonstrated in the repeat myelogram and the histologic examination of the arachnoid in these animals. In all animals the cisterna magna cerebrospinal fluid iodine concentrations were significantly higher on repeat myelography ($P < .02$, Wilcoxan Rank Sum Test) sometimes by a factor of 100.

Effect of Hydration

Cisternal cerebrospinal fluid and serum iodine concentrations were compared in animals that had myelography after an overnight fast and in animals that were hydrated with 75 ml/h dextrose in water for 4 hours starting 30 min prior to myelography. The hydrated animals in general had greater serum iodine concentrations than the dehydrated ones, indicating a more rapid transfer of the contrast medium from the cerebrospinal fluid to blood, but the differences were not statistically significant [1]. The results suggest that the increased incidence of backache observed after myelography in dehydrated patients [1] may be related to the persistence of metrizamide intrathecally. In all animals in this study, the cisternal cerebrospinal fluid iodine concentrations after myelography were negligible. Therefore, the greater incidence of headache, nausea, and vomiting that is observed in patients undergoing myelography while dehydrated [1] was not attributable to a greater intracranial concentration of contrast medium in these patients. Dehydration may, however, increase the risk of seizures or a fatal complication from myelography in animals with arachnoiditis [2].

## Discussion

Normally aqeuous myelographic contrast media injected into the lumbar subarachnoid space is eliminated directly through the arachnoid into the vascular circulation, perhaps by absorption through the arachnoid villi (Pacchionian bodies) in the lumbar root sheaths, which histologically appear similar to the intracranial arachnoid villi [7, 8]. Normally little myelographic contrast medium reaches the cranial cisterns in the contrast medium is injected into the lumbar subarachnoid space and if the animal is injected into the lumbar subarachnoid space and if the animal is positioned to minimize the gravitation of contrast medium toward the cranial cisterns. If, however, the normal route of excretion is blocked, for example, by arachnoiditis, a tumor or possibly by spinal stenosis, of if the animal is dehydrated, or positioned so that gravity promotes the flow of contrast medium toward the cranial cisterns, larger amounts of contrast medium reach the cisterns around the brain. Therefore, in clinical lumbar myelography, the amounts of the contrast medium reaching the cranial cisterns probably depend on the patient's position and hydration and condition of the lumbar sac. Possibly some side effects and complications of myelography may be minimized by promoting the rapid excretion of the contrast medium to the blood and preventing the accumulation of contrast medium into the cranial cisterns.

*Acknowledgment.* These studies were supported in part by an NIH grant no. 5 RO1 NS 14274-03.

## References

1. Eldevik OP, Haughton VM, Nakken KO (1978) Effect of dehydration on the side effects of metrizamide myelography. Radiology 129:715–717
2. Eldevik OP, Haughton VM, Ho KC (1978) Effect of dehydration on the acute and chronic complications of iocarmate myelography, an experimental study. Radiology 129:713–715

3. Eldevik OP, Haughton VM (1978) Risk factors in complications of aqueous myelography. Radiology 128:415–416
4. Eldevik OP, Haughton VM, Sasse EA (1980) Effect of dehydration on the elimination of aqueous myelographic contrast medium from the subarachnoid space. Invest Radiol 15:155–157
5. Eldevik OP, et al. (1980) Excretion of aqueous myelographic contrast medium in animals undergoing a repeat myelogram. Invest Radiol 15:507–510
6. Eldevik OP, et al. (1980) Elimination of aqueous myelographic contrast media from the subarachnoid space. Invest Radiol 15:S260–S263
7. Gomez DG, Potts DG, Deonarine V, Reilly KF (1973) Effects of pressure gradient changes in the morphology of arachnoid villi and granulations of the monkey. Lab Invest 28:648–657
8. Hassin GB (1930) Pacchionian bodies of the spinal arachnoid. Acta Neurol Psychiatr 13:65–78
9. Skalpe 10 (1977) Adverse effects of water-soluble contrast media in myelography, cisternography, and ventriculography. A review with special reference to metrizamide. Acta Radiol [Suppl] 355: 359–370

# Experimental Model of Neurotoxicity Study of Water-soluble Contrast Media

M. Gioux, P. Arne, J. Paty, and J.M. Caille

In spite of recent progress in neuroradiology with water-soluble contrast media, some neurological disturbances have been described in man [1]. Our aim is to describe an animal experimental model for studying Central Nervous System (CNS) toxicity with such media, after subarachnoid injection.

Spontaneous brain electrical activity (EEG), is a classical index for studying brain toxicology [5].

Evoked potentials, following external stimulation, may be recorded at differents levels, on a sensory pathway, and may help to demonstrate the effects of these substances on conduction and synaptic transmissions [7].

Using such a model it is possible to analyze the action of these substances, and to predict their adverse reactions in clinical use.

## Method

The preparation (Fig. 1) used is the rabbit chronically implanted with electrodes for recording over long periods. The injection cannula is opened into the cerebrospinal fluid. These implantations were made stereotaxically, using Sawyer's [8] reference points.

The electrodes were placed in the following structures: two cortical electrodes at the level of the somatomotor and visual cortex; two thalamic electrodes in the ventropostero-lateral nucleus and the lateral geniculate body. The electrical connection was to a connector cemented to the skull.

A sealable canula was permanently implanted in the same way, passing into the arachnoid spaces above the olfactory bulb. The substances to be tested were injected by this canula without interrupting the electrical recording.

Recordings were carried out in rest conditions. We measured the electrical activity from the four implanted electrodes. These were monopolar recordings with respect to the ear reference. This activity was amplified and recorded on magnetic tape. The ECG of the animal was recorded at the same time, and the synchronizing signals when stimuli were delivered. Data were analyzed later, using an intertechnique PLURIMAT S signal analyzer, which studied:

1. Spontaneous brain activity or EEG between the stimulation sequences
2. The evoked potentials obtained by averaging the EEG after the stimuli

Eight rabbits were studied by this method. Eight recordings were carried out during and after injection of four contrast media: metrizamide 2, Dimer X 1, iopamidol 2, ioglunide 3.

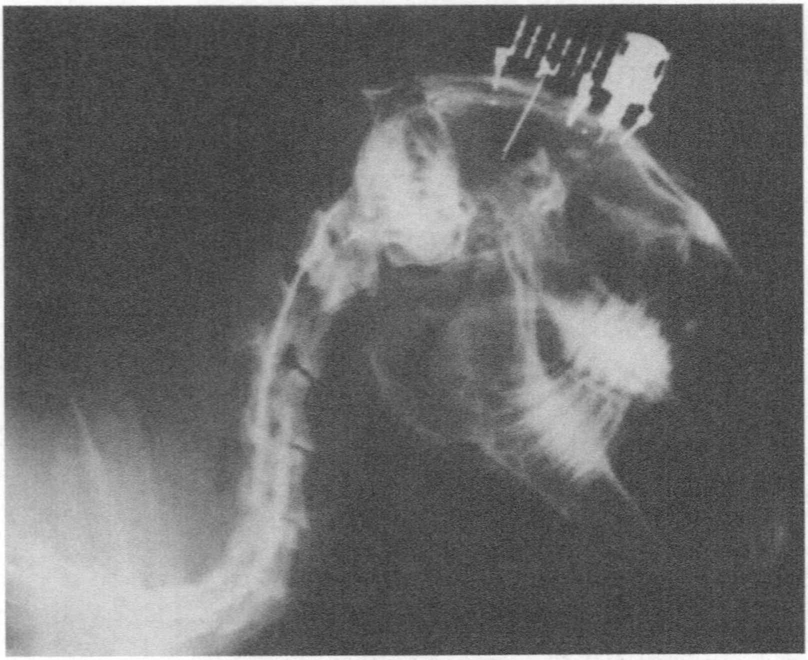

**Fig. 1.** X-ray of implanted rabbit with cortical and thalamic electrodes, after injection of contrast medium via sealable canula

## Results

### Spontaneous Electrical Activity or EEG

This may be shown in two ways: the variations in potential difference with time (rhythms) may be recorded from the different electrodes. This *polygraphic study* either analyzes the fundamental frequencies of the rhythms, or by *spectral analysis* represents the energies of the different frequency bands.

*Polygraphic Study (Conventional EEG).* The continuous tracing reveals certain changes:

Slowing of the rhythms after injection of contrast with the appearance of high voltage slow waves, during which, basal activity disappears,

Epileptic seizures (Fig. 2) occur, with or without clinical manifestations, and are characterized by sharps beginning in the thalamic regions,

Marked cerebral changes before the animal's death. The tracing shows large paroxyms, then burst suppression before ensuing electrical silence.

*Computerized EEG.* This is a quantitative study of the different frequencies (sinusoidal) which make up the EEG. There are obtained by a Fast Fourier Transform of the recorded electrical signals. The sequence of frequency spectra shows certain changes with time:

Reduced frequency of spontaneous basal rhythm (5 Hz)

Increase in low frequencies (left side of diagrams)

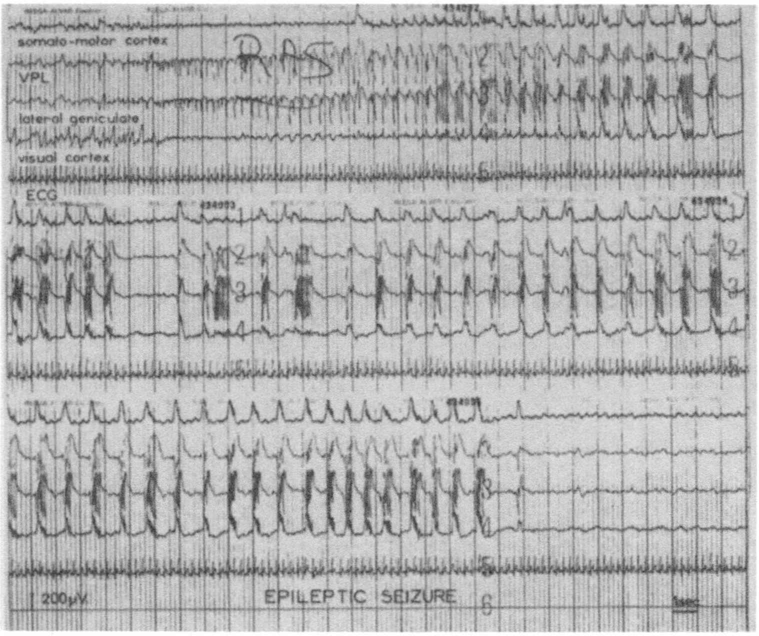


**Fig. 2.** Epileptic seizure in polygraphic study, beginning in thalamus

The changes are, however, different, according to the contrast injected.

*A quantitative study* can be made of these spectra for statistical analysis. The energy content in certain characteristic frequency bands is measured: 0.5–2.5 Hz; 2.5–4.5 Hz, etc.

The percentage energy of these bands with respect to the total spectrum energy gives the index. We calculate the mean index at different times of the recording: before injection, 30 min after injection of solvent, 30 min, 1 h, 2 h, and 3 h after injection of substance. Using these six indices we are able to study the quantitative changes in the frequencies.

1. On the basis of the total group mean
2. For each of the recordings, in order to see the differences between the different substances injected

1. Averaged indices for all substances used show general slowing of electrical activity (increase in 0.5–2.5 Hz band) after injection of solvent or contrast. The difference is, however, greater after contrast and reaches significance at 0.001, whereas the others are not significant. This slowing disappears rapidly when solvent is injected but continues to develop after contrast. The slowing of electrical activity recorded from the four structures is maximal 1–2 h after injection of substance. This is shown by increase of the 0.5–2.5 Hz index and by complementary lowering of the 4.5–6 Hz index.

2. We then studied the changes of two indices (0.5–2.5 Hz and 6–16 Hz) from a single somatomotor cortical electrode for the different substances injected (equal to 150 mg iodine altogether). For some (metrizamide: ME – ioglunide: AG) shift toward the low frequencies is obvious. For others (Dimer X : DX – iopamidol : IO) this change is less

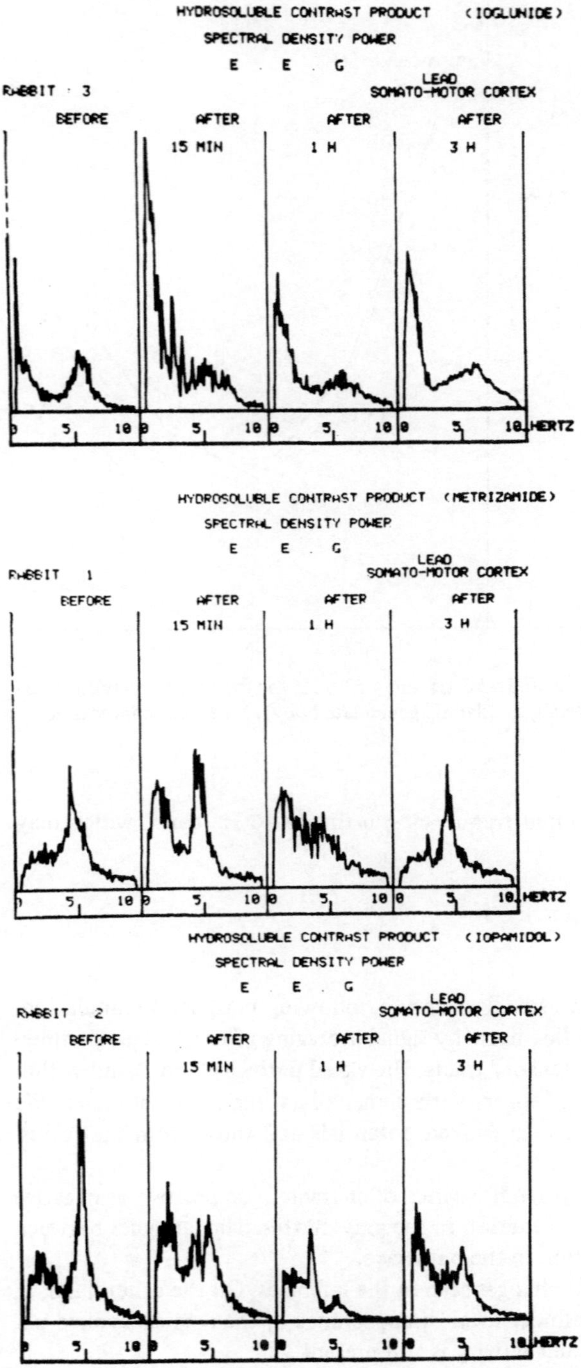


**Fig. 3.** Frequency spectra at different times in relation to the injection. The frequencies are shown on the horizontal axis (0.5–10 Hz) and their energy on the vertical. The lead is the somatomotor cortex; and three drugs were injected

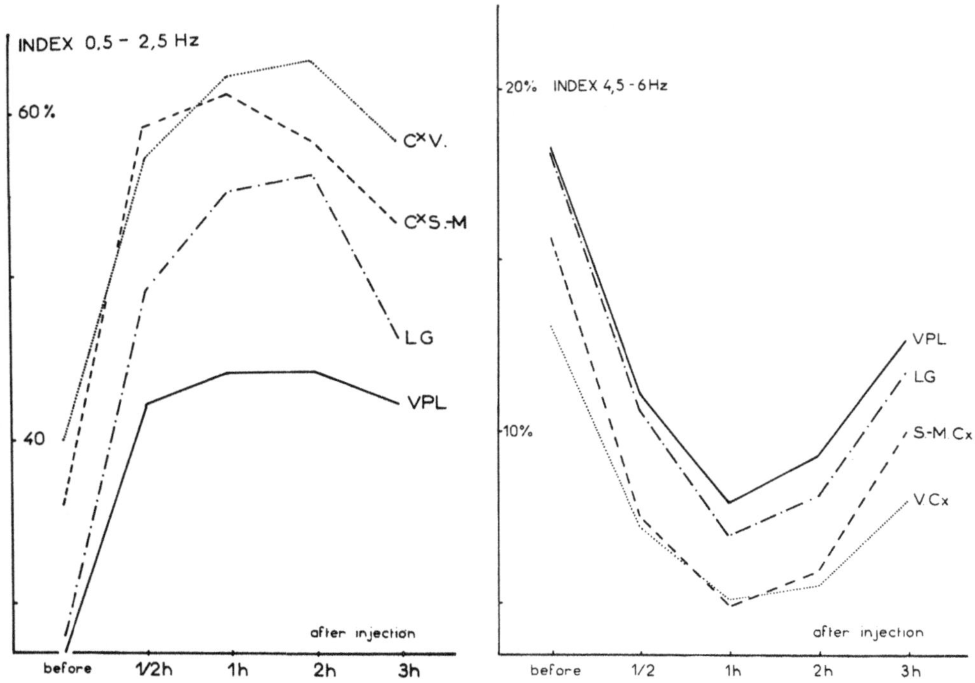


**Fig. 4.** Changes in the mean frequency bands: 0.5–2.5 Hz and 4.5–6 Hz for the four leads (visual cortex, somatomotor cortex, ventroposterolateralis and lateral geniculate body), for all substances used

marked and shows a light return of rapid frequencies in the 6–16 Hz band, which may account for their convulsant effect.

## Evoked Potentials

There is the electrical response of a central structure following peripheral stimulation. This signal is extracted from the baseline noise by signal averaging after repeated peripheral stimulation. We have studied two sensory tracts: the visual pathway, short, and within the brain; and the somesthesic tract, longer, with a medullary then central route. We measured for these two routes the cortical evoked potentials and those from the corresponding thalamic relays.

Each evoked potential is made up from a series of characteristic positive or negative spikes. The spikes represents synaptic function in the gray matter. The latencies between spikes are the result of signal conduction in the pathways.

There are no stable or significant changes seen in the latencies. On the other hand, in the somesthesic system, there is an almost total disappearance of the cortical evoked potential after injection, although thalamic activity is still present.

Injection of solvent produces no change in the visual system, whereas contrast triggers an increase of the cortical evoked potential, followed by a decrease. In the thalamic nucleus (VPL) there is a similar increased amplitude, but appearing later.

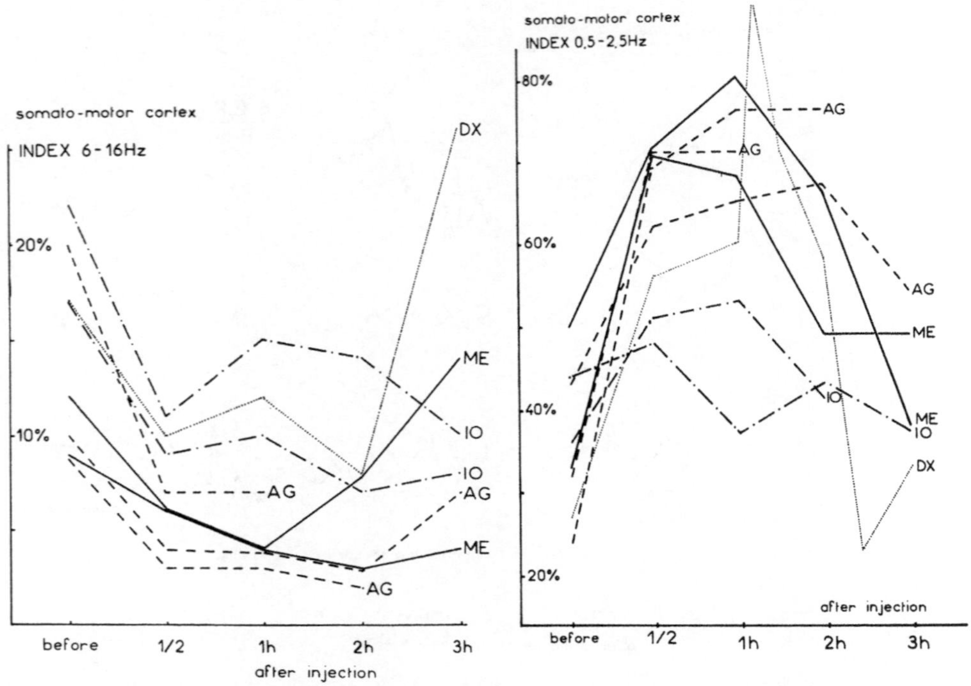


**Fig. 5.** Changes in two mean frequency bands in the somatomotor cortex, for each injection of contrast

## Conclusion

This experimental model demonstrates definite changes when contrast media are injected. These effects may be analyzed statistically. On the other hand, it is a simple preparation, which lies between human clinical observation and more fundamental studies at cellular level.

The results obtained show:

An increase in low frequency activity; this effect was also seen when solvent was used, which may be due to metabolic effects and not necessarily indicate a toxic effect.

Weakened evoked potentials from the cortex, indicating a lowering of signal/noise ratio; this may be due to increased basic noise following weakening of cortical synchronizing signals, or decreased signal strength [6].

A subcortical action triggering epileptic seizures at thalamic level as well as interrupting thalamocortical conduction.

An action essentially on the gray matter, which agrees with reflexologic [4] or intracellular studies [3].

Finally, we have shown different actions according to the substance used, both in frequency analysis of spontaneous activity, and the changes with time of these frequency spectra. It is possible in this way to build up activity profiles of the different substances and grade them in relation to each other.

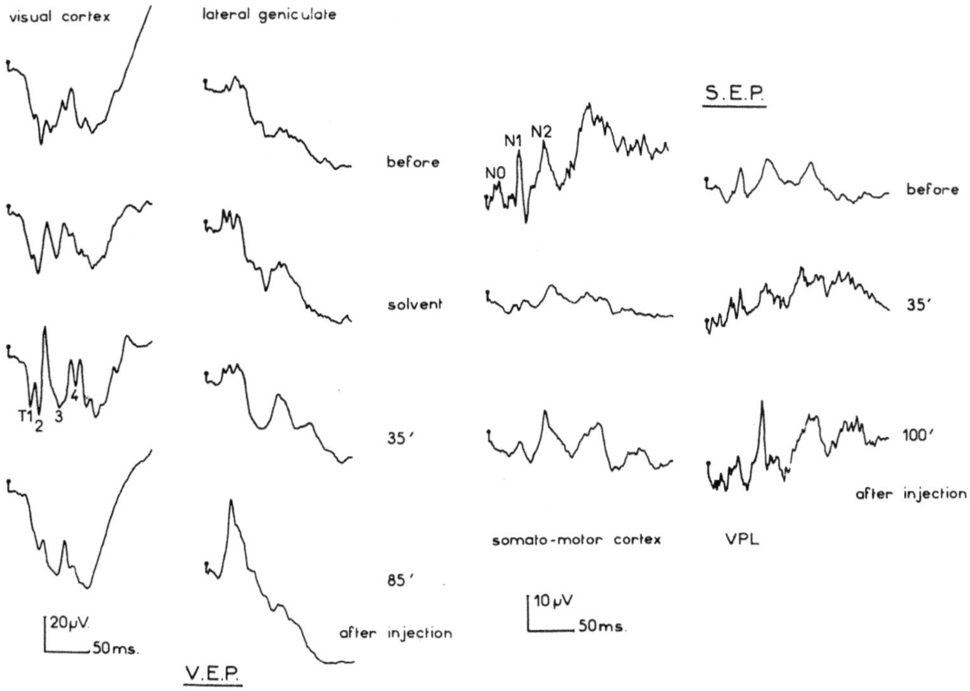


**Fig. 6.** Evoked potentials by visual or somesthesic stimulation from the cortex and thalamus, after injection of metrizamide

## References


1. Caille JM, Guibert-Tranier F, Howa JM, Billerey A, Calabet A, Piton J (1980) Contamination encéphalique par la métrizamide après myélographie. J Neuroradiol 7:3–12
2. Grossman RI, Marder E, Davis KR, Traveras JM (1981) The effect of metrizamine on synaptic transmission. The American Society of Neuroradiology, Chicago, 4–10 April 1981
3. Hershkowitz N, Bryan NR (1981) Intracellular effects of radiographic contrast agents. The American Society of Neuroradiology, Chicago, 4–10 April 1981
4. Hilal SK (1977) Effect of isotonic contrast agents on spinal reflexes in the cat. Radiology 122: 149–155
5. Mellerio F (1964) L'electroencéphalographie dans les intoxications aiguës, 1 vol. Masson, Paris
6. Oftedal SI (1973) Effect of water soluble contrast media on cortically evoked potentials in the cat. Acta Radiol [Suppl] 335:133–142
7. Paty J, Corcelle L, Faure JMA (1974) Visual evoked response and antimalarial drugs. XIIth ISCERG Symp. 20–22 may 1974, The Haye.
8. Sawyer CH (1954) The rabbit diencephalon in stereotaxic coordinates. J Comp Neurol 101:801–824

# Immediate and Delayed Neurotoxicity of Newly Synthesized Contrast Media Demonstrated by EEG Sequential Analysis

R.E. Gonsette

## Introduction

It appears from the literature that minor side effects as well as serious adverse reactions are usually observed 6–12 h following metrizamide intrathecal injections.

The parenchymal penetration of intrathecally injected contrast media (CM) into the spinal cord as into the brain tissue is not an unexpected phenomenon. The time frame over which this penetration occurs has been demonstrated in animals by CT scan [3] and autoradiography [2]. It has been confirmed in man [1] and helps to explain delayed occasional toxic encephalopathy or limb myoclonus.

Using histological techniques, immediate brain tissular reactions were observed for as long as 72 h after pericerebral injections of CM in the guinea pig, and it was suggested by us in 1971 [4] that clinical untoward reactions are likely to occur during this limited interval of time.

The influence of CM on the brain physiology can be investigated by electroencephalographic recordings (EEG) but, for technical reasons, continuous monitoring of cerebral bioelectric activities is quite impossible using standard techniques. EEG samples are therefore taken at regular intervals of time and transient or brief bioelectrical changes can be missed.

The widespread use of electronic computers opens new possibilities in mass screening and monitoring of electrical brain activities. Screening requires the maximum amount of information to be extracted both as regard basic structures and specific shapes of sequences. Monitoring continuously extracts from the signal a number of basic parameters whose evolution in time is presented in a synthetic and immediate form.

The transformation of time to frequencies and the presentation of spectral patterns in perspective offer a practical and comprehensive picture of the EEG evolution in time. Using this recent technique, we looked for possible differences between metrizamide and newly synthetized CM, concerning their immediate and/or delayed neurotoxicity.

## Material and Methods

Effects of anesthesia on the EEG are well known and experiments were therefore conducted on unanesthetized restrained guinea pigs. The animal is placed on a table with its head and four limbs firmly fixed in order to avoid movement artifacts.

Four bipolar electrodes are inserted into the cleaned skull in the frontal and parietal regions of both hemispheres, and care is taken not to penetrate the internal part of the bone.

A burr hole (1 mm diameter) is made with a dentist's drill in the prefrontal region, adjacent to the sagittal suture, without damaging the dura mater. The CM is injected with a microsyringe through a short beveled needle placed in contact with the orbital base of the skull. Thereafter the burr hole is occluded with surgical bone wax to prevent escape of the CM. In those conditions, the CM is distributed in the basal cisterns and over the entire surface of the brain. In order to keep the CM in the intracranial cavity, the animal is placed in supine position with its head lowered.

EEG sequential analysis is performed using a standard OTE Galilleo Berg-Fourier analyzer. Experimental conditions, with special regard to external stimuli, are exactly the same for each animal.

The following compounds were tested: Ioserinate (Schering), metrizamide (Nyegaard), Iopamidol (Bracco), Ioglunide (Guerbet), MP 8000 (Mallinckrodt), and Iohexol (Nyegaard).

## Results

It was first confirmed with this technique that saline (0.2 ml) in concentration equimolar to 300 mg/I/ml CM solutions failed to produce any changes for as long as 12 h. In opposition, meglumine hydrochloride provoked an early increase in the 2–5 Hz band that persisted for 6–8 h.

Ioserinate, a dissociable meglumine salt, provokes early epileptic fits and subsequent death of the animals after pericerebral injection of 0.05 ml 280 mg/I/ml solutions. The results confirm the high neurotoxicity of previous dissociable CM.

Injections of 0.2 ml metrizamide at a concentration of 400 mg/I/ml failed to produce any immediate changes. Delayed high voltage slow waves were sometimes observed and low amplitude hypersynchronous activities occurred in a few animals (Fig. 1a, b).

Iopamidol induces early typical epileptic discharges. They are observed quite systematically after injection of 0.2 ml 400 mg/I/ml solutions. A normal EEG frequency pattern is rapidly restored and remains unchanged thereafter. However, we learned from prolonged recordings that delayed epileptic seizures can be observed after 6 or 8 h with possible fatal results (Fig. 2a, b).

Injection of 0.2 ml Ioglunide 400 mg/I/ml solutions failed to produce any change of the EEG frequency pattern. Increase in the 0.5–6 Hz band and low voltage fast activities were sometimes observed. Epileptogenic seizures were never detected (Fig. 3a, b).

MP 8000 solutions with an iodine content higher than 300 mg/I/ml were not available. After injection of 0.2 ml of these solutions, we did not observe any changes on the EEG frequency analysis.

Injections of 0.2 ml Iohexol solutions with an iodine concentration of 400 mg/ml produced early but transient increase of the 5–10 Hz band. After injections of 0.3 ml, these early changes were more pronounced but always shortlasting and high voltage discharges or epileptic seizures were never observed (Fig. 4a, b).

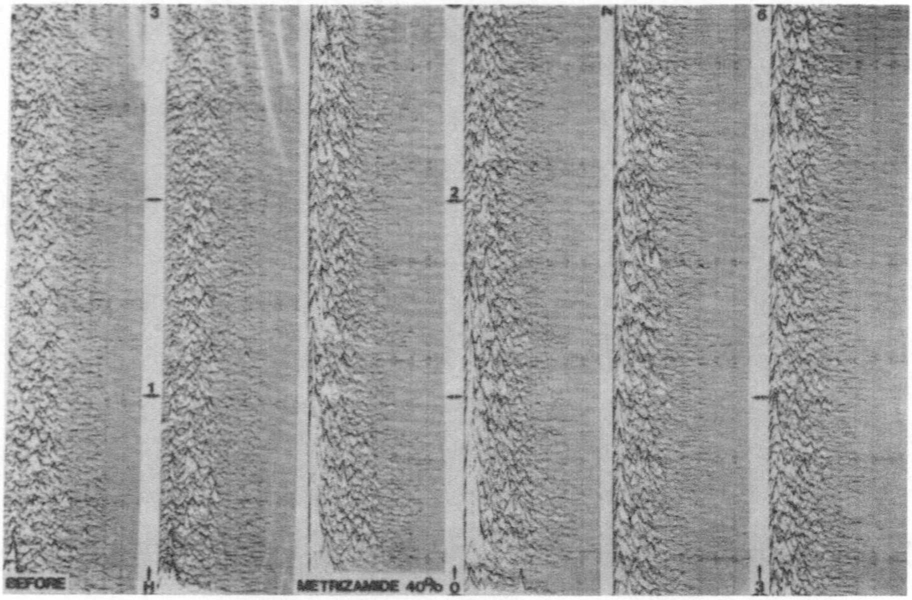


**Fig. 1a.** EEG sequential analysis after pericerebral injection of 0.2 ml metrizamide 40% iodine: no changes

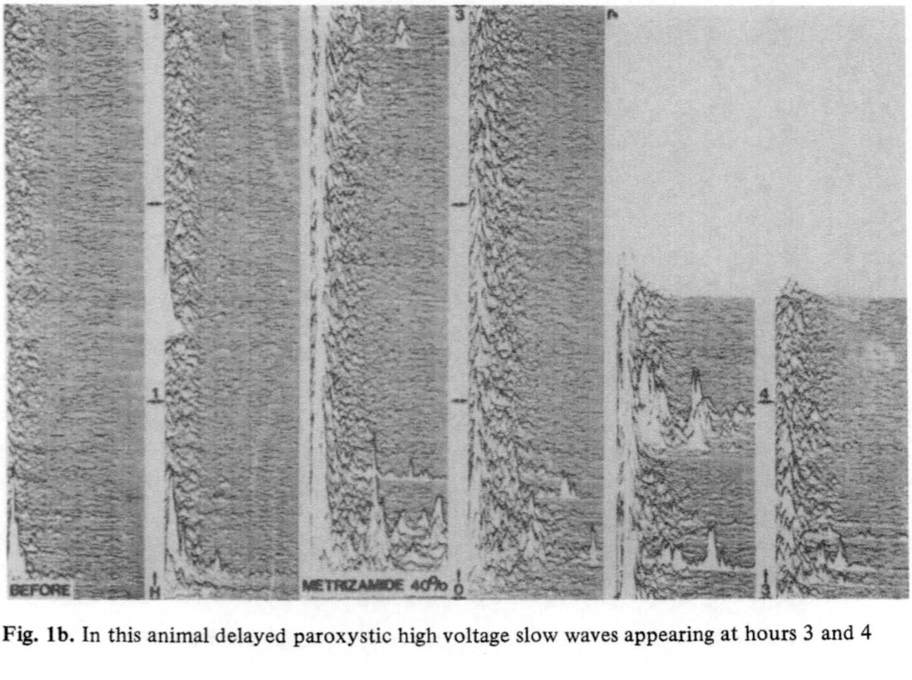


**Fig. 1b.** In this animal delayed paroxystic high voltage slow waves appearing at hours 3 and 4

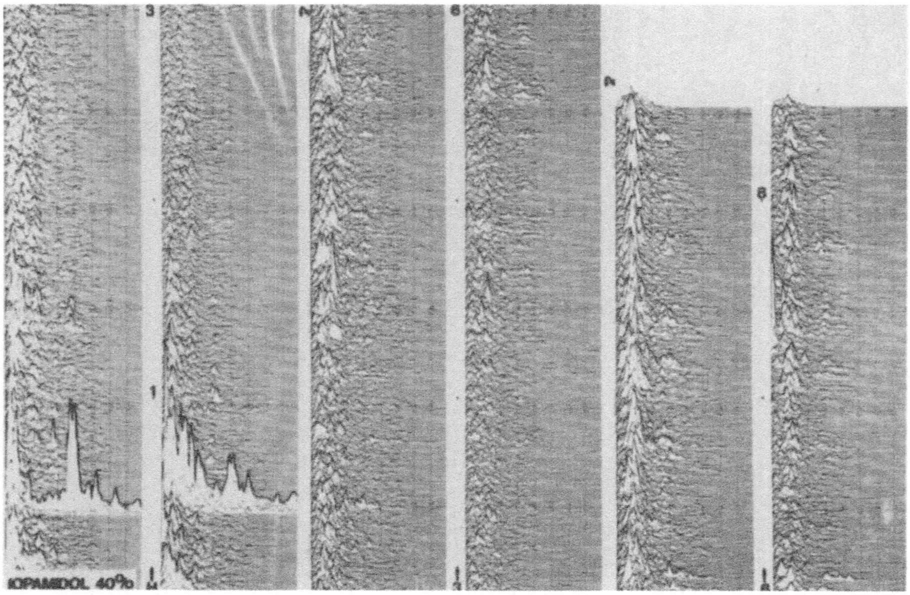


**Fig. 2a.** Pericerebral injection of 0.2 ml Iopamidol 40% iodine: epileptic fits after 30 min and normal recording thereafter

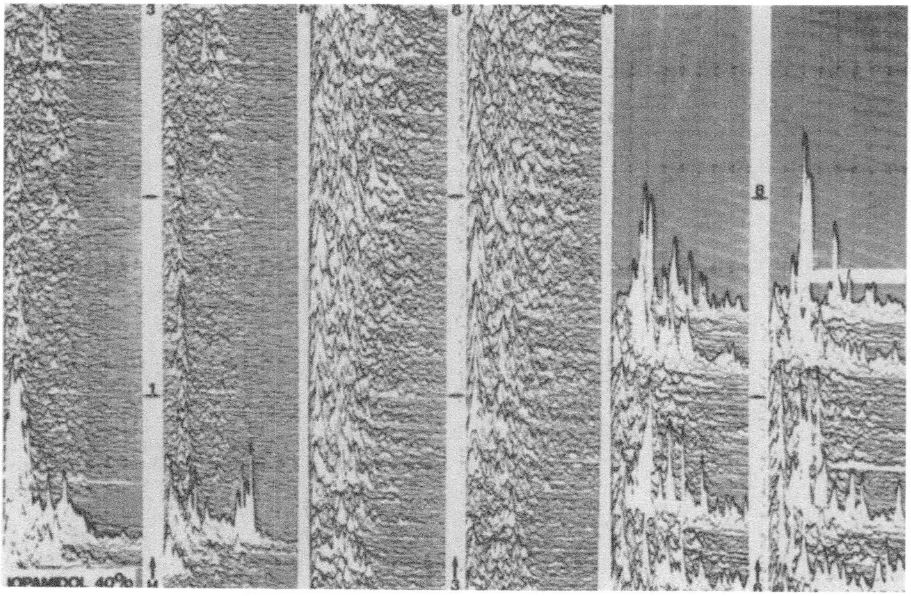


**Fig. 2b.** In this animal reappearance of epileptic fits, status epilepticus, and death after 6 h

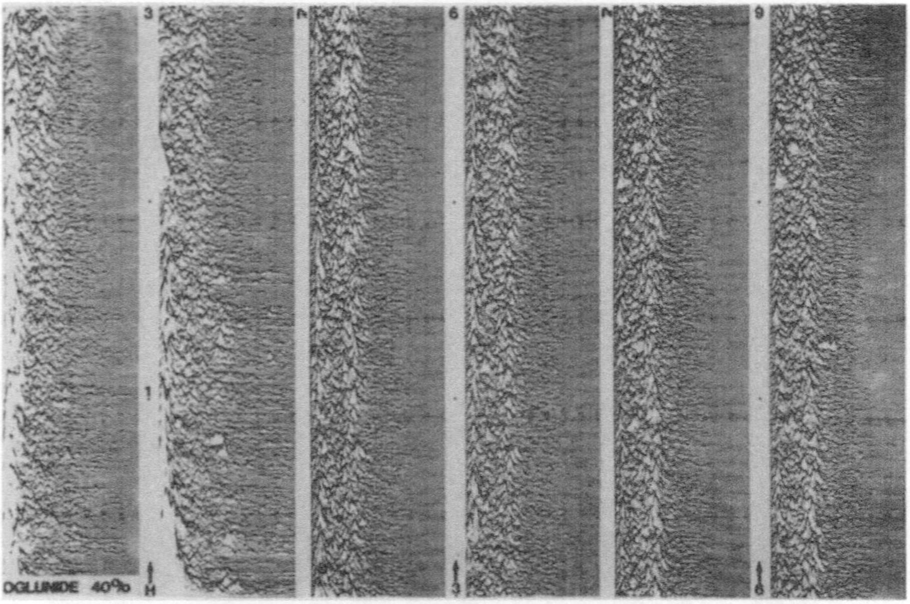

**Fig. 3a.** Pericerebral injection of 0.2 ml Ioglunide 40% iodine: normal EEG sequential analysis for 9 h

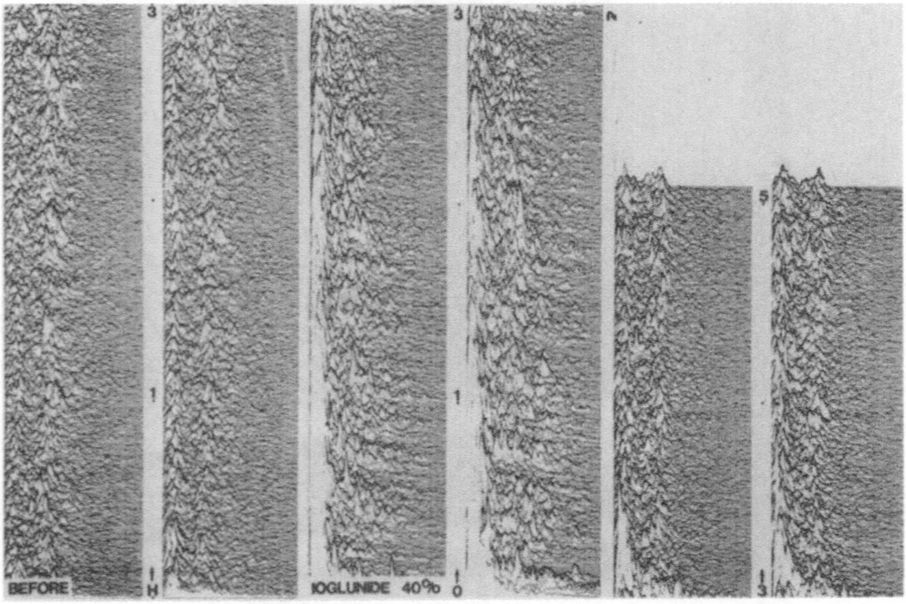

**Fig. 3b.** In this animal: mild power increase of the 0.5–4 Hz band during 2 h 30 min

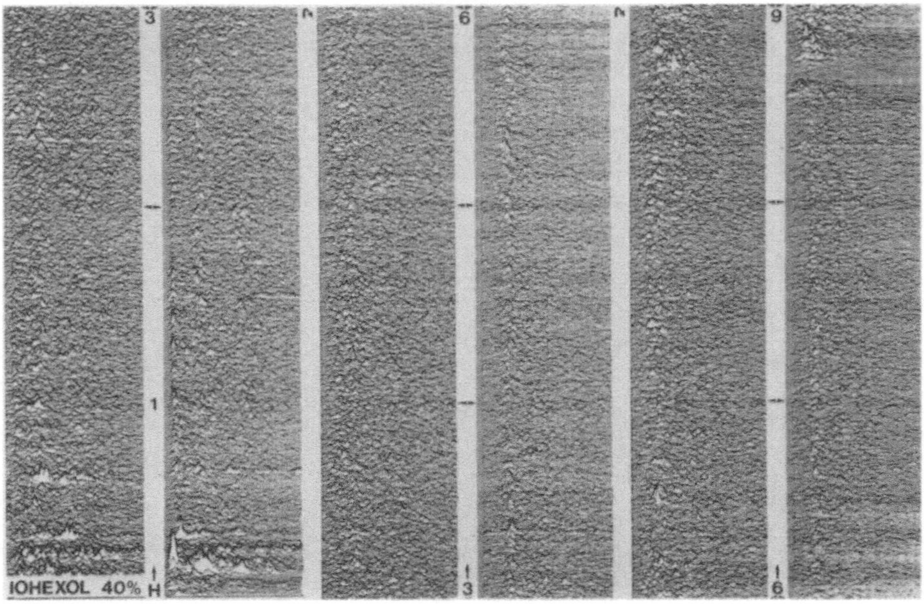


**Fig. 4a.** Pericerebral injection of 0.2 ml Iohexol 40% iodine: transient power increase of the 0.5–8 Hz band for 5 min

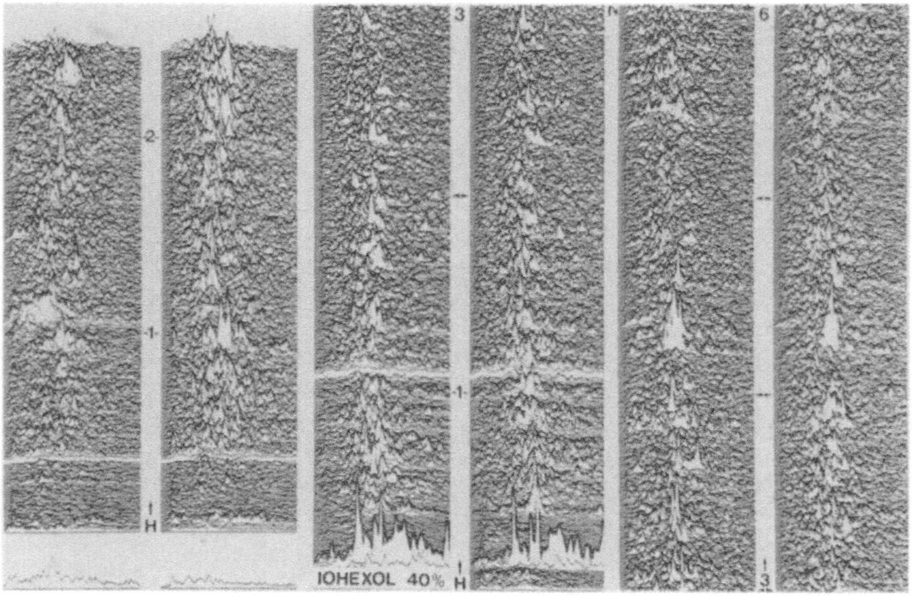


**Fig. 4b.** Pericerebral injection of 0.3 ml Iohexol 40% iodine: transient but definite power increase of the global 0.5–16 Hz band, normal recording thereafter

## Discussion

Sovak et al. [7] recently included the EEG spectrum analysis in their testing battery of new CM. Continuous monitoring of EEG frequency analysis for 10–12 h provides new insights into the neurotoxicity of CM since delayed as well as immediate effects on brain electrophysiology are detected.

Using standard EEG recordings, we were unable to demonstrate any effect of metrizamide on brain potentials in the guinea pig, whereas the monitored frequency analysis demonstrated slow waves bursts like those sometimes observed in patients following metrizamide investigations.

The possible epileptogenicity of Iopamidol, previously demonstrated [5] was confirmed. Moreover, delayed status epilepticus appeared potentially lethal.

MP 8000 seems promising but further experiments with more concentrated solutions will be needed.

Ioglunide and Iohexol provoke mild immediate changes if any and delayed reactions were never observed. With this technique, the two CM appear therefore to have the lowest neurotoxicity and to be potentially useful as intrathecal radiopaque agents in man.

Our preliminary clinical experience with Ioglunide will be published elsewhere [6], but when compared to metrizamide, minor side effects were less frequent. Intracranial presence of the CM was demonstrated in 45 patients. No psychoorganic syndromes were observed and EEG changes occurred in only 3.5% of the patients (57 controls). The percentage of subjective reactions and EEG changes in this group of patients was definitely lower than that generally accepted following metrizamide investigations conducted in the same clinical conditions.

## Conclusion

Monitored EEG spectral analysis makes it possible to observe cerebral bioelectric activities evolution in time. Delayed effects of CM on the EEG can be detected and this technique provides new criteria for the screening of CM. More clinical correlations will be needed but it is suggested that the subjective and objective tolerance of a new CM not producing delayed effects on the EEG is better than that of previous contrast agents.

## References


1. Caille JM, Guibert-Tranier F, Howa JM, Billerey J, Calabet A, Piton J (1980) Cerebral penetration following Metrizamide myelography. J Neuroradiol 7:3–12
2. Drayer BP, Rosenbaum AE (1977) Metrizamide brain penetrance. Acta Radiol [Suppl] 355: 280–293
3. Dubois PJ, Drayer BP, Sage M, Osborne D, Heinz ER (1981) Intramedullary penetrance of Metrizamide in the dog spinal cord. Amer. J. Neurorad. 2:313–317
4. Gonsette R (1971) An experimental and clinical assessment of watersoluble contrast medium in neuroradiology. A new medium – Dimer X. Clin Radiol 22:44–56
5. Gonsette RE, Brucher JM (1980) Neurotoxicity of novel water-soluble contrast media for intrathecal application. Invest Radiol 15:254–259
6. Gonsette RE, Liesenborgh L (to be published) Ioglunide: a new contrast medium for myelography and cisternography (Animal experiments and preliminary clinical experience).
7. Sovak M, Ranganathan R, Johnson M (1980) Spectral analysis of lapine EEG: neurotoxicologic evaluation of new nonionic contrast media. Invest Radiol 15:452–456

# The Effect of Myelographic Contrast Media on the Arachnoid

V.M. Haughton

The need to develop a sensitive assay for postmyelographic arachnoiditis was apparent when Autio [2] and Ahlgren [1] detected arachnoiditis complicating clinical iocarmate myelography.

We developed a model of lumbar myelography in monkeys, which have a cauda equina and subarachnoid space like man's so that lumbar puncture can be performed safely and reliably below the conus medullaris and contrast medium can be pooled in the caudal sac as in clinical myelography. In initial studies, it was shown that postmyelographic arachnoiditis could be detected and quantitated 3 months after the initial experimental myelogram in a repeat myelogram and in anatomic sections of the dura and arachnoid. The severity of myelographic changes of root sheath obliteration and dural sac constriction correlated well with histologic evidence of arachnoid fibrosis. Furthermore, the experimental results in the monkey model have correlated well with the clinical investigations of aqueous media.

## Materials and Methods

Bonnet, macaque, and nemestrina monkeys are utilized in the study. All animals undergo quarantine and testing for mycobacterial and intestinal parasites prior to being used in experiments. The procedure for myelography is a follows: The animal is fasted overnight and premedicated with phencyclidine hydrochloride and atropine. Its back is shaved and disinfected and the animal is then placed prone on a myelographic table tilted 15° head-end up. Lumbar puncture is performed at the L3–4 interspace with a disposable 22-gauge needle under fluoroscopic monitoring. After 1.2 ml cerebrospinal fluid are removed for routine tests, the test myelographic contrast medium is injected intrathecally. Radiographs are obtained at 1 and 5 minutes following injection to verify the subarachnoid placement of the contrast medium and to visualize the root sheaths and arachnoid sac. The needle is then removed and the animal is placed in sitting position in a primate restraint chair for 16 h.

Twelve weeks later, the myelogram is repeated and then the animal is sacrificed. The dural sac and its contents are removed, fixed, stained, and examined by light and electron microscopy.

Postmyelographic changes in the arachnoid are determined by comparing the first and the subsequent myelograms. The changes in the root sheaths, dural sac, and nerve roots that are characteristic of arachnoiditis are scored on a scale of 0 to 36. The scoring system, described in detail elsewhere [6], consists of grading nine sites (L4, L5, L6, left and right nerve root sheaths, and arachnoid sac) 0 for normal; 1 for questionable arachnoiditis; 2 for mild arachnoiditis; 3 for moderate; and 4 for severe.

This histologic changes of chronic arachnoiditis are scored also on a scale of 0 to 36. The degree of fibrosis on nine different sections taken between L3 and L6 are scored 0 for normal to 4 for severe.

## Results

The dose response curves for arachnoiditis from several aqueous myelographic contrast media were studied (Fig. 1). Thirty-six monkeys had myelography with different concentrations of metrizamide, iocarmate or iohexol. For both metrizamide and iocarmate, more severe arachnoiditis could be demonstrated as the concentration of the myelographic contrast medium increased (V.M. Haughton, unpublished work). For iohexol in concentrations up to 370 mg I/ml, no arachnoiditis could be demonstrated. The chance that the dose response with metrizamide or iocarmate occurred fortuitously was less than 5% (Wilcoxan Rank Sum Test).

Arachnoiditis from different approved and experimental myelographic contrast media were compared (Fig. 2). Thirty-two monkeys were used for these studies. Control animals having an intrathecal injection of either isotonic saline or autologous cerebrospinal fluid had histologic scores for arachnoiditis ranging from 0 to 8. Four animals having iocarmate myelography had scores ranging from 9 to 28 (V.M. Haughton, 1978, unpublished work). The differences between the control and iocarmate scores were significant at the 5% level (Wilcoxan Rank Sum Test). Histologic arachnoiditis scores for the other four agents (metrizamide, ioglunide, iopamidol, and iohexol) ranged up to 7, 8, or 12 units. The differences between the scores in these four contrast agents and controls did not differ significantly.

In other experiments, aqueous contrast media and blood were not synergistic in producing postmyelographic arachnoiditis (V.M. Haughton, unpublished work). Prophylactic intrathecal methylprednisolone had no significant effect on postmyelographic arachnoiditis [4]. Arachnoiditis did not seem to be caused by hyperosmolality alone in the subarachnoid space [5].

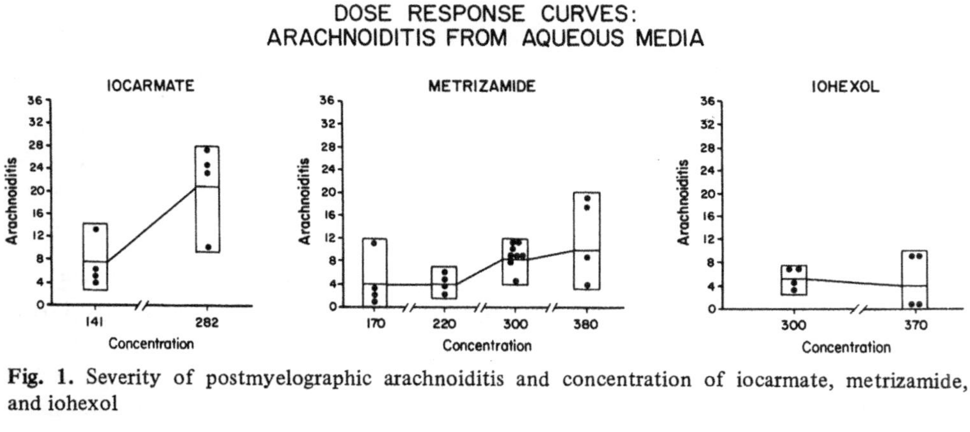


**Fig. 1.** Severity of postmyelographic arachnoiditis and concentration of iocarmate, metrizamide, and iohexol

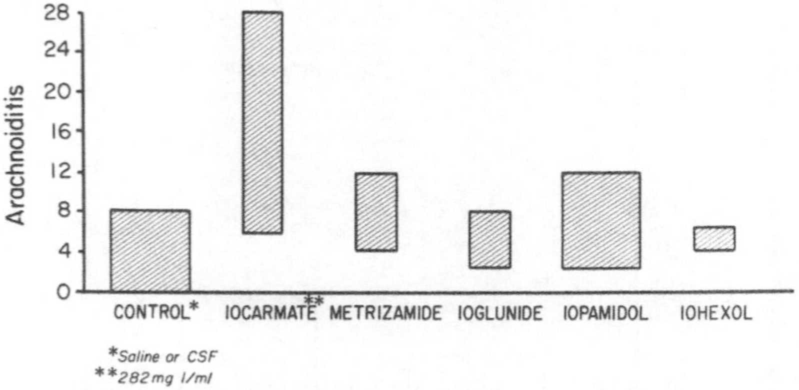


**Fig. 2.** Severity of postmyelographic arachnoiditis and type of contrast medium. Metrizamide, ioglunide, iopamidol, and iohexol were used in a concentration of 300 mg I/ml, iocarmate in a concentration of 282 mg I/ml

The effect of arachnoiditis on the safety of myelography in the monkeys was also studied. It was noted (Fig. 3) that animals having had previous myelograms had a higher incidence of seizures or fatal complications from myelography with aqueous media than animals undergoing their first myelogram. When the animals were classified according to the severity of arachnoiditis evident on the terminal myelogram (Fig. 4), the risk of seizures of arachnoiditis increased. Other effects of arachnoiditis on the monkeys include

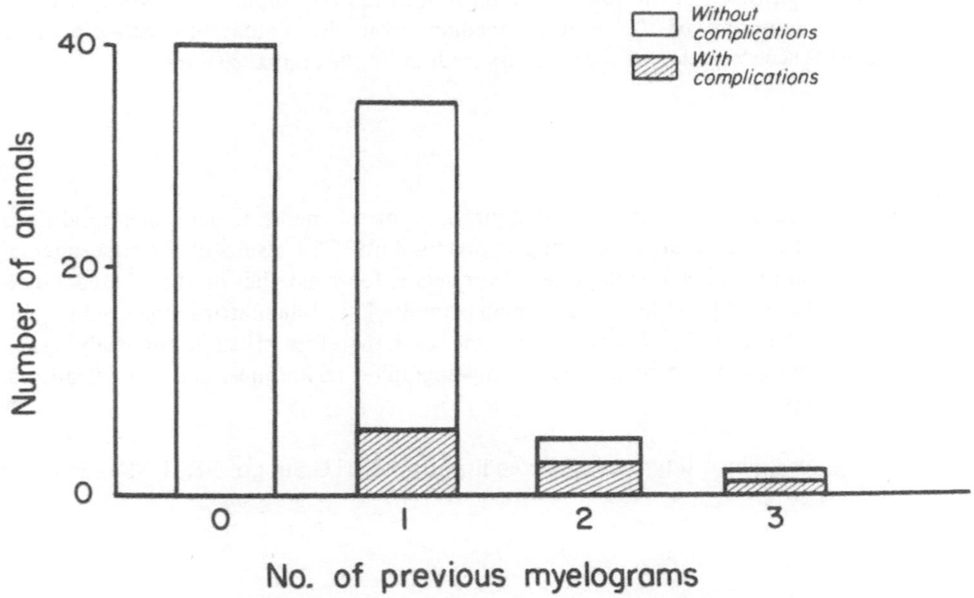


**Fig. 3.** Proportion of animals with acute complications (seizures, death) of myelography in relation to the number of previous myelograms

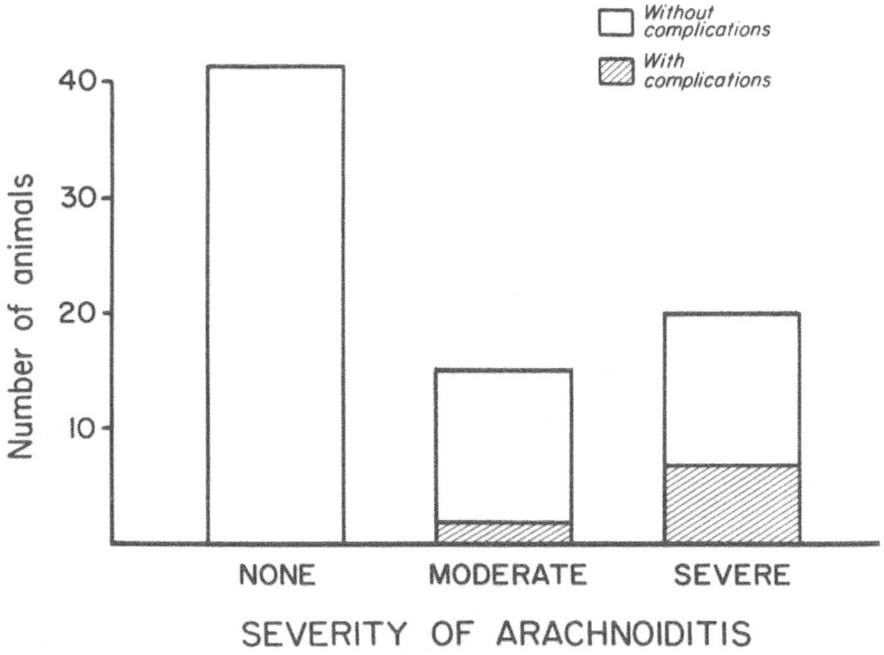


**Fig. 4.** The risk of acute complications in experimental lumbar myelography in animals with an without arachnoiditis

neuromuscular atrophy in the lower extremities (Haughton, unpublished work) delayed physiologic elimination of the contrast medium from the lumbar subarachnoid space [3] and greater accumulation of the contrast medium in the cranial cisterns.

## Discussion

The experimental studies indicate that aqueous contrast media under some conditions produce a serous inflammation resulting in arachnoiditis. The results of the experimental myelography correlated well with clinical experience. Iocarmate has produced arachnoiditis both in patients [1] and in the subhuman primates [7] while metrizamide used in judicious amounts has not [7, 9]. The primate model is therefore effective for studying experimental myelographic contrast media, myelographic techniques, and the intrathecal toxicity of drugs.

*Acknowledgment.* This study was supported in part by NIH Grant no. 5 R01 NS14274-03.

## References


1. Ahlgren P (1973) Long term side effects after myelography with watersoluble contrast media: Conturex, Conray, Meglumine 282, and Dimer-X. Neuroradiology 6:206–211
2. Autio E, Suolanen J, Norrback S, Slatis P (1972) Adhesive arachnoiditis after lumbar myelography with meglumine iothalamate. Acta Radiol [Diagn] 12:17–24
3. Eldevik OP, et al. (1978) Excretion of aqueous myelographic contrast media in animals undergoing a repeat myelogram. Investigative Radiology 15:507–510
4. Eldevik OP, et al. (1978) Ineffectiveness of prophylactic intrathecal methylprednisolone in myelography with aqueous media. Radiology 129:99–101
5. Haughton VM, et al. (1977) Arachnoiditis following myelography with water-soluble agents: The role of contrast medium osmolality. Radiology 125:731–733
6. Haughton VM, et al. (1978) Severity of postmyelographic arachnoiditis and concentration of meglumine iocarmate in primates. AJR 130:313–316
7. Haughton VM, et al. (1978) Comparison of arachnoiditis produced by meglumine iocarmate and metrizamide myelography in an animal model. AJR 131:120–132
8. Haughton VM, Ho KC (1980) The risk of arachnoiditis from experimental nonionic contrast media. Radiology 136:395–397
9. Skalpe IO (1976) Adhesive arachnoiditis following lumbar radiculography with water-soluble contrast media. A clinical report with special reference to metrizamide. Radiology 121:647–652

# Comparative Experimental Study of Contrast Media in Neuroradiology

J. Cahn, M.G. Borzeix, R. Cahn, J.P. Akimjak, M. Labos, J. Angignard, and J.P. Brizard

## Introduction

Iodinated contrast media are injected in human beings in order to reveal the organic origin of functional disturbances. It is well known that most water-soluble contrast media used in neuroradiology elicit epilepsia when directly applied to the nervous tissue subarachnoidally or intraventricularly [2]. Moreover, uncomfort, nausea, and headache are often associated in man with lumbar myelography. Finally, late sequelae may follow such intrathecal use of contrast media such as cell proliferation in CSF [6] and risk of arachnoiditis [5]. Most of the experimental studies have been performed on normal animals; however, it is important to outline the fact that these contrast media are given to people presenting a disease; at brain level, they are mainly suffering from trauma and tumor. In this way, contrast media have been injected to rabbits exhibiting EEG disturbances due to a traumatic-induced cerebral edema. Contrast media are also administered into cerebral arteries for arteriographic exploration; this situation has been mimicked in rats in which the possible deleterious effect has been revealed by a BBB breakdown allowing the extravasation of Evans blue within the brain parenchyma. Finally, the risk of arachnoiditis so as the cellular reaction in CSF have been carried out in adult Cynomolgus monkeys (*Macaca irus*) after intrathecal injection of contrast media.

## Material and Methods

### In the Rat

The experiment was performed in 120 male SD rats. The different contrast media were injected into the internal carotid artery, a previous i.v. injection of Evans blue enabling the extent of the BBB breakdown to be determined.

### In the Rabbit

The experiment was performed in 21 male rabbits. An experimental traumatic edema was performed according to the method of Borzeix et al. [1]. Cortical EEG was continuously recorded after i.v. injection of contrast media so that the tissular iodine content was determined in both "control" and injured hemispheres.

### In the Monkey

The experiment was performed in nine adult *Macaca irus* (Cynomolgus). Contrast media were injected by the intrathecal route (L4–L5). Cellular proliferation was studied by means of CSF punctures and brain histological examination was carried out 15 days later.

## Results

### In the Rat

According to the dosage given, Telebrix 38 induces a BBB breakdown (Figs. 1–2b) and also causes neurological symptoms (clonotonic convulsions) to originate ending with four exitus for the biggest volume. For 0.6 and 1.2 ml, Hexabrix also elicits an extravasation of Evans blue within the brain tissue but of less importance than that with Telebrix 38 (Figs. 1–2c). Finally, Iopamidol 300 has no deleterious effect upon BBB as shown in Figs. 1–2a.

### In the Rabbit

The i.v. injection of contrast media is followed by iodine entry into brain parenchyma under conditions of cerebral edema, this entry being very similar to Telebrix 38 and Iopamidol 370. But the injection of the latter does not change in any way the edematous electrocortical activity whereas Telebrix 38 i.v. injection leads to a reduction in $\beta$ rhythms proportion.

### In the Monkey

The CSF cell count exhibits a striking increase after intrathecal administration of metrizamide whereas it is less marked with Iopamidol 300, this cell proliferation being mostly related to the occurrence of eosinophilic polymorphonuclears. Morever, neurological symptoms such as nausea and clonic seizures occur after metrizamide injection whereas they do not appear with metrizamide. Light and electron microscopic examinations (from Foncin, J.F. – Ecole Pratique des Hautes Etudes – Paris 1981) reveal that deep cortical

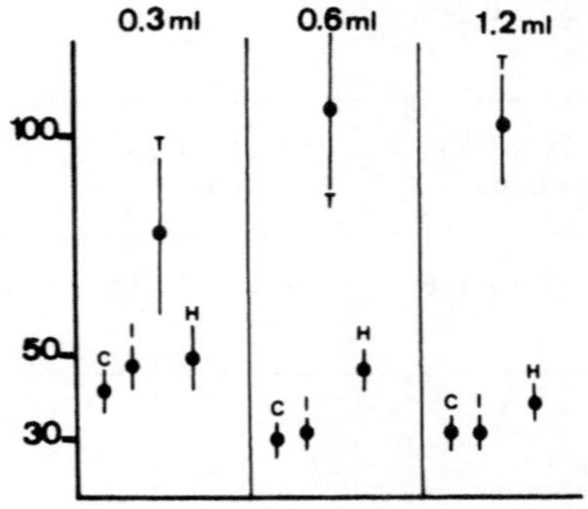


Fig. 1. Evans blue content ($\mu g.g^{-1}$ left hemisphere)

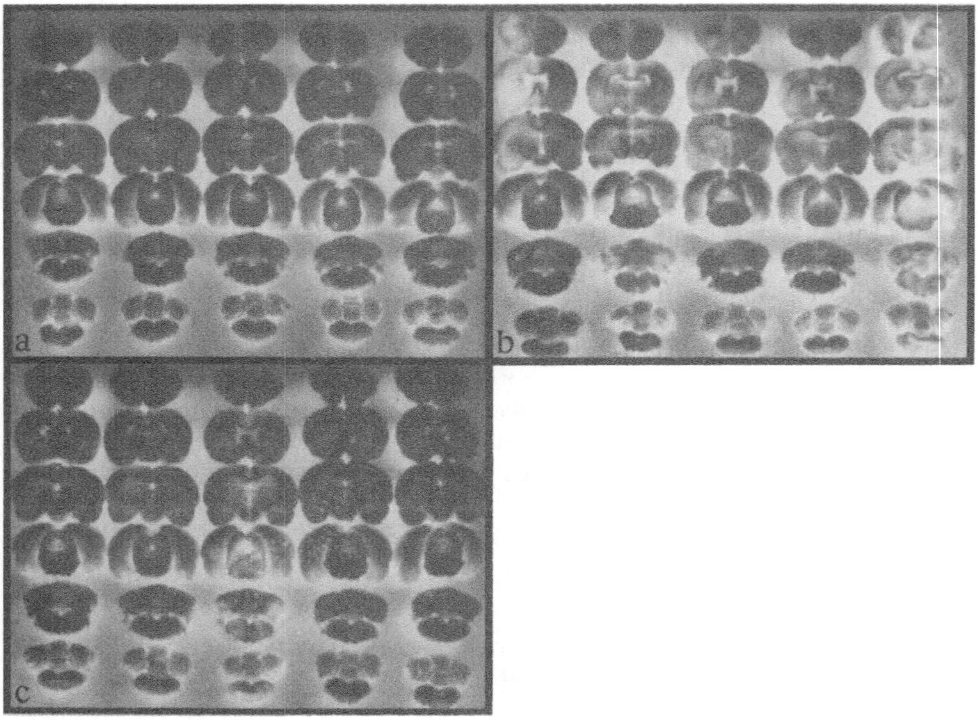

**Fig. 2a–c.** Brain slices after intra-arterial injection of contrast media. **a** Iopamidol 300 (300 mg iodine). **b** Telebrix 38 (380 mg iodine). **c** Hexabrix (320 mg iodine)

**Table 1.** Iodine cerebral content in case of traumatic-induced cerebral edema in rabbits

| Series | | Doses iodine mg · kg$^{-1}$ | Iodine cerebral content (µg per g brain tissue): Control hemisphere | Iodine cerebral content (µg per g brain tissue): Edematous hemisphere |
|---|---|---|---|---|
| Control + iodine (Telebrix 38) | | 760 | 2.55 ± 0.240 | – |
| Cerebral edema | Iopamidol 370 | 740 | 5.66 ± 1.055<br>$P = 0.05$ | 15.21 ± 1.735<br>$P = 0.0005$ |
| | Telebrix 38 | 760 | 5.31 ± 1.556<br>$P$* | 14.99 ± 5.013<br>$P = 0.05$ |

*P*; level of statistical significance according to Student's *t*-test
* NS; not significant

**Table 2.** Effect of i.v. injection of contrast media on the relative proportion of rhythms

| Series | | Spectral EEG analysis (FAT system) Relative time occurrence for $\beta$ (%) |
|---|---|---|
| Control | | 29 |
| Cerebral edema | | 25 |
| Cerebral edema | Iopamidol 370 | 26 |
| | Telebrix 38 | 21 ($P = 0.03$) |

*P*; level of statistical significance according to Student's *t* test

layers have a normal aspect in all cases but a marginal fibrous gliosis exists, more marked in metrizamide-injected monkeys (Fig. 3a). On the contrary, in Iopamidol 300-injected monkeys the fibrosis as well as the cell infiltration of the arachnoid is less pronounced (Fig. 3b).

## Discussion

From these experiments, it has been shown that the intra-arterial injection of iodinated compounds can lead to a BBB breakdown, the extent of which seems to be related to the iodine amount under conditions of traumatic-induced cerebral edema in rabbits; the intracerebral entry of iodine is not concomitant with any change in the previously observed ECoG disturbances with Iopamidol 370; on the contrary, a similar quantity of Telebrix 38 favors the drop in $\beta$ rhythms, thus leading to an aggravation of the edematous ECoG symptomatology. The risk of arachnoiditis has been largely investigated in animals during the past decade and is diminishing since new kinds of contrast media have been synthetized. One of these new compounds is metrizamide, but in man the occurrence of acute encephalopathy after lumbar myelography is still described [7]. Besides these transient and acute phenomena, more prolonged signs of intolerance have been observed, such as cell proliferation in the CSF [6] and occurrence of arachnoiditis [3–5]. A recent study by Haughton [4] in pigtail monkeys reveals that 12 weeks after a lumbar injection of Iopamidol 300, ioglunide, or metrizamide there is no more fibrosis of the arachnoid than in control animals receiving a similar volume of autologous CSF; only a severe arachnoiditis is noticed with meglumine iocarmate. In our experimental conditions, the cell proliferation in the CSF as well as the fibrous gliosis is markedly less pronounced with Iopamidol 300 as compared to that observed with metrizamide. The difference noticed with the results from Haughton et al. may be related to the different animal species because it is well known that Cynomolgus are the most reactive monkeys to intrathecal injection of contrast media. Our histological examination is also localized to the brain whereas Haughton's

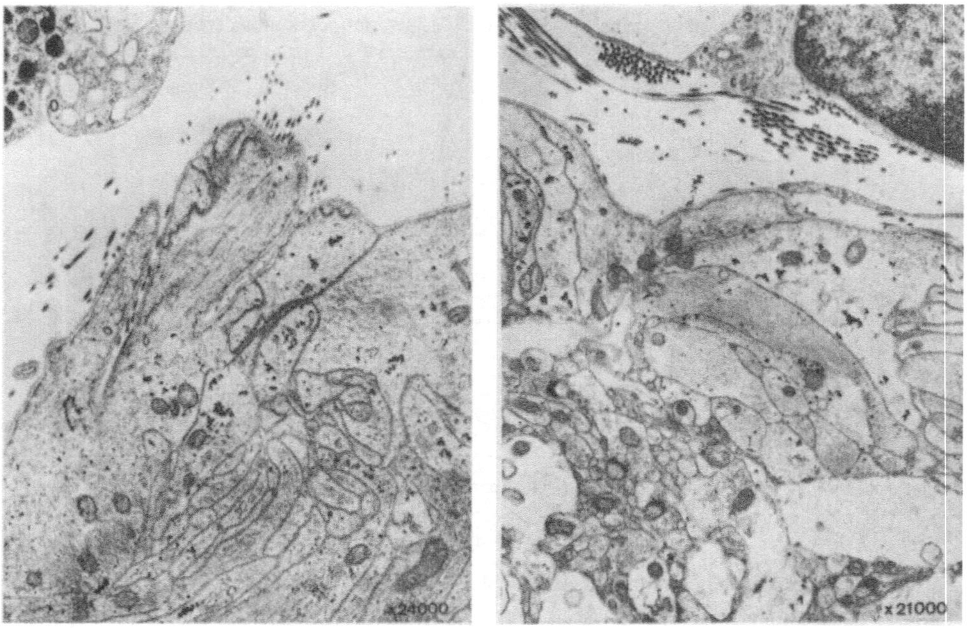


a b

**Fig. 3.** Electron microscopic pictures of the upper part of the cerebral cortex near the longitudinal cerebral fissure. The irregular cortical surface reveals a marked marginal fibrous gliosis in a metrizamide-injected monkey (**a**) whereas no important change in the cortical structure can be seen after intrathecal injection of Iopamidol 300 (**b**)

histologic score was performed at the spinal cord level. From all the results obtained in this experiment it can be concluded that Iopamidol 300 is safer than other iodinated contrast media studied as reference drugs (Telebrix 38, Hexabrix, metrizamide).

## References

1. Borzeix MG, Labos M, Cahn J (1972) A propos d'un modèle experimental d'oedème cérébral pour l'étude des substances agissant sur le débit sanguin et/ou le métabolisme cérébral. Agressologie 13/4:257–260
2. Grepe A, Widen L (1973) Effects of cisternal application of metrizamide. An experimental investigation in dogs in $N_2O$ analgesia with and without Halothane. Acta Radiol [Suppl] 335:119–124
3. Haughton VM, Khang-Cheng-Ho, Larson SJ, Unger GF, Correa-Paz F (1978) Comparison of arachnoiditis produced by Meglumine Iocarmate and Metrizamide myelography in an animal model. AJR 131:129–132
4. Haughton VM, Khang-Cheng-Ho (1980) The risk of arachnoiditis from experimental nonionic contrast media. Radiology 136/2:395–397
5. Skalpe IO (1976) Adhesive arachnoiditis following lumbar radiculography with water-soluble contrast agents. A clinical report with special reference to Metrizamide. Radiology 121:647–651
6. Svare A, Taller K (1973) Lumbar myelography with Metrizamide. An Evaluation of 15 cases. Acta Radiol [Suppl] 335:387–390
7. Vallat JM, Leman JP, Demarti D, Dumas M, Pascaud JL (1981) Encéphalographie aigüe après myélographie lombaire à la Métrizamide. Nouv Presse Med 10/15:1241–1243

# Changes in the Cerebrospinal Fluid Pressure After Intrathecal Injection of Contrast Media in Rabbits

B. Carlborg, P. Maly, K. Golman, T. Almén, and C. Lindqvist

## Introduction

It has recently been reported that intrathecal injection of nonionic contrast media into cisterna magna of rabbits resulted in both excitative and depressive effects when the doses were increased sufficiently [1]. The severity of the excitative effects was not only dose dependent but varied with the compound tested.

Figure 1 shows effects produced by intrathecal injection of the nonionic contrast media metrizamide, iopamidol, and iohexol at a dose of 1 ml/kg and a concentration of 370 mg I/ml. The score given shows that metrizamide produced general excitation with the animals having at least one general epileptic fit within 3 h after the infusion.

Iohexol produced no excitative effects.

Iopamidol produced significantly more excitative effects than iohexol, but significantly less than metrizamide.

The effects were found to have a maximum between 1 and 1 ½ h after the intrathecal injection. At this time after the injection, the contrast medium is almost no longer visible on the radiograph and the contrast medium concentration is only about 20% of the initial

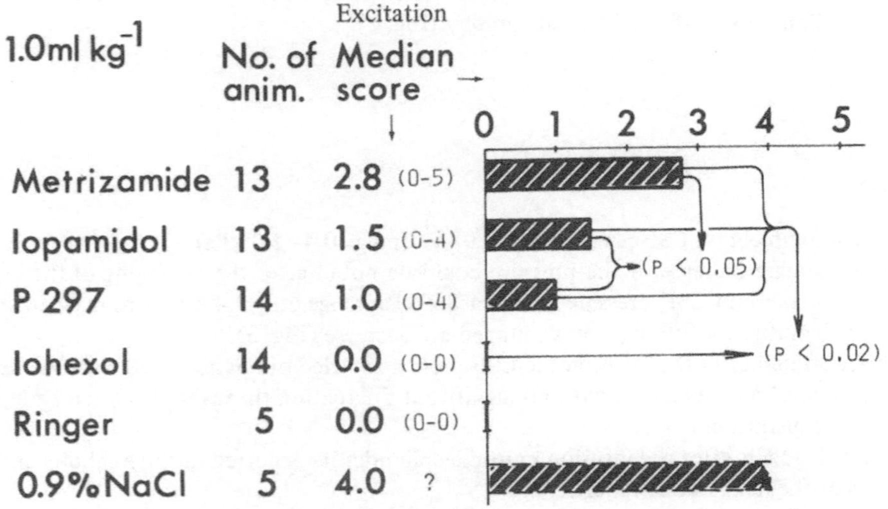


**Fig. 1.** Excitative effects produced after intrathecal infusion of nonionic contrast media (1 ml/kg) in rabbits

concentration. The effects therefore might be attributable to additional factors rather than the contrast medium per se.

Possibly an increase in CSF pressure might be a causative factor because a considerable CSF pressure rise must be expected when injecting a volume equal to the whole subarachnoid space relatively fast.

The aim of the present investigation was to examine the changes in the cerebrospinal pressure during and after injection of an nonionic contrast medium. Metrizamide, the most viscous of the above-mentioned contrast media was chosen for the investigation.

## Method

Five rabbits, weighing 1.5–2.2 kg, were used. The animals were anesthetized with pentobarbital, tracheotomized, and ventilated by a respirator. Arterial blood gases were repeatedly determined during the experiment. The cerebrospinal fluid pressure ($P_{CSF}$) was measured via a craniotomy. A metallic cannula (ID 0.8 mm) with a short plastic adaptor mounted on top was inserted into the lateral ventricle. The cannula was coupled to a microtip pressure transducer. The total volume in the pressure measurement system was about 20 $mm^3$. The central venous pressure ($P_{CV}$) was recorded in the internal jugular vein. The arterial blood pressure ($P_A$) was measured in the femoral artery. All pressure measurements were performed simultaneously. The integrated mean values of $P_{CSF}$ and $P_{CV}$ were calculated from the graphic recordings.

The rabbit was placed horizontally on a table with the head fixed. The $P_{CSF}$, $P_{CV}$, and $P_A$ were measured with Millar microtip transducers PC 350 5F with a diameter of 1.67 mm, and a volume displacement of $1 \times 10^{-3}$ $mm^3$/13.3 kPa (Millar Instruments Inc., Houston, Texas, USA).

The microtip transducers were coupled to a specially designed amplifier. The output signals from the amplifier were simultaneously recorded on an ink jet recorder [Gould Brush 4000]. For further methodological details see [2].

Metrizamide 370, 1 ml/kg body weight, was infused at a rate of 0.4 ml/min into the cisterna magna after suboccipital puncture (Butterfly G25). Subarachnoid position of the contrast medium was confirmed by radiography (Fig. 2).

## Results

### CSF Pressure

The median preinjection CSF pressure was 0.9 kPa (range 0.4–1.3 kPa).

An immediate increase of the pressure could be noted after the beginning of the infusion. The maximum CSF pressure (median 8.2 kPa, range 6.8–9.4 kPa) was reached at the end of the infusion, followed by an immediate decrease (Fig. 3).

About 30 min after the infusion the CSF pressure leveled out at about 30% above the preinjection level and remained without significant fluctuation throughout the remaining 2½ h of the registration period.

Within 1–2½ h after the infusion multiple epileptic fits occurred in three rabbits and local jerks of the head in one rabbit.

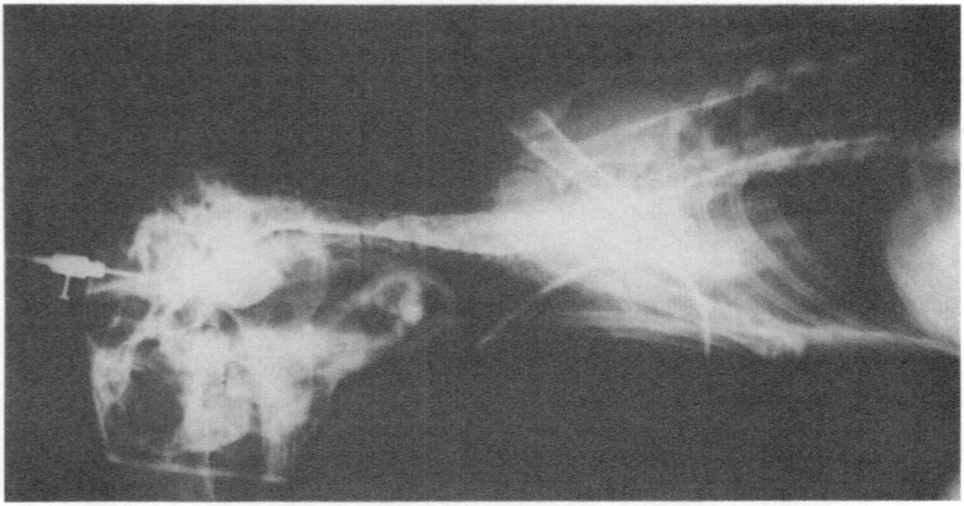

**Fig. 2.** Radiograph showing the correct position of the contrast medium in the subarachnoid space. The cannula positioned in the left ventricle for pressure recording can also be seen

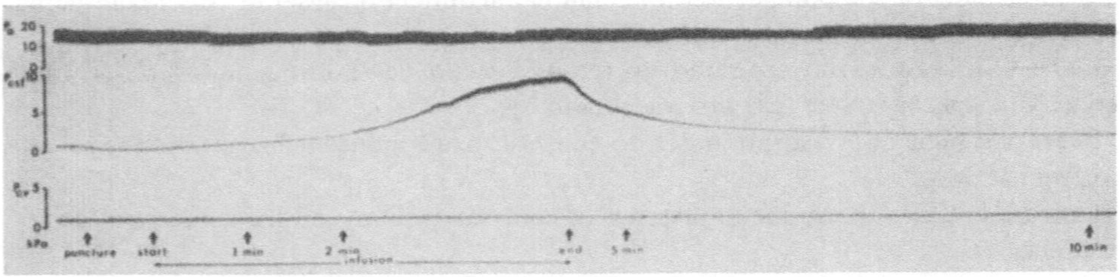


**Fig. 3.** Typical pressure recording pattern during and after the infusion. $P_{\mathrm{CV}}$, central venous pressure; $P_{\mathrm{a}}$, arterial pressure; $P_{\mathrm{CSF}}$, cerebrospinal fluid pressure. All values in kPa

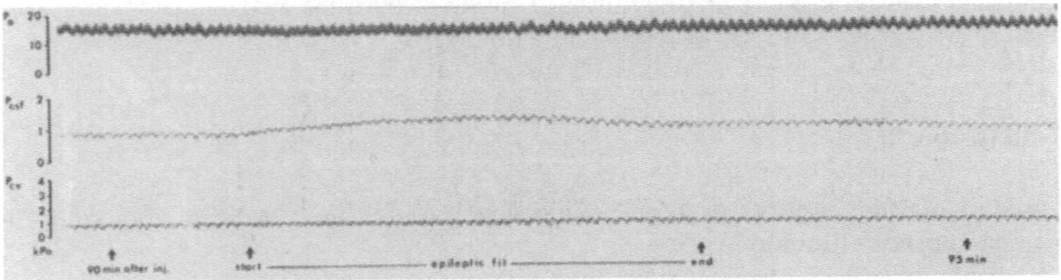


**Fig. 4.** Typical pressure recording pattern during an epileptic fit in a rabbit. $P_{\mathrm{CV}}$, central venous pressure; $P_{\mathrm{a}}$, arterial pressure; $P_{\mathrm{CSF}}$, cerebrospinal fluid pressure. All values in kPa

Concomitantly with the epileptic fit the CSF pressure increased by 0.5 kPa (median value, range 0.2–0.9 kPa) (Fig. 4).

### Vascular Pressure

During the infusion and the epileptic fits changes in the central venous pressure and arterial pressure did not exceed values of 0.3 kPa and 2.7 kPa, respectively.

## Discussion

Davson et al. [3] have shown that injecting artificial CSF at a rate of 0.4 ml $\times$ $min^{-1}$ produces a sevenfold increase in the CSF pressure.

In accordance with these results, we obtained, using a more viscous solution, a ninefold increase of CSF pressure at the same infusion rate.

In similar experiments in dog, using *ionic contrast media*, it has been found [5] that a secondary increase in CSF pressure (5 kPa) started 30 min after the injection. The CSF pressure remained elevated during the 2-h observation period. Convulsions started in the secondary phase of elevated CSF pressure. The incidence of the convulsions was, however, dependent on the examined ionic contrast media. Such a secondary phase of elevated CSF pressure was not found in the present study, using nonionic contrast medium and a fourfold dose. The elevation of CSF pressure during an epileptic fit in our study was only about 50% of the preinjection level and can hardly be a causative factor considered in relation to the 900% increase during the injection.

The CSF pressure did not return to the preinjection level during the 3-h observation period. One may speculate that this was caused by:

1. Decreased bulk CSF resorption due to contrast media-induced changes of the CSF absorptive pathways
2. Increase in CSF volume due to presence of contrast medium and the consequent osmotic effects
3. General edema of the brain cells caused by shifts in osmolality and changes in composition of ions normally present in CSF

Most likely perhaps is a combination of all three factors.

A significant fall of the arterial pressure following subarachnoid injection of ionic contrast media was observed both by Melartin in dogs [4] and Salvesen in rabbits [5]. Using a nonionic contrast medium (metrizamide 0.5 ml/kg), Salvesen could not find any significant changes in $P_A$. Our study, using 1 ml/kg of the same medium have confirmed this.

## Conclusion

The CSF pressure is elevated above preinjection level for more than 3 h after contrast medium infusion (1 ml/kg).

Excitative effects of the contrast media do not seem to be related to CSF pressure at the time of excitation as this pressure is smaller than the pressure during the first ½ h after the injection, when no excitation can be noted.

*Acknowledgment.* Supported in part by the Medical Research Council, University of Lund, Sweden.

## References

1. Maly P, Olivecrona H, Gustafson C, Salvesen S, Almen T (1981) Excitation and depression after intrathecal injection of contrast media in non-anaesthetized rabbits. Presented at the International Congress of Radiology, Brussel, June
2. Carlborg B (1981) On physiological and experimental variation of the perilymphatic pressure in the cat. Acta Otolaryngol 91:19–28
3. Davson H, Hollingsworth G, Segal MB (1970) The mechanism of drainage of the cerebrospinal fluid. Brain 93:665–678
4. Melartin E (1970) Intracisternal toxicity of angiographic contrast media. Thesis, TURKU University, Finland
5. Salvesen S (1973) Suboccipital injection of metrizamide to anaesthetized and unanaesthetized rabbits. Acta Radiol [Suppl] 335:93–101

# Adverse Effects From Contrast Media: Preliminary Results Obtained with an Experimental Model

U. Salvolini, U. Pasquini, A. Molinari, and P. Tirone

## Introduction

The use of intravenous contrast for enhancing the images of computerized tomography (CT) of the brain dates back to early clinical trials of the method (Ambrose, 1973). We have been doing brain CT since 1975, and have now collected a total of over 28 000 cases; of these, about two-thirds were examined with intravenous contrast.

From the beginning we made a number of observations on the CNS effects of contrast media, which we presented as a communication to the French Society of Neuroradiology in 1978.

The first observation was the occurrence of epileptic seizures of the motor type following large intravenous doses of contrast in some patients with prerolandic lesions (particularly the brain metastases).

The second observation was the evolution toward porencephalia of many patients in whom the diagnostic procedure had revealed an area of irregularly increased density after c.e. due to unstable cerebromalacia. We interpreted these findings as reflecting damage to the blood-brain barrier affording the passage of contrast from the blood stream to the extravascular brain compartment (brain parenchyma), in accord with Gado et al. [1].

There was a good deal of discussion about the brain tissue damage produced by extravasated contrast material. At the same time, other authors [2] denied any such damage and reported using very high dosages (up to 80 g iodine per patient) without adverse effects.

Meanwhile, a recent paper [3] offered evidence that one characteristic peculiarly responsible for such untoward effects was the high osmolarity of contrast solutions, which produces physiochemical modifications of the erythrocytes and causes injury to the endothelial barrier of brain capillaries. Hyperosmolarity, however, is not the only toxic mechanism attached to contrast media: we certainly must consider a chemotoxic effect specifically connected with the chemical structure of these molecules whose hydrophobic sites interact with enzyme proteins and penetrate lipid barriers.

We must also consider a bioelectrical effect (related to the ionic separation of the saline solution that results in severe upset of the extracellular ionic balance and consequent disturbance of such bioelectrical phenomena as depend on ionic movements, therefore the membrane potentials and nervous impulse conduction). In theory we can classify the adverse effects of contrast media as reflecting an *anatomical* or a *functional* damage. Anatomical damage consists essentially of alteration of the blood-brain barrier, which may be transitory or permanent [4] and reflects a morphological alteration of intracellular tight junctions.

Functional damage is reflected by alteration of CNS parenchymal functions, again transitory or permanent. In terms of neurotoxicological aspects of the study of functional damage, much importance is attached to behavioral studies [5] and to electrophysiological exploration.

Going back now to clinical reality, we must say that we have noticed certain behavioral changes after rapid intravenous infusion of a saline contrast at a high dosage (3 ml/kg), particularly in children: namely a very high incidence of motor restlessness, nervousness, anxiety, and crying spells without apparent motive; all these disorders occurred very shortly after dosing and were reported through careful questioning of the patients.

## Experimental

Starting from these personal observations and from the data found in published papers, therefore, we developed an experimental method for testing the effects of various vascular contrasts, at different dosages, in laboratory animals with a damaged blood-brain barrier.

## Materials and Methods

Adult rats were given rapid intravenous injections of the following contrast media at high dosages (iodine 600 mg/kg) at the rate of 10 ml/h:

1. *Acetrizoic acid:* sodium salt solution, iodine 300 mg/ml
2. *Diatriozoic acid:* meglumine salt solution, iodine 306 mg/ml
3. *Iopamidol:* nonionic solution, iodine 300 mg/ml

Shortly before these treatments, a reversible lesion of the blood-brain barrier was produced in each animal by the method of Rapoport and Thompson [4] to ensure the passage of contrast medium into the brain parenchyma.

Control animals were prepared with the same reversible lesion and then infused with an equal volume of physiological salt solution. Each test group consisted of five rats.

Each contrast medium was administered to two groups of animals, which were sacrified respectively 7 and 28 days after dosing. Meanwhile, at 24 h of dosing and again every 7 days afterward, the animals were examined as follows:

Behavioral study: motor coordination assessed by the rota-rod test, and spontaneous activity measured with a movement counter

Daily water and feed consumption, and animal weight growth

Recovery time from barbiturate anesthesia

At termination (7 or 28 days after dosing in the two groups) each animal was tested for impermeability of the blood-brain barrier to Evans blue injected intravenously.

## Results

### Behavioral Tests

Behavioral tests of motor coordination revealed that some animal fell of the rota-rod only in the groups treated with acetrizoic acid and diatrizoic acid salts. Motility tests revealed

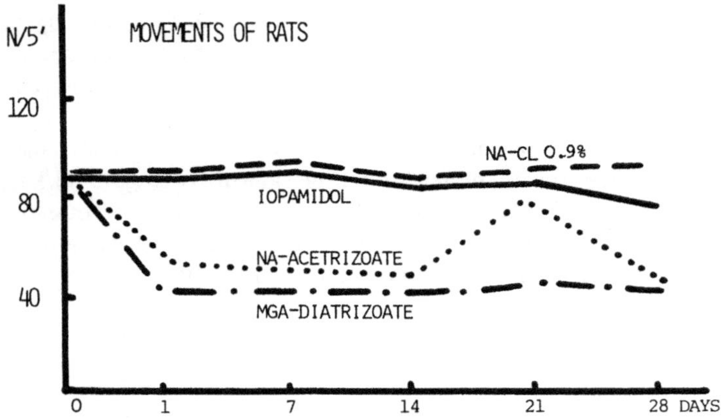


**Fig. 1.** Motility in rats treated with two acid salts, Iopamidol, and a control group

no changes in individual animals at different test times; but there was a statistically significant difference (reduced motility) between animals treated with the two acid salts and the control group, both at 24 h and at 7 days of dosing. No such difference was found in the group treated with Iopamidol (Fig. 1).

### Clinical Examinations

There were no significant variations of water and food consumption or of animal weight.

### Recovery From Anesthesia

There was a significant increase of recovery time from barbiturate anesthesia, in the group treated with acetrizoic and diatrizoic acid salts; no significant difference was found in the group treated with Iopamidol (Fig. 2).

### Autopsy

There were no differences between treatment groups in terms of brain aspect, morphology, or weight. With the Evans blue test, animals treated with physiological salt solution or with Iopamidol revealed no areas of abnormal permeability; those treated with acetrizoic acid salt showed mild permeabilization of the blood-brain barrier in the group examined at 7 days; and those treated with diatrizoic acid salt showed very slight permeabilization in the group examined at 28 days.

## Addendum

Two additional animals per product were treated with double doses of contrast medium (iodine 1200 mg/kg) and tested in the same way. There were no significant differences from control values in the animals treated with Iopamidol. The animals treated with

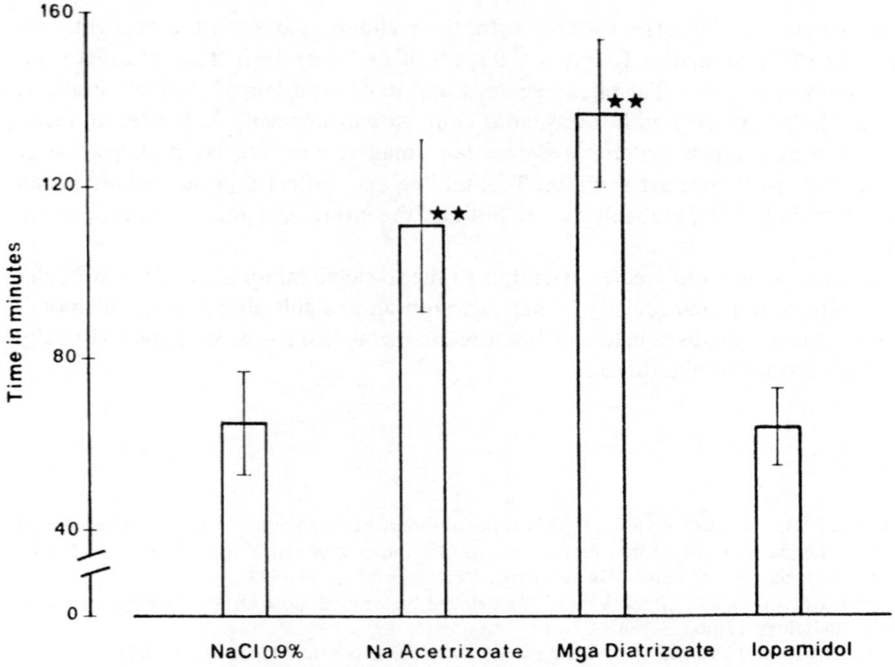

**Fig. 2.** Recovery from anesthesia in rats treated with two acid salts, Iopamidol, and a control group

either acetrizoic or diatrizoic acid salt showed a marked reduction of spontaneous activity and likewise marked increase of recovery time from anesthesia. Only those treated with acetrizoic acid salt showed a loss of motor coordination. Permeability to Evans blue was definitely increased by acetrizoic acid treatment and to a lesser extent diatrizoic acid.

## Conclusions

Our preliminary experimental results confirm that intravascular administration of a contrast medium is not biologically indifferent – indeed, it brings out at least one of the possible toxic mechanisms of such products, namely permeabilization of the blood-brain barrier. Next, our study confirms that the tolerability of a contrast medium is greater, the lesser its hyperosmolarity (nonionic contrasts).

Last, tolerability is definitely influenced by dosage, as suggested in the "Addendum" section of this paper.

Conversely we have nothing to say at present about the effects of contrast media on the brain itself, even though there are valid indications that these substances are not "indifferent." For all these reasons we feel encouraged to continue our experimental work, especially in regard to possible brain damage from contrast media in the presence of an altered blood-brain barrier.

To this end it may prove useful also to verify such findings after injection of the contrast into cerebrospinal fluid, since the CSF-brain barrier is much less selective than the blood-brain barrier. In this respect we can offer the preliminary observation of slightly reduced density of brain matter found in CT scans made 24 or 36 h after intrathecal injection of nonionic contrast. The phenomenon seems to be dose dependent and transitory. In one patient, re-examined with intravenous contrast enhancement 72 h after an intrathecal injection of contrast material, we detected a massive but irregular impregnation of the brain cortex with contrast medium. This finding may reflect a prolonged alteration of the blood-brain barrier, probably caused both by the intrathecal and by the intravascular contrast.

These results command greater attention to the so-called minor risks of intravascular contrast administration, particularly in patients with an unstable alteration of the blood-brain barrier and major disturbance of brain tissue metabolism – as is characteristically the case with cerebrovascular disease.

## References


1. Gado MH, Phelps ME, Coleman RE (1975) An extravascular component of contrast enhancement in cranial computed tomography. Part I: the tissue-blood of contrast enhancement. PartII: contrast enhancement and the blood-tissue barrier. Radiology 117:589–597
2. Haymann LA, Evans RA, Hinck VC (1980) Delayed high iodine dose contrast computed tomography. Radiology 136:677–684
3. Grainger RG (1980) Osmolality of intravascular radiological contrast media. Br J Radiol 53:739–746
4. Rapaport SI, Thompson MK (1975) Opening of the blood-brain barrier (BBB) by a pulse of hydrostatic pressure. Biophys J 15:326a
5. Brimblecombe RW (1979) The use of behavioral and neuropharmacological methods in toxicology. J Pharmacol Methods 2:91–96

# First Round Table: Concluding Remarks

R.E. Gonsette

The increasing interest in the neurotoxicity of CM is mostly due to the development of metrizamide cisternography and the resulting progress in the diagnosis of basal and cranio-vertebral junction lesions.

The good, but still imperfect, tolerance of this new CM had the effect of giving incentive to research based on original and more sensitive experimental models.

This Round Table shows that, in spite of numerous meetings and congresses, there is still something to be learned about the neurotoxicity of CM.

Their influence on brain histological structures as well as their incidence on the neurophysiological functions basically remain the experimental parameters.

In this field, continuous EEG monitoring for as long as 12 h using the frequency analysis technique seems important progress. This new experimental approach not only provides original insight into the effects of CM on brain electrophysiology but makes it possible to detect delayed EEG changes. There is reasonable hope that it will help to understand some of the untoward reactions observed in man.

The factors influencing the elimination of CM from the CSF as well as their distribution in the subarachnoid spaces are under extensive study. Indeed, a better understanding of CM resorption dynamics will explain some of the differences existing between various CM, when minor side effects are concerned.

Influence of CM on animal behavior will possibly cast some light on the difficult problem of psychic disturbances observed after intrathecal use of CM. This is a very difficult approach but the animal models already developed seem very promising.

A new and interesting avenue is the development of experimental models stimulating the BBB lesions so frequently observed in clinical neuropathology. These techniques allow a better appreciation of the brain capillary toxicity, and they will be a useful tool when screening CM with a lower toxicity for cerebral angiography in high-risk patients.

Some of the papers presented during this session are based on experimental techniques currently used in neurophysiological studies: chronically cannulated animals, chronic intracerebral electrodes, cells cultures. They certainly will play a great part in elucidating the mechanisms underlying CM neurotoxicity but it must be borne in mind that in order to draw useful conclusions from experimental studies, they have to stick as close as possible to daily clinical conditions.

The papers presented during this session demonstrate that progress is still possible in synthesizing better CM and these studies are an important contribution in making neuroradiological investigations safer and safer.

# The Stream of Metrizamide in the Subarachnoid Spaces in Relation to Adverse Effects of Cisternography

N. Kobayashi, Y. Saito, and T. Miyashita

Nonionic hydrosoluble contrast material metrizamide is available for cisternography with conventional X-ray technique, but convulsive seizure must not be neglected as a severe side effect. We have encountered ten cases of convulsive seizure, in 88 cases of cisternography. The stream of contrast material in the subarachnoid spaces is discussed in reference to the severe side effect.

## Technique of Cisternography

Our technique of cisternography is briefly mentioned. We employ the following methods to get the best images in cisternography with minimal iodine content and minimal quantity of contrast material (Fig. 1).

To examine the sellar region and the frontal cranial fossa, contrast material is administered by lateral C1-C2 puncture, keeping the patient in prone position. For the examination of the posterior fossa, contrast material is injected by the same root with supine position, and for the cerebellopontine angle region, suboccipital puncture is available, keeping the patient in lateral decubitus position.

We call the first maneuver "anterior cisternography", the second, "posterior cisternography", and the third, "lateral cisternography".

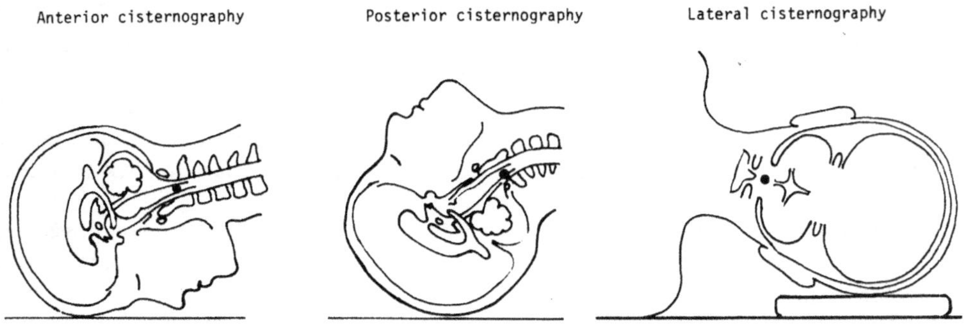


**Fig. 1.** Position of head and needle in cisternography

## Materials and Methods

Eighty-eight cases of cisternography were performed by the technique mentioned above (59 anterior, 21 posterior, and 8 lateral cisternographies). In these studies 6.0–9.0 ml contrast material with 190–210 mg/ml iodine content is mainly used, but for the cases of lateral cisternography, 3.0–5.0 ml contrast material with 250–270 mg/ml iodine content is used to opacify the internal auditory canal.

The side effects of anterior cisternography and the stream of contrast material during cisternography are compared.

## Results

Headache, nausea, vomiting, and fever were noticed with almost the same frequency as in cervical myelography, and they were extremely less severe than that of pneumoencephalography, but ten cases of generalized convulsive seizure were experienced in all 88 cases. In all ten cases, convulsive seizures occurred after anterior cisternographies.

In anterior cisternography, contrast material entered into the interpeduncular and the suprasellar cisterns through the prepontine cistern, and flowed anteriorly into the interhemispheric fissure, and laterally into the sylvian fissures (Fig. 2).

Opacification of the basal cisterns in anterior cisternography is classified into several types (Fig. 3).

In most of the cases with large suprasellar masses or postoperative arachnoid adhesion, much of the contrast material flowed into the sylvian fissures. The type in which most of contrast material precipitated into the frontal tips was seen mainly in the cases with prominent cerebral atrophy. In other cases, the sylvian fissures and the interhemispheric fissure are well opacified with various degree. In the last type, contrast material flowed into the upper frontal to the central areas in the interhemispheric fissure along the pericallosal sulcus and other cortical sulci. Most of the cases of convulsive seizure presented this type, and in the cases of convulsion, a large amount of contrast material was seen in the upper frontal interhemispheric fissure.

No contrast material was noted in the lateral surface of the frontal and the parietal lobes on X-ray films.

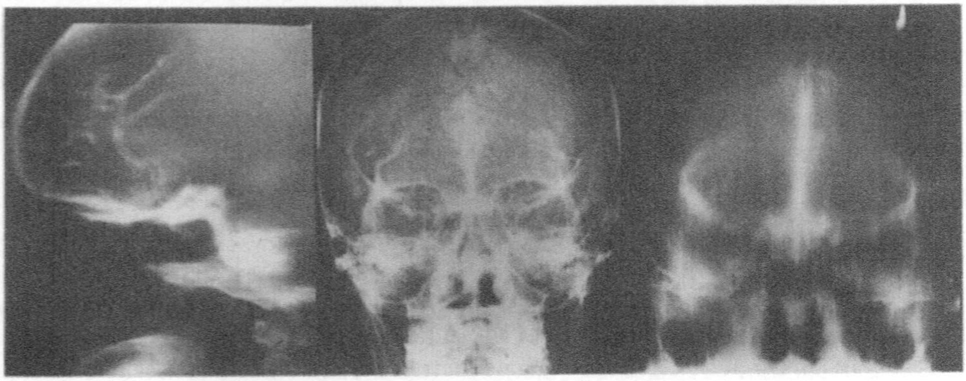

**Fig. 2.** Anterior cisternography (a case of small pituitary adenoma)

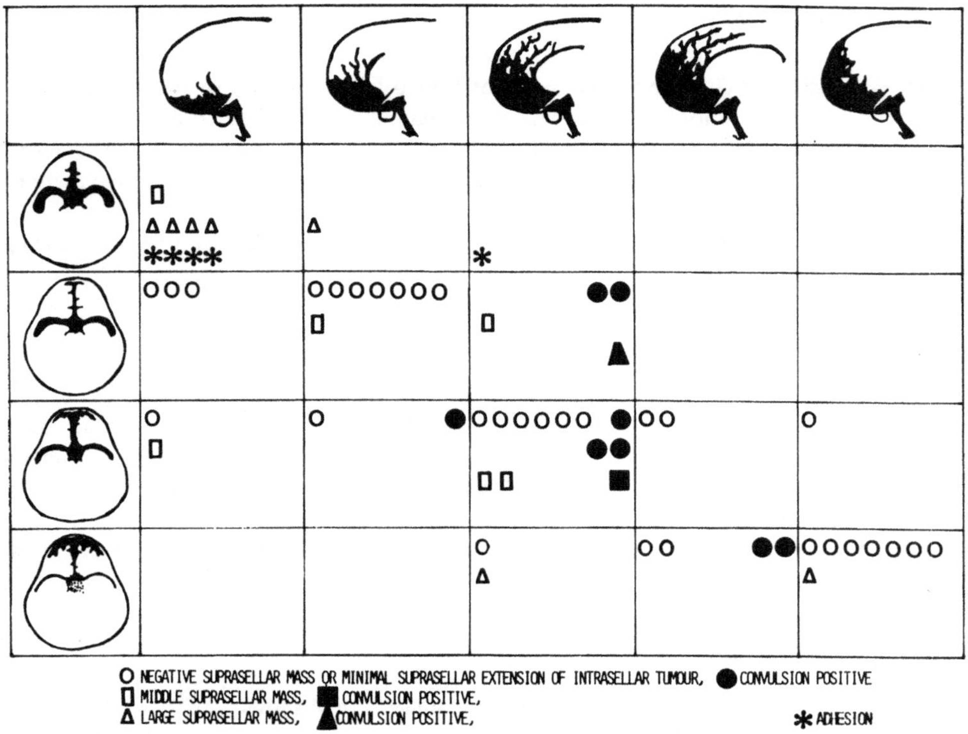


**Fig. 3.** Types of anterior cisternograms and intracranial lesions

In posterior cisternography, contrast material was precipitated into the posterior surface of the cerebellar hemispheres without extension of the patient's neck, but contrast material passed not only into all the subarachnoid spaces in the posterior fossa, but also into the fourth ventricle with backward tilting of the head (Fig. 4). Only a little contrast material accumulated in the galenic or the quadrigeminal cistern flowed into the occipital region along calcarine and the parieto-occipital fissures, then into the parietal region along the pericallosal sulcus, and laterally into the retropulvinar cisterns. There is not so much contrast material in the interhemispheric fissure as in anterior cisternography, and little contrast material is seen in the lower or outer surface of the occipital or parietal lobes.

In lateral cisternography, the lateral cerebellar surface, the cerebellopontine angle cisterns, and the ambient cistern were opacified in order, and leakage of contrast material into the temporal fossa through the tentorial incisula was recognized.

## Discussion

The stream of metrizamide in the basal cisterns is affected by its gravity in cisternography, which is more prominent than that of CT cisternography with lower concentration of iodine, by lumbar puncture. The stream of contrast material in the subarachnoid spaces is affected by the position of the head and also by the degree of cerebral atrophy, existence

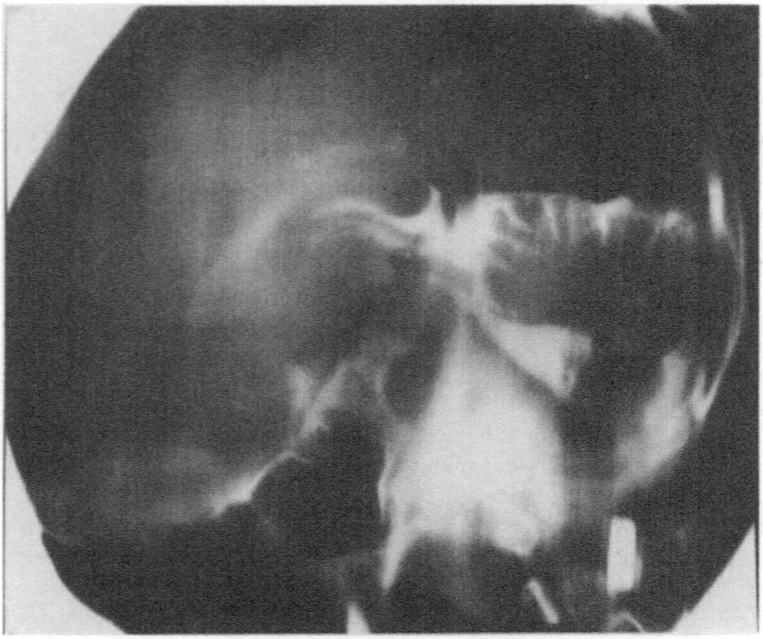

**Fig. 4.** Normal posterior cisternogram taken with head tilting backward

of mass, the velocity of the injection of contrast material, and iodine concentration of contrast material. Furthermore, in the supine or prone position, constrast material moves relatively free in the interhemispheric fissure along the cortical sulci, which might be the cause of convulsive seizure.

Metrizamide cisternography with conventional X-ray films is excellent for evaluating anatomical details of the basal cisterns [1–5], compared with CT cisternography, and less complicated and less invasive than pneumoencephalography, if there is no convulsive seizure. I hope that contrast material will be developed for use in the subarachnoid spaces more safely, but if the examination is performed paying attention to the stream of contrast material in subarachnoid spaces, the frequency of convulsions will be diminished.

## References


1. Grepe A (1977) Cisternography with metrizamide of the posterior fossa following lateral C1-C2 puncture. Acta Radiol [Suppl] 355:257–268
2. Hall K, McAllister VL (1980) Metrizamide cisternography in pituitary and juxtapituitary lesions. Radiology 134:101–108
3. Roberson GH, Ellis G, Brismer J, Taverus JM (1977) Cisternography with metrizamide and hypocycloidal tomography. Acta Radiol [Suppl] 355:314–322
4. Sartor K, Richerts S (1979) Konventionell-radiographische und computerassistierte Zysternographie der hinteren Schädelgrube mit Metrizamid. ROEFO 130:472–478
5. Sortland O, Nornes H, Djupesland G (1977) Cisternography with metrizamide in cerebellopontine angle tumors. Acta Radiol [Suppl] 355:345–356

# Use of the New Hydrosoluble Contrast Materials (Metrizamide and Iopamidol) in Tomodensitometric Exploration of the Subarachnoid Spaces and Cisterns

C. Manelfe, A. Bonafe, and J. Prere

Tomodensitometric exploration of the subarachnoid spaces required the preliminary introduction of a totally resorbable hydrosuluble contrast material, calling in clinical practice for either metrizamide or iopadmidol.

Our comparative study covered 88 cisternographies, 47 with iopamidol and 41 with metrizamide. The pathology in 50 patients related to the sella, in 14 to the posterior fossa, and in 11 to the craniospinal junction; there were ten cases of rhinorrhea of cerebrospinal fluid and three of normal pressure hydrocephalus. The 47 computerized cisternographies using iopamidol included 26 men and 21 women ranging in age from 9 to 70 years with a mean age of 41 years. The mean volume of contrast material, injected by the lumbar route, was 6.17 ml (range 4–12 ml) with an iodine concentration of 200 mg/ml.

The 41 computerized cisternographies with metrizamide included 19 men and 22 women whose ages ranged from 16 to 72 years with a mean age of 39 years. Their mean weight was 70 kg. The mean volume injected was 5 ml, at an iodine concentration of 170–200 mg/ml.

All 88 patients were subjected to clinical surveillance for 48 h after cisternography, and any complications noted were classified as early (occurring in the first 6 h) or late (from 6 to 48 h). Recovery was uncomplicated for 64 patients (35 with iopamidol and 29 with metrizamide). Complications were dominated by headaches, which occurred in 25.5% of the patients with iopomidol and 29.26% of those with metrizamide. Their early (11 cases) or late (12 cases) onset was not influenced by the nature of the contrast material injection.

In descending order of frequency, the next complication was vomiting, noted in five cases with iopamidol and nine cases with metrizamide. It occurred twice in isolation and once with an early headache, but was usually (11 cases) associated with late headaches. Electrical tolerance was checked in 44 patients, and in the majority there was no change of electrogenesis, 33 control EEGs showing no anomaly. Slow waves of the theta type with variable distribution (frontal, temporal or posterior) were recorded in 11 cases. Neither clinical seizure or epileptic discharges were observed.

Opacification of the cisternal spaces with metrizamide or iopamidol does not show much difference between the two products in quality of image or in clinical and elctrical tolerance.

# Adverse Reactions to Myelography with Metrizamide in Children

H. Petterson, Ch. R. Fitz, D.C.F. Harwood-Nash, S.H. Chuang, and E. Armstrong

The adverse effects of metrizamide myelography are well documented, especially experimentally and in adults [1]. There are also several reports of adverse effects in infants and children, but the materials in these reports have been fairly small [2].

The purpose of the present investigation was therefore to define the character, frequency, and severity of adverse reactions in children, and to define the circumstances during the procedure that might have an impact on these reactions. A detailed report of this investigation is in print [3].

## Material and Procedures

The material consisted of 246 consecutive patients that had metrizamide myelography performed at the Hospital for Sick Children, Toronto, during a 1½-year period 1977–1979. There were 130 girls and 116 boys. The ages varied between 16 days and 19 years (mean 8 years), and the weights between 2.5 and 80 kg (mean 32 kg).

The examinations were performed under general anesthesia in 52% of the cases and under local in 48%, the type of anesthesia mainly depending on the patient's age. Sedation used in 18 cases was Nembutal or Valium, and as seizure prophylaxis, Phenobarbital or valproic acid was used. In 28 cases no sedation or seizure prophylaxis was used at all. Lumbar puncture was performed in almost all cases, most of them at the level L2–L4. The needle size varied between 20 and 22 gauge. The volume of metrizamide injected varied between 1.6 and 15 ml and the concentration varied between 170 and 250 mg iodine/ml. The total amount given varied between 270 and 3400 mg iodine, depending on the patient's age and size. The extension of the diagnostic concentration of metrizamide varied from the lumbar level to the basal cisterns.

## Methods

During and after the examination all procedure data and all adverse reactions were recorded in a special protocol. The procedure data considered were age, sex, anesthesia, sedation, seizure prophylaxis, needle size, puncture site, radiologic findings, and for the metrizamide its concentration, total amount, and the cranial extension. In the present investigation, the data from the procedure and all adverse reactions observed were reviewed. A trial was done to find the circumstances during the procedure that might have had an impact on the frequency and severity of the reactions.

**Table 1.** Adverse Reactions

| Type | No. of cases |
|---|---|
| Nausea and vomiting | 98 |
| Headache | 53 |
| Fever 38°–39° | 10 |
| Leg and/or back pain | 5 |
| Dizziness | 4 |
| Rash | 2 |
| Diplopia | 1 |
| Decreased level of consciousness | 1 |
| Irregular heart beats | 1 |
| Seizures | 2 |

## Results

Adverse reactions occurred in 143 cases (58%). The type and frequency of these reactions are given in Table 1. The most common reactions were nausea and vomiting, headache, and fever. Infants and small children obviously have difficulties in expressing their problems and irritability at these ages was recorded as headache.

An attempt was made to classify the reactions as mild, moderate, or pronounced, depending on the severity and duration of the nausea and vomiting, headache and irritability, fever, leg and back pain, dizziness, and rash. According to this classification, 33% of all patients had a mild reaction, 18% had a moderate reaction and 8% a pronounced reaction. Four patients (1.6%) were regarded as having severe reactions (diminished consciousness, diplopia for a long time, and in two cases seizures).

*The mild reactions* increased in frequency with increasing age; otherwise there were no significant changes between patients with no or mild reactions concerning the procedure data. On the whole, the mild reactions were of the same frequency and type that should be expected after a lumbar puncture alone – the post lumbar puncture syndrome as described in detail by Tourtelotte et al. [4]. Thus, there was no causal relation between the metrizamide injected and the mild reactions.

Concerning *the moderate and pronounced reactions,* none of the following procedure data had any impact on the reactions: sex, type of anesthesia, sedation, seizure prophylaxis, needle size, puncture site, radiologic finding, or concentration of metrizamide injected.

On the other hand, we found that the frequency and severity of the moderate and pronounced reactions increased with age and with the total amount of metrizamide given and its cranial extension in the spinal canal. But a larger amount of metrizamide had been given to the older children, because of their larger size. Thus, the relation between age, total amount of metrizamide, and type and severity of reactions must be analyzed further. Therefore, the amount of metrizamide per kilo body weight was calculated. It was found that the older children received significantly less metrizamide per kilo body weight than the small children. However, most of the effects are probably CNS reactions [5]. Therefore, the dose given per kilo brain was also calculated, and the brain weight according to age taken from Copoletta and Wobach [6] and Laroche [7]. It was then found that the older children got significantly more metrizamide, and more in the same proportion as the increased frequency of reactions. But, the brain surface area or the volume of the subarachnoid space might be as good or better parameters as the brain weight to express the size of the CNS. All these parameters are functions of the age of the child, given a normal brain development, and therefore, a statistical analysis of the total amount of metrizamide given to those with and without reactions within each age group was performed. Using the Mann-Whitney U Test, it was found that in most age groups, the amount given to those with a moderate and severe reaction was significantly larger than that given to those with a mild or no reaction (Fig. 1). There was no significant difference between those who had a moderate and pronounced reaction.

Concerning the *severe reactions* there was no significant difference in the patients with severe reactions compared with those with moderate or pronounced.

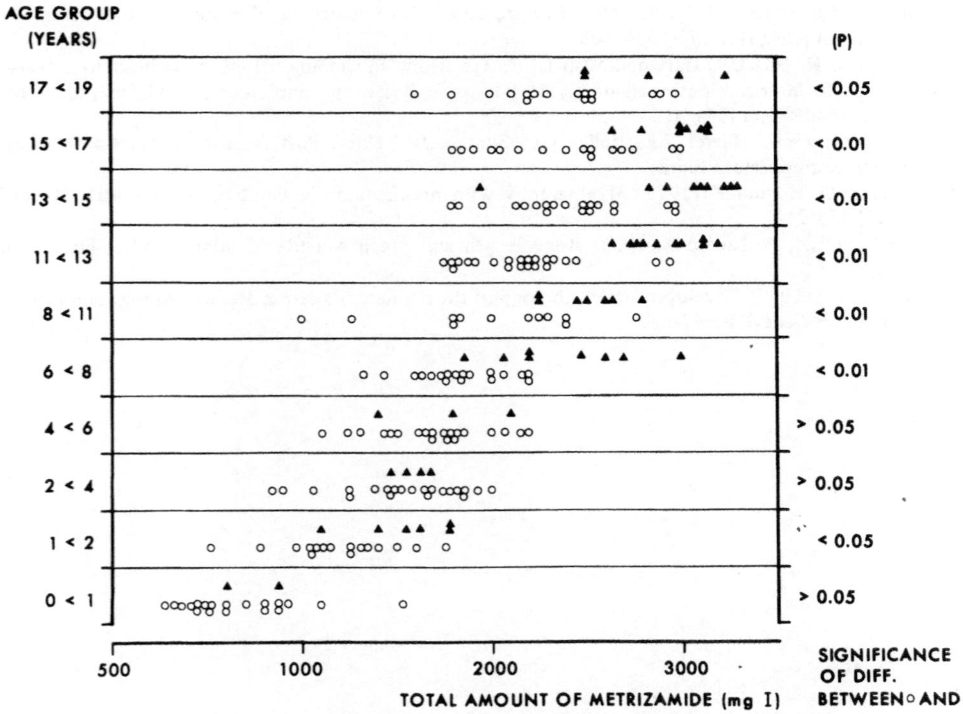


**Fig. 1.** The total amount of metrizamide given, according to age and to severity of reaction. ○, patients with no or mild reaction; ▲, patients with moderate or pronounced reactions. The figure also gives the significance of the difference in dose within each age group to those with no or mild reactions and to those with moderate or pronounced reactions respectively

## Conclusions

1. Adverse reactions to metrizamide myelography occurred in 58% of all cases in pediatric material.
2. The majority of the reactions (33%) were mild. They were caused by the lumbar puncture and were not related to the metrizamide.
3. The frequency of moderate (18%) and pronounced (8%) reactions was directly correlated to the total amount of metrizamide within each age group, and to the cranial extension of the examination in the spinal canal.
4. The severe reactions were rare (1.6% of all cases). There was nothing concerning the clinical history or procedure data that distinguished the patients with severe reactions from those with moderate or pronounced.
5. The appropriate amount of metrizamide given should be related to the child's age (and hence to the size of the CNS) and not to the size or weight of the child.

## References


1. Almén T, Golman K (1979) Pharmacology and toxicology of some intrathecal contrast media. In: Socket JF, Strother CM, New techniques in myelography. Harper & Row, Hagerstown, p 8
2. Fitz CR, Harwood-Nash DCF, Barry JF, Byrd SE (1977) Pediatric myelography with metrizamide. Acta Radiol [Diagn] [Suppl] 355:102
3. Pettersson H, Fitz CR, Harwood-Nash DCF, Armstrong E, Chuang SH (to be published) Adverse reactions to Metrizamide myelography in infants, children and adolescents. I. General and CNS effects. Acta Radiol [Diagn]
4. Tourtellotte WW, Haerer AE, Heller GL, Somers JE (1964) Post lumbar puncture headaches. Thomas, Springsfield, Illinois
5. Sortland O, Hovind K (1977) Myelography with metrizamide in children. Acta Radiol [Diagn] [Suppl] 355:211
6. Copoletta LM, Wobach SD (1933) Body length and organ weights of infants and children. Am J Pathol 9:55
7. Laroche JC (1977) Developmental pathology of the neonate. Excerpta Medica, Amsterdam Princeton London Geneve New York

# Iopamidol, a New Nonionic Contrast Medium for Myelography and Sacculoradiculography: A Review of 800 Cases

E. Signorini, E. Ciorba, and N. Caputo

Iopamidol was used at iodine concentrations of 200, 300, and 370 mg/ml for dorsolumbar and cervical myelography and radiculography by injection into the lumbar CSF space.

We performed cervical myelography in 75 cases (72 with iodine 370 mg/ml and three with iodine 300 mg/ml); dorsolumbosacral myelography in 116 cases (82 with concentration 370, 32 with 300, and 2 with 200); and sacculoradiculography in 609 cases (287 with concentration 370, 297 with 300, and 25 with 200).

On the strength of radiological results obtained in these trials with the various concentrations of test product we recommend using the iodine concentration of 200 mg/ml only for sacculoradiculography, with the understanding that some roentgenograms may not prove fully satisfactory on account of rapid dilution of the contrast in CSF.

In our opinion the iodine concentration of 300 mg/ml is best for sacculoradiculography in that it always yields X-ray pictures of excellent quality with perfect visibility of the smaller structures (radicular pouches), even with very small doses of contrast. The same concentration (iodine 300 mg/ml) produces technically perfect roentgenograms also in myelography of the cone and cauda equina segments and of the lower and intermediate segments of the dorsal spine, particularly in the presence of total block or major stenosis of the spinal canal.

As for exploration of the upper dorsal and cervical spine, and of course of the craniovertebral hinge, we definitely recommend the iodine concentration of 370 mg/ml. With the 300 mg/ml formulation, indeed, one can never be sure of obtaining consistently good results; nor can this be obviated merely by increasing the dose of contrast. In planning myelography or radiculography, in addition to the suitability of contrast in terms of picture quality, one must take into account the incidence and type of attendant complications; this parameter was indeed the essential criterion of evaluation that led to the abandonment of ionic contrast media despite the remarkably good quality of roentgenograms obtained with them. The overall incidence of side effects in our series of observations was 18% between immediate (painful paresthesia) and early complications (headache, nausea, vomiting, nuchal rigidity, photophobia, fever, collapse, and convulsive seizures). If we recalculate percentages of side effects according to the segments of spinal canal being explored and the iodine concentrations used we get the following:

| Procedure | Iodine concentration | Percent side effects |
|---|---|---|
| Sacculoradiculography | 200 mg/ml | 8.00% |
| | 300 mg/ml | 8.44% |
| | 370 mg/ml | 22.37% |

| Procedure | Iodine concentration | Percent side effects |
|---|---|---|
| Dorsal myelography | 300 mg/ml | 15.00% |
| | 370 mg/ml | 18.75% |
| Cervical myelography | 370 mg/ml | 47.2 % |

The detailed study of side effects encountered in contrasted examinations relative to the two fundamental parameters of assessment (iodine concentration of the contrast medium and segment of spinal canal being explored) yields some extremely interesting results [1]. As for concentration there is a definite increase of complications with increasing iodine content per unit of volume: if we go back to our own breakdown per type of examination we can see quite clearly that the incidence of complications increases with increasing concentration of the contrast material. This circumstance makes it mandatory to use the least concentrated preparation for each type of examination with the only exception of sacculoradiculography, where the 200 and 300 mg/ml iodine concentrations give practically the same percentage of side effects – hence the advisability of using iopamidol 300 for sacculoradiculography, since the quality of roentgenograms obtained with this concentration is definitely superior.

As for the level of spinal canal being explored, we find a higher incidence of side effects in connection with cervical myelography than in dorsolumbar myelography, with the exception of the 370 mg/ml concentration which produces more side effects in dorsolumbar than in dorsal spine examinations. This apparent discrepancy may be explained, however, by the fact that the bulk of our experience in the field of sacculoradiculography with the more concentrated contrast (iodine 370 mg/ml) was accumulated in the early stage of our work, when we used large doses of product. In summation therefore, the highest incidence of complications was seen in cervical myelography with Iopamidol 370 (47.2%). To understand this finding we must bear in mind that cervical myelography by the lumbar approach invariably involves the flooding of intracranial cisterns by contrast material, and this alone produces a large crop of headaches and other subjective and objective symptoms. On the other hand, cervical myelography is an important diagnostic procedure, not easily replaced by other methods: thus for instance, cervical myelography with gas or fat-soluble contrast certainly does not produce fewer or lesser side effects – enough so as to justify the use of water-soluble contrast even at the cost of a high incidence of side effects.

Aside from sheer numbers, also, we must consider the qualitative aspects of such complications, which were seldom severe or alarming with Iopamidol. In fact, most patients complained only of headache, rarely associated with nausea and vomiting; only a few showed evidence of radicular irritation; and very few experienced dizziness, convulsions (one case), fever, or tachycardia. Remarkably, there was not a single instance of mental confusion, which is reported to occur with some frequency with metrizamide.

Also the amount of contrast-injected influences the incidence and severity of complications. Both in overall terms and relative to each concentration, indeed, there was a definite relationship between increasing dose volumes and increased incidence and severity of the side effects. Clearly, therefore, one should use the smallest amount of contrast solution of the appropriate concentration consistent with reliable diagnosis.

The problem of complications is particularly relevant in the study of lumbosacral disk hernias by sacculoradiculography, since in a great many cases a definite diagnosis of disk hernia can be made on the strength of clinical findings and other nonradiological methods, sacculoradiculography representing a confirmatory procedure more than anything else. Accordingly, radiological diagnosis for lumbosacral disk hernia appears justified only if the incidence and the severity of side effects is truly negligible; otherwise the injection of contrast in the CSF should be avoided. For our part we have tried to reduce side effects in patients examined for suspected lumbosacral disk hernia by developing a procedure that requires very small doses (1.5–2 ml) of contrast medium (iodine 300 mg/ml) and the making of roentgenograms with a horizontal tangent beam with the patient in a horizontal lateral, and semiprone decubitus. This method affords excellent exposure of the anterolateral margin of the dural sac and of the whole length of radicular pouches, with very good visibility of alterations caused by herniated disks.

We have used this technique in a total of 57 patients over the last 2 months, and we have seen a drastic reduction of side effects – only two cases of mild headache lasting a few hours.

## References

1. Signorini E, Ciorba E, Pelliccioli GP, et al. (1979) First experiences with the clinical use of a new hydrosoluble nonionic contrast medium, Iopamidol, in the study of the subarachnoid space. Rays 4:47–68

# Ioglunide: A New Contrast Medium for Myelography and Cisternography (Animal Experiments and Preliminary Clinical Experience)

R. E. Gonsette and L. Liesenborgh

## Introduction

Since 1972, metrizamide (Amipaque) has been extensively used for the opacification of perimedullary and pericerebral spaces, and there is a general agreement that the neurotoxicity of this new contrast medium (CM) is definitely lower than that of previous ionic iodinated compounds.

Nevertheless, it appears from our personal experience and from a recent publication by Bertoni et al. [1] that, in addition to minor side effects (headaches, nausea, vomiting), more severe reactions have been described. Even if the incidence of epileptic seizures is very low, transient EEG changes are rather frequently observed (14%–35%) [8], according to the site of injection, and the penetration of metrizamide into the pericerebral cisterns. Transient neurological deficits [6], as well as psychoorganic syndromes [7, 9], have been reported by different authors, and their frequency must not be underrated.

It seems evident therefore that metrizamide is far from nontoxic and for this reason, there is an increasing interest for new CM with a lesser biological activity. Our results with newly synthetized CM have been recently published [2], and the aim of this paper is to report our experimental results and our preliminary clinical experience with Ioglunide, a nonionic substance synthesized by the Guerbet Laboratories.

## Material and Methods

The chemical formula of Ioglunide is given in Fig. 1. The reduction of neurotoxicity of this new nonionic CM is presumably due to the substitution of a more hydrophilic *N*-hydroxy-ethyl-carbamyl radical in the triiodobenzene ring. This compound was experimented in our laboratory in aqueous solution as soon as 1977. These unpublished pre-

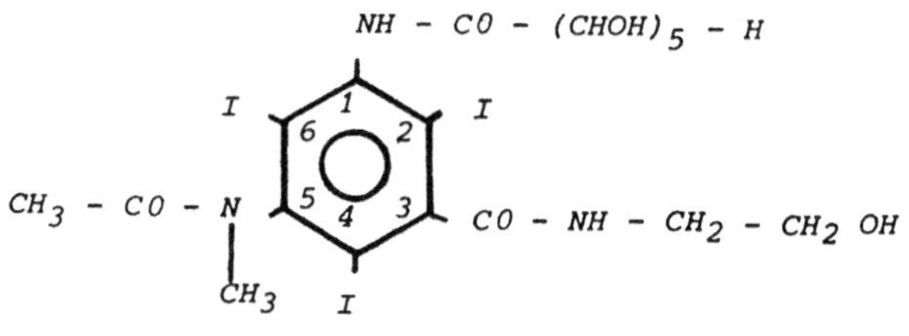


**Fig. 1.** Chemical formula of Ioglunide

liminary results were encouraging but it soon appeared that the sugar substituent was cleaved off on heating, and consequently that the CM must be dispensed as a lyophilized powder. The good tolerance of Ioglunide was confirmed with the EEG and corticospinal evoked potentials techniques in monkeys by Hilal et al. in 1978 [5].

More recently, using the monitored EEG frequency analysis, we observed that delayed changes (6–8 h) were definitely less marked for Ioglunide than for metrizamide and other similar CM. This prompted us to investigate the neurotoxicity of the lyophilized form with a view to a possible better clinical tolerance in man.

The neurotoxicity of Ioglunide was evaluated in the guinea pig according to the techniques currently used in our laboratory. Influence on the brain electrophysiology was determined by usual EEG recordings and EEG frequency analysis. The brain cellular toxicity was observed in optic and electron microscopy.

## Experimental Results

No tissular damage and no inflammatory reactions were observed in optic microscopy after pericerebral injection of 0.1 ml 300 mg/iodine/ml solution Ioglunide. Histological reactions observed in electron microscopy compared to metrizamide and Iopamidol are summarized in Table 1.

The cellular toxicity of Ioglunide seems very close to that of metrizamide, and it must be stressed that both CM produce histological reactions. For that reason, they cannot be considered as biologically "inert" toward the central nervous system (CNS). It appears that Iopamidol is slightly more toxic since mild neuronal alterations were observed. Those reactions are probably related to the more pronounced irritative activity of Iopamidol.

Epileptogenic activity of Ioglunide, metrizamide, and Iopamidol was determined on conventional EEG recordings after pericerebral injections of highly concentrated solutions

**Table 1.** Comparative brain tissular toxicities. Pericerebral injections in the guinea pig 0.1 ml, 300 mgI/ml (electron microscopy)

| Substances | Time interval | Perivasc. | Edema Cell. | Edema Intercell. | Neurone changes |
|---|---|---|---|---|---|
| Metrizamide | 24 h | ± | 0 | 0 | 0 |
| | 48 h | + | 0 | 0 | 0 |
| | 72 h | 0 | 0 | 0 | 0 |
| Ioglunide | 24 h | ± | 0 | 0 | 0 |
| | 48 h | + | ± | 0 | 0 |
| | 72 h | ± | 0 | 0 | 0 |
| Iopamidol | 24 h | ++ | + | ± | + |
| | 48 h | + | ± | 0 | 0 |
| | 72 h | + | 0 | 0 | 0 |

(400 mg I/ml). The epileptogenic threshold of the three CM (pericerebral injections in the guinea pig) are:

| | Maximal amount without EEG changes |
|---|---|
| Metrizamide | 0.30 ml |
| Ioglunide | 0.30 ml |
| Iopamidol | 0.08 ml |

Metrizamide did not produce any changes. After injection of Ioglunide, sporadic slow waves and fast activities spindles were observed. As reported before, Iopamidol in amounts as low as 0.1 ml provoked epileptic seizures in the same experimental conditions.

A better discrimination of the three CM was obtained by the EEG frequency analysis, monitored for as long as 12 h. As reported elsewhere [3], delayed reactions were observed with Iopamidol and metrizamide, whereas Ioglunide failed to produce any changes in the 0.5–16 Hz band.

In conclusion, the immediate CNS tolerance of Ioglunide is quite similar to that of metrizamide, but its delayed effects on the EEG are definitely less marked, if any.

Finally, it must be remembered that it has recently been demonstrated by Haughton and Ho [4] that the incidence of arachnoiditis with intrathecal Ioglunide in monkeys was the same as it was in the control animals.

## Clinical Experience

Our animal experiments being in favor of an Ioglunide better tolerance, a preliminary clinical investigation was conducted in agreement with the Guerbet Laboratories.

Intrathecal injection of Ioglunide was performed by lumbar or suboccipital puncture with 22 gauge needles in 62 patients. Myelographies were performed using iodine concentration of 280 mg/I/ml and injecting a volume of 5 ml for cervical and lumbar investigations, and of 10 ml for total myelographies. A concentration of 170 mg/I/ml in a volume of 10 ml was used for CT scan cisternographies. The doses of iodine ranged therefore from 1.7 to 2.8 g. After all procedures, patients were asked to remain in bed with their head slightly elevated (15°–20°) for 6 h.

Follow-up neurological examinations were performed at 8, 24, and 48 h and patients were questioned in regard to current minor side effects and other symptoms not specifically requested. They were checked particularly for disturbances of consciousness and/or orientation, lack of concentration, perceptual disorders, dizziness, etc.

EEG (57 patients) and EEG frequency analysis (20 patients) were performed before and 8 or 24 h after the radiological procedure.

The number of investigations performed is as follows:

| | |
|---|---|
| Myelographies | |
| Lumbar | 21 |
| Dorsal | 3 |
| Cervical | 18 |
| Ventriculographies | 3 |
| CT scan | |
| Cisterno | 14 |
| Cervical | 3 |
| Total | 62 |

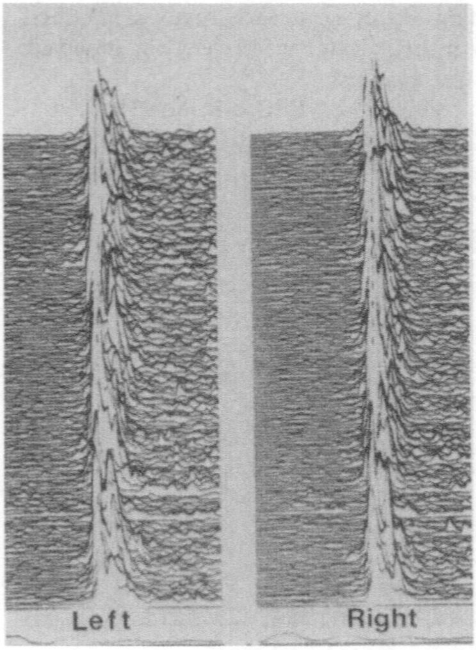


**Fig. 2a.** Normal EEG sequential analysis, 24 h after intrathecal injection of 10 ml Ioglunide 28%

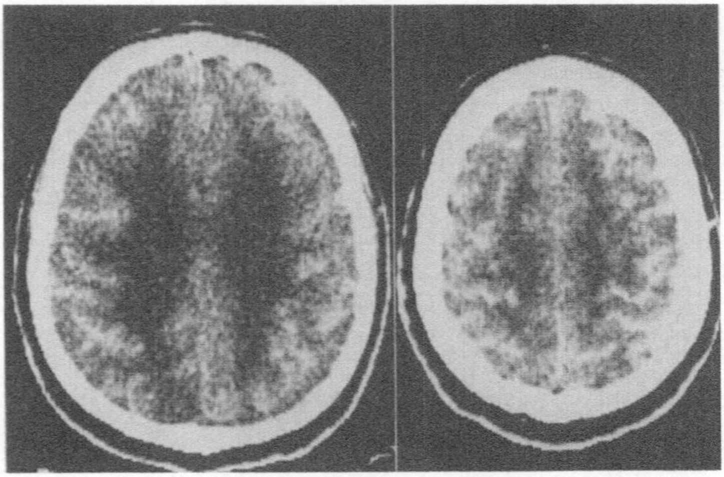

**Fig. 2b.** A definite intracerebral penetration of the CM is demonstrated on the CT scan in this patient

In 66% of the patients, the upper part of the spinal cord or the pericerebral cisterns were investigated and the CM was therefore directly in contact with the brain tissue. Moreover, CT scan performed 24 h after lumbar myelographies revealed the presence of CM around the brain in some patients (Fig. 2a, b).

Side effects are listed in Table 2. According to our experience, minor side effects are less marked for Ioglunide, and until now mental disturbances were not observed, even after cervical myelographies or CT scan cisternographies.

The better tolerance of Ioglunide was also confirmed on EEG controls (Table 3). It appears that the incidence of EEG changes (3.5%) is definitely much lower than that observed after intrathecal injection of metrizamide (14%–35%).

**Table 2.** Ioglunide side effects (57 evaluable patients)

| Investigations | No patients | Headache | Nausea | Backache | Psych. Disturb. |
|---|---|---|---|---|---|
| Myelographies | | | | | |
| Lumbar | 19 | 3 | 1 | 3 | – |
| Dorsal | 3 | 1 | – | – | – |
| Cervical | 16 | 4 | 1 | – | – |
| Ventriculographies | 3 | – | – | – | – |
| CT scan | | | | | |
| Cisternogr. | 13 | 1 | – | – | – |
| Cervical | 3 | – | – | – | – |
| Total | 57 | 9 (16%) | 2 | 3 | 0 |

**Table 3.** Ioglunide (EEG controls) latency: 8 h, $n$ = 31; 24 h, $n$ = 26

| EEG Before | After | M.[a] Lumbar | M.[a] Cervical | M.[a] Dorsal | Cist. CT sc. | V.[b] | Total | |
|---|---|---|---|---|---|---|---|---|
| N1 | N1 | 21 | 14 | 3 | 6 | – | 44 | |
| Pat | Pat | 1 | 3 | 1 | 3 | 3 | 11 | |
| N1 | Pat | – | 1 | – | – | – | 1 | 3.5% |
| Pat | ↗ | – | – | – | 1 | – | 1 | |
| Total | | 22 | 18 | 4 | 10 | 3 | 57 | |

[a] Myelography; [b] Ventriculography

## Conclusion

According to our animal experiments, the brain cellular toxicity of Ioglunide is the same as that of metrizamide and less marked than that of Iopamidol.

The main interest of this new CM is its virtual absence of immediate or delayed effect on the brain electrical activity. Compared to other CM, Ioglunide seems therefore to have the lowest neurotoxicity.

The absence of delayed effects on the EEG in animals prompted us to investigate its clinical tolerance. A preliminary experience in 62 patients indicates that minor side effects as well as EEG changes are definitely less frequent. Mental disturbances were not observed.

According to the generally accepted percentage of side effects and EEG changes following metrizamide injection, the number of patients investigated seems already sufficient to support the conclusion that Ioglunie indeed represents an important advance in myelography and cisternography.

## References


1. Bertoni JM, Schwartzman RJ, Van Horn G, Partin J (1981) Asterixis and encephalopathy following Metrizamide myelography: investigations into possible mechanisms and review of literature. Ann Neurol 9:366–370
2. Gonsette RE, Brucher JM (1980) Neurotoxicity of novel water-soluble contrast media for intrathecal application. Invest Radiol 15:254–259
3. Gonsette RE (to be published) Immediate and delayed neurotoxicity of newly synthesized contrast media demonstrated by EEG sequential analysis.
4. Haughton VM, Ho KC (1980) The risk of arachnoiditis from experimental nonionic contrast media. Radiology 136:395–397
5. Hilal SK, Dauth GW, Hess KH, Gilman S (1978) Development and evaluation of a new water-soluble iodinated myelographic contrast medium with markedly reduced convulsive effects. Radiol 126:417–422
6. Picard L, Vespignani H, Vieux-Rochat P, et al. (1979) Serious neurological complications of Metrizamide myelography. Report of 8 cases. J Neuroradiol 6:3–14
7. Richert S, Sartor K, Holl B (1979) Subclinical organic psychosyndromes on intrathecal injection of Metrizamide for lumbar myelography. Neuroradiology 18:177–184
8. Ropper AH, Chiappa KH, Young RR (1979) The effect of Metrizamide on the electroencephalogram: a prospective study in 61 patients. Ann Neurol 6:222–226
9. Schmidt RC (1980) Mental disorders after myelography with Metrizamide and other water-soluble contrast media. Neuroradiology 19:153–157

# Second Round Table: Discussion

J.M. Caille

The four papers studied established clinical side effects after myelography or cisternography using either metrizamide or Iopamidol.

These two products are not entirely without neurotoxic effects. Side effects are more frequent at higher dosage: for children the dosage is calculated according to age and not body weight.

In adults, the most frequent clinical complications are headaches (20%–30% of cases), vomiting (15%–20%), and the appearance of slow waves EEG.

These studies have not dealt with changes in consciousness which, however, occur relatively often when metrizamide is used.

There seems to be no significant difference between metrizamide and Iopamidol if one considers the frequency of headaches and vomiting and the quality of the radiological image.

Although these contrast media represent major progress, they are not without neurotoxic effects, and it is essential:

To consider carefully the indications for myelography

To use a perfect technique

To reduce the total quantity of iodine injected as much as possible.

# Section D:
# Effects on the Kidney

# Kidney: Pharmacology of Contrast Media

G.T. Benness

## Physiology

Water accounts for 60% of the body weight of normal man, varying inversely (10%) with the presence or absence of fat [14]. Body water is distributed between the intracellular (40%) and the extracellular (20%) spaces. The transcellular space well be ignored in this review. Water moves between these spaces to balance osmotic and hydrostatic pressures. The movement of solutes is restricted by cell membranes and is mediated by active transport processes. The extracellular space may be further subdivided into a plasma (or vascular) component and an interstitial fluid component. Water and solutes distribute themselves freely between these compartments by diffusion, without the constraint of crossing cell membranes. The diffusion of solutes is influenced, to varying degrees, by factors such as molecular weight and protein binding. One quarter of the cardiac output perfuses the kidneys, providing a renal blood flow of 1250 ml/min or, expressed as renal plasma flow, 600 ml/min. Blood passing through the glomeruli produces a filtrate equivalent to 125 ml/min of plasma of 116 ml/min of water. Solutes are removed from and added to the filtrate by active tubular transport processes. The movement of solutes is accompanied by the passive movement of water in response to osmotic effects. The proximal tubule is the principal site of water reabsorption. In health, the final concentration of the filtrate is adjusted during its passage through the distal segments of the nephron, by the action of antidiuretic hormone, in response to the overall hydration status. The range of water reabsorption varies from 110 to 115 ml/min, leaving a residual urinary output of 6.0–0.5 ml/min. Fluid restriction (hydropenia) or fluid loading (hydration) produce a small increase or decrease in plasma osmolality. The normal plasma osmolality 300 mO/kg may increase to 305 mO/kg with hydropenia or decrease to 295 mO/kg with hydration. Solute loading may artificially increase the plasma osmolality to 310 mO/kg. Renal plasma flow and glomerular filtration rate are largely unchanged under these conditions. However, tubular reabsorption of water does vary. The dehydration status controls water reabsorption from the distal tubule and solute output is constant, while urinary flow rate and osmolality are inversely related.

With solute loading, the elevation of plasma osmolality produces an increase in filtered solute load. If tubular reabsorption is limited or tubular secretion of the loading solute is significant, there will be an increase in the amount of solute passing down the proximal tubule. This osmotic load will limit reabsorption of water from the proximal tubule. An overall increase in water and solute excretion occurs. This produces an osmotic diuresis, characterized by a higher urinary flow rate with an intermediate osmolality [15]. In disease, following extensive loss of renal substance, the remaining renal tissue continuously produces urine of this type [17]. Injected contrast medium acts as a loading solute. Changes in solute and water reabsorption, under varying conditions of fluid restriction and solute loading, are the basic physiological events i.v. urography [2, 6, 16, 18].

## Contrast Media

All water-soluble contrast media are distributed between the vascular and interstitial compartments. Following injection equilibration is rapid. Plasma half-life and excretion half-life are approximately 60 and 30 min respectively. No metabolism of the CM is recorded. Excretion is principally by glomerular filtration and secondarily into the alimentary tract by passive transport.

Urographic contrast media have evolved remarkably in 50 years. With these changes, the iodine content of the molecule increased from one to three atoms, the toxicity decreased more than tenfold, and the recommended adult dose was increased. Dimer and trimer molecules with six and nine atoms per molecule have been developed and tested [1]. A monoacid "dimer", Ioxaglate, has been developed (Guerbet), tested [9], and marketed in Europe. In addition, nonionic agents, metrizamide (Nyegaard) and Iopamidol (Bracco), have been tested as urographic agents but are not marketed for the purpose [8, 11].

Ionic contrast media are prepared as water-soluble salt solutions, in combination with sodium and/or methylglucamine; sometimes calcium and magnesium are included in small quantities. Many are understandably confused by the range of preparations available.

## Dose

Plasma level of solute and glomerular filtration rate are the primary factors influencing the rate of renal excretion of solute. Cattell et al. [6] clearly demonstrated the relationship between plasma contrast media concentration, dose, and rate of administration. A rapid injection produced twice the initial plasma concentration of contrast medium compared with an infusion of an equal dose.

The influence of dose on plasma contrast medium concentration, urinary solute output, urine flow rate and osmolality, and final urinary iodine concentration is important. Plasma contrast concentration is dose and time dependent. There is an initial rapid increase then decrease in plasma concentration with mixing and a further decrease due to excretion. Glomerular filtration of contrast medium produces a marked increase in urinary solute output. Urine flow rate increases in proportion to urinary solute output, and an inverse relationship between solute output and urinary osmolality is demonstrated. Finally urinary contrast concentration increases with dose to a maximum value [2]. Current radiological practice supports the administration of 300 mgI/kg in patients with normal renal function. Children have received "high dose" urography for a considerable time. In renal disease, with reduced glomerular function, it is necessary to increase the dose, to maintain adequate glomerular filtration of the contrast medium [17].

## Drug

There is now wide acceptance that the sodium salts of contrast media produce a better urogram than methylglucamine salts [2, 7, 13]. With the methylglucamine salts, the urinary solute output is greater, there is a greater increase in urinary flow rate and a greater reduction in urinary osmolality; that is, a greater osmotic diuresis. The net result is a lower urinary iodine concentration with methylglucamine salts.

The basis for this effect lies in the different renal handling of the sodium and methylglucamine cations. Methylglucamine is not metabolized and is excreted entirely by glomerular filtration with no tubular reabsorption. Following glomerular filtration sodium undergoes extensive tubular reabsorption.

Recent developments in contrast media present further aspects for consideration. Iodamine (Squibb) is excreted by glomerular filtration and renal tubular secretion. The latter is not really significant at plasma concentration levels achieved in clinical studies [3]. However, osmotic diuresis is related purely to solute output, and is independent of the mode of renal excretion [15]. Thus it is unlikely that the maximum urinary contrast concentration obtainable with iodamide will be greater than that with iothalamate or diatrizoate. Until matched human comparison studies are available, final judgment must be reserved.

The future possibilities with monoacid dimer and nonionic molecules are exciting. Osmotic diuresis is greatly reduced. This has been shown to produce considerably higher maximum urinary iodine concentrations [8, 9, 11, 18].

## Dehydration

As described earlier, the hydropenic subject produces more concentrated urine. These observations have led to the recommendation of overnight fluid restriction but this practice has been questioned. Experimental evidence weighs in its favor. Fry et al. [10] and Sherwood et al. [17] showed that, while overnight fluid restriction did not reliably dehydrate the patient, the initial state of hydration influences the subsequent urographic quality. Cattell et al. [6] showed that dehydration increased the urinary concentration of diatrizoate when care was taken to control dehydration. Webb et al. [18] showed clearly that diuresis, by substances other than CM (including water), leads to a marked reduction in urinary iodine concentration. On balance, it seems that routine overnight fluid restriction will lead to an overall improvement in urographic results in uncompromised patients.

## Nephrogram and Pyelogram

The physiological factors discussed may be applied to optimize the nephrographic and pyelographic phases of IVU. The nephrogram density has both a plasma and tubular component. The plasma contribution is purely dependent on contrast medium concentration and is established by the dose and rate of administration. The tubular contribution is determined by the plasma contrast concentration and by the renal function [16, 17]. Analysis of the nephrogram density by computed tomography confirms this observation [4] and further analysis shows additional dependence on fluid restriction (Benness et al. unpublished) and type of contrast medium [5] (Benness et al., unpublished).

The pyelogram is dependent on complete filling of the collecting system with an adequate concentration of contrast medium in the urine. Filling will be greatest at high urine flow rates. Urinary iodine concentration increases with increasing dose up to a maximum of about 300 mgI/kg. Further increases in dose are self-defeating as the associated osmotic diuresis leads to lower urinary contrast concentration [2, 17]. Although adequate distension of the collecting system is important, the urinary contrast concentration has a greater effect on pyelographic density.

With diminished renal function, nephrographic and pyelographic quality can be improved by injecting a larger dose of contrast media to elevate the plasma contrast concentration. This will partly compensate for reduction in glomerular filtration or tubular concentration. Further fluid restriction will not improve quality and is specifically contraindicated. Perhaps the newer lower osmolality contrast agents will have a specific application in this area.

## References


1. Benness GT (1970a) Urography with the iothalamate dimer and trimer. Australas Radiol 14:416
2. Benness GT (1970b) Urographic contrast agents. A comparison of sodium and methylglucamine salts. Clin Radiol 21:150
3. Bollerup AC, Hesse B, Stiness E (1975) Renal handling of iodamine and ditrizoate. Evidence of active tubular secretion of iodamide. Eur J Clin Pharmacol 9:63
4. Brennan RE, Curtis JA, Pollack HM, Weinberg I (1979a) Sequential changes in the C.T. numbers of the normal canine kidney following intravenous contrast administration. I. The renal cortex. Invest Radiol 14:141
5. Brennan RE, Curtis JA, Pollack HM, Weinberg I (1979b) Sequential changes in the C.T. numbers of the normal canine kidney following intravenous contrast administration. I. The renal cortex. Invest Radiol 14:239
6. Cattell WR, Fry IK, Spencer AG, Purkiss P (1967) Excretion urography. I. Factors determining the excretion of Hypaque. Br J Radiol 40:561
7. Dacie JE, Fry IK (1971) A comparison of sodium and methylglucamine diatrizoate in clinical urography. Br J Radiol 44:51
8. Evill CA, Benness GT (1974) Metrizamide as a non-ionic urographic agent. A comparison with sodium iothalamate and its dimer. Invest Radiol 9:434
9. Evill CA, Benness GT (1978) Urographic excretion studies: preliminary results with a six iodine, singly ionising sodium salt P 286. Invest Radiol 13:325
10. Fry IK, Cattell WR, Spencer AC, Purkiss P (1967) The relation between Hypaque excretion and the intravenous urogram. Br J Radiol 40:572
11. Golman K, Almen T (1976) Metrizamide in experimental urography. IV. Effects of renal contrast media on urinary solutes. Acta Pharmacol 38:120
12. Pearson MC, Gilkes R, Hall JH, Boultbee JE, Saxton HM (1971) Sodium or methylglucamine? A comparison of iothalamates in urography. Br J Radiol 44:55
13. Pitts RF (1968) Physiology of the kidney and body fluids, 2nd edn. Year Book Medical, Chicago
14. Rapoport S, Brodsky WA, West CD, Mackler B (1949) Urinary flow and excretion of solutes during osmotic diuresis in hydropenic man. Am J Physiol 156:433
15. Saxton HM (1969) Urography. Br J Radiol 42:321
16. Sherwood T, Doyle FH, Brechenridge A, Dollery DT, Steiner RE (1968) Intravenous urography and renal function. Clin Radiol 19:296
17. Webb JA, Fry IK, Cattell WR, Cummack B, Jewell SE (1978) The effect of osmotic diuresis on urinary iodine concentration using contrast media of differing osmolality. Br J Radiol 51:106

# Nephrotoxicity of Uroangiographic Contrast Media

J.F. Moreau

Problems in nephrotoxicity of water-soluble iodinated uroangiographic contrast media (CM) are either old fashioned or up to date, according to the way by which they are handled. More and more, renal ultrasonography, when reliable, is taking the place of IVU in one of its most classical but dangerous indications: the differential diagnosis between obstructive and nonobstructive renal insufficiencies (RI). This change in approach should lead to a reduction in the number of anuric accidents, which are mainly observed in non-obstructive azotemic patients [11]. On the other hand computerized tomography and angiographic procedures requiring large amounts of CM are more and more extensively indicated. Nowadays, these examinations should provoke more nephrotoxic accidents than conventional IVUs [5, 15].

## Clinical Description of Nephrotoxic Accidents

The intravascular injection of CM may induce one of the following three renal functional effects ([11] Moreau, 1981, unpublished work): (1) no effect, which is the usual consequence in patients with normal renal function or in patients with mild RI. The renal tolerance of the conventional CM is excellent, when the kidneys are normal. Even very high doses of iodine, rising to 3 g/kg b.w., do not significantly damage the kidneys. This allows complex procedures, such as transcatheter embolizations. (2) Renal functional impairments induced by CM are usually mild to moderate. As they are painless, they are discovered only by daily dosages (serum creatinine, proteinuria, diuresis output). Their prognoses are good even if a transient oliguria occurs, (3) Anuria needing intensive care are rare: less than 200 cases in the literature [11]. Usually, significant increase of se creatinine and oliguria appears by 24 h after the injection. The peak rise in the functional abnormalities is mostly observed between the 2nd and the 5th days [4, 6, 11]. If no intercurrent complications occur, anuric accidents have a good prognosis: preinjection renal function returns within 2 weeks or less and there are no sequelae, except in a few cases of preexisting near end-stage RI.

Older et al. [12] recently described a persistent nephrogram as an aid to early detection of post-IVU oligoanuric accidents occurring without acute systemic hypotension. There is no satisfactory explanation of this unreliable and inconsistent symptom. A few cases of anuria are atypical because they start late, and/or they recover late, and/or recover with sequelae. Other nonnephrotoxic processes, able to induce a renal failure by themselves or to potentialize the nephrotoxic effects of CM, must be discussed. They are mainly cardiovascular collapses, resulting from the CM general toxicity or from a coincidental acute cardiac failure. Anuria complicating angiographies can result from a traumatic dissection of the arterial trunk or from diffuse blood clots or atheromatous embolisms, both inducing renal ischemia.

## Predisposing Factors

Several predisposing factors of nephrotoxicity must be recounted, because they enable preventive measures to be defined.

### Types of Nephropathy

No case of IVU-induced oligoanuria has been reported in the literature in which the preexisting RI was due to mechanical obstruction of the urinary tract. Previous chronic RI secondary to parenchymal renal diseases seems to be a necessary predisposing condition. While the risk of nephrotoxic accidents increases with increasingly severe preexisting RI, the two are not absolutely related. The appraisal of what types of nephropathy are the most sensitive is still beyond our means. Nephrotoxic accidents can occur whatever the nephronic structural component prominently involved in the underlying nephropathy (glomerulus, tubule, interstitium, vessel). However, the renal tolerance to CM decreases markedly when the underlying nephropathy involves the small cortical vessels [13]. For that reason kidneys of patients with diabetic nephropathy (Kimmelstiel-Wilson's syndrome) are at high risk [12, 13]. But diabetes mellitus does *not* increase the nephrotoxic risk when the kidneys are normal, except if the patient is treated by metformine [14].

### Hydration

Excluding myeloma, the role played by dehydration has been controversial during the past decade. Anuric accidents can occur in normally hydrated patients [11, 13]. Dehydration is not the prominent factor of nephrotoxicity expected to prevent serious accidents. However, it appears likely that dehydration makes old patients and infants more sensitive to high doses of CM injections. The treatment of the water balance disorders in dehydrated patients and the normal hydration of other patients, excluding diuretics, are safe prevention measures prior to injections of CM [2].

### The Dose of Iodine

It is amazing that only a few papers give precise details about the doses of CM injected in patients developing nephrotoxic accidents. For that reason, notions of threshold of nephrotoxicity and of overdose level cannot actually be defined. According to Mudge [11] the range of iodine doses known to induce anuria is 5–145 g. The dose should be related to the body weight. The smallest dose of iodine known for inducing a posturographic anuria is 0.27 g/kg [13]. The serious effects of relatively small doses should lead to a discussion of the roles played by eventual obesity, severe parenchymal atrophy, single kidney, in making an actual overdosage at the renal level easier.

Associated severe renal and hepatic functional impairments were expected to enhance the nephrotoxic effects of high doses of iodine. In oliguric patients, a large amount of the dose injected is excreted by extrarenal pathways, mainly by the bile. Uroangiographic CM are not more aggressive for the kidney if the patient has a severe hepatic cirrhosis, contrary to the biliary contrast media [3, 8]. Some original data can be found in retrospective studies made in transplanted patients [9] and in patients with chronic RI submitted for high doses of CM during the first years of the decade (Moreau et al., 1981, unpublished work). There is no significant relationship between the amount of iodine injected and the development of anuric accidents. Many patients (2/3) receiving very high doses of iodine up to 1.2 g/kg b.w. and more, did not develop severe functional impairment, often in spite of severe underlying RI. No truly significant relationship between the type of underlying nephropathy, the amount of iodine injected, the risk of nephropathy, the risk of accident, and the possibility of functional sequelae has been clearly established. There is no clear-cut threshold of nephrotoxicity. Every patient seems to have their own threshold. The dose of iodine would influence the severity of the functional impairment only. For that reason, the adequate dose is the smallest dose giving all the diagnostic data expected from the examination. The problem of angiographies can be quite easily handled [7]. Usually the risk of overdosage is not closely related to the amount of iodine required for the angiograms themselves but to that of preinjection tests, often underestimated.

IVU pose more difficult problems, which can be fortunately solved by ultrasound. Reliable ultrasonography allows the patients to be classified into one of the two following groups: (a) low-risk group of patients with obstructive RI: they can receive a dose up to 1 g iodine/kg b.w. (b) high-risk group of patients with nonobstructive RI; useless IVUs are obviously contraindicated; remaining indicated IVUs should be done with a moderate dose, around 0.4 g iodine/kg b. w.; additional doses may be secondarily injected until the diagnostic questions have been answered. This rule is applicable to CT. If the amount of iodine injected appears very large and eventually dangerous, hemodialysis or peritoneal dialysis are helpful for a fast epuration of the blood.

### Repetition of the Doses

Iterative injections of CM enhance the nephrotoxic risk [11, 13]. Ten years ago, at the Necker Hospital, renal arteriographies were notorious for being very dangerous in azotemic patients. In fact, the anuric accidents resulted from too short a delay between a previous IVU and the arteriography. No anuric accident occurred when a 5-day interval policy between two examinations requiring CM was respected.

### The Types of Iodinated Molecules

The nephrotoxic properties of the four conventional triiodinated ionic CM (salts of diatrizoic, iothalamic, ioxitalamic, metrizoic acids) are practically similar. In animal experiments, the new low osmolar molecules have a low nephrotoxicity. Until now, the nephrotoxic effects of ioxaglic acid and of iopamidol in humans do not seem to be higher than those of conventional media. But they can induce nephrotoxic effects [10]. However, a lower nephrotoxicity or, at least, a similar nephrotoxicity already appears to be a reasonable expectation.

## Pathogenic Hypotheses

The mechanism of CM nephrotoxicity remains almost unknown. Several hypotheses have been discussed.

### Tubular Obstruction by Casts or Crystals

Anuric accidents in dehydrated patients with hyperproteinuric myeloma can occur spontaneously by coagulation of the Bence Jones protein in the tubular lumen. CM potentialize the coagulation of proteins [11]. But anuric accidents of IVU in myeloma result much more from the diet than from the coagulation effect. This is demonstrated by the efficiency of a large hydration. Tubular obstruction by protein casts such as Tamm-Horsfall protein in newborns probably explains only a very small minority of nephrotoxic accidents [11]. Anuric accidents of cholecystographic agents must result from a precipitation of uric cristals in the the tubular lumina, the consequence of an hyperuricosuric effect [3, 8, 13]. A prophylactic alkalinization of the urine has been proposed in order to prevent postcholecystographic anuria. The uricosuric effects of conventional CM are much too trivial to play a major role in uroangiographic CM nephrotoxicity [11].

### The So-Called "Osmotic Nephrosis"

Osmotic nephrosis (ON) consists of large reversible vacuoles of the cytoplasm of the proximal tubular cells [10]. As in hyperosmolar solutions of sugars but also as in rheomacrodex, iodinated CM can induce this lesion which narrows the tubular lumina. Several studies demonstrate that there is a lack of correlation between the extent of ON and the intensity of the possibly associated renal functional impairment. Diffuse ON are mostly but not consistently seen in azotemic patients submitted for high doses of iodine. However, diffuse ON can be seen without renal functional impairment. Conversely, anuria can develop without associated ON. Therefore, the theory of CM nephrotoxicity based on a mechanical tubular obstruction by cytoplasmic swelling can be abandoned. The new ionic or nonionic low osmolar molecules of CM are able to induce all degrees of ON. This data confirms that neither hyperosmolality nor the cation methylglucamine are responsible for inducing ON. ON might result from the pinocytosis phenomenon. The CM molecules, eventually bound to albumins in the tubular lumina, should be absorbed by the cytoplasmic lysosomes through the brush border. This could explain the high frequency of ON in patients with the nephrotic syndrome. ON are never observed in normal kidneys. An underlying nephropathy – but not a renal functional impairment – seems to be a necessary condition. Conventional CM are supposed to be neither excreted nor absorbed by the tubules in humans. The tubular metabolism varies according to the animal species [11]. The development of ON in humans could signify that CM molecules have a tubular excretion or reabsorption only when the cells are previously damaged. The tubular nephrotoxicity is also proven by changes in enzymuria and lysosomuria. The potential relationship between enzymuria and ON has still not been studied. The inability to induce ON in rat kidneys leads to a reappraisal of the choice of the most appropriate animal for experimental studies.

### Hemodynamic and Hematologic Changes

Whatever the hemodynamic changes observed in experimental animals [1, 11], there is no evidence that nephrotoxic accidents result from ischemia in humans. Even after major angiographies, the hemodynamic changes are neither prolonged, nor consistent. Significant hemodynamic changes occur only in a very small minority of patients submitted for IVU. The ischemic factor related to the red cells aggregation also plays no prominent role. We never observed microembolisms in the samples of renal tissue examinated after injections of CM, even when they were biopsied after severe functional impairments. Hemodynamic and hematologic disorders probably play a major role in a few cases of postangiographic RI. Associations with other factors are probable.

The role played by dehydration has been treated previously. Recently the emphasis has been made on the role played by a loss of sodium that CM could provoke [13]. According to Thurau and Boylan, anuria would result from a stimulation of the renin angiotensin system by the sodium and chlorine balance abnormalities. Therefore, the preventive treatment of anuria should be an increased sodium intake. The validity of the hypothesis applied to CM has still not been proven. The loss of sodium provoked by CM injections is probably not large and not long enough for a significant stimulation of the macula densa.

### Glomerular Injury

Histological examinations of renal tissue fail to demonstrate a specific symptom of glomerular injury by CM. Massive and transient proteinuria has been described after angiography [1, 11]. Proteinuria is not consistently concomitant with reduced glomerular filtration.

### Immunological Theory

Antibodies against CM have been found in one case of posturographic anuria [11]. CM have been suspected to provoke acute rejections in transplanted kidneys [11]. This is not confirmed by all series [9]. There is no decisive argument supporting an immunological theory of CM nephrotoxicity.

## Conclusion

There is no prospective evidence that the use of CM will decrease in the present decade. Therefore the emphasis must be made on studies of nephrotoxicity of CM. These studies still pose unsolved problems:

1. Determination of the best clinical approach to the CM nephrotoxicity in humans – what are the best parameters? When do they have to be studied? How to criticize the signification of the results?
2. Determination of the best model for animal experiments. This problem is urgent on account of the difficulties of studies in humans. What is the best animal? Is it possible to select universal standards, allowing the validity and the consistency of the results to be controlled? What is the best cost-effective animal?

Objective studies should avoid overestimations of the nephrotoxic risk (often carelessly used for promoting new "nonaggressive" examinations) or underestimations (often carelessly used for the opposite aims). The problem of CM nephrotoxicity should worry people more about CT than conventional radiology. A better selection of the patients undergoing IVU or angiography, a more exacting study of the patient's background, a better understanding of what kind of diagnostic helps CM can give, a more flexible determination of the adequate doses, should tremendously decrease the rate of nephrotoxic accidents. Another source of improvement should come not only from new media but also from other fields of research, for instance digital imaging.

*Acknowledgment.* This work was supported in part by INSERM grant ATP 78–102.

## References


1. Almen T (1971) Toxicity of radiocontrast agents. In: International encyclopedia of pharmacology and therapeutics, vol 2/76. Pergamon Press, Oxford, pp 443–550
2. Eisenberg RL, Bank WO, Hedgock MW (1981) Renal failure after major angiography can be avoided with hydration. AJR 136:859–861
3. Ganeval D, Grunfeld JP, Franco D, Moreau JF, Daniel F (1975) Complications rénales des opacifications biliaires. J Radiol Electrol Med Nucl 56:616–618
4. Harkonen S, Kjellstrand CM (1977) Exacerbation of diabetic renal failure following intravenous pyelography. Am J Med 63:939–946
5. Hayman LA, Evans RA, Fahr LM, Hinck VC (1980) Renal consequences of rapid high dose contrast CT. AJR 134:553–555
6. Krumlouski FA, Simon N, Santanam S, Del Grego F, Roxe D, Pomaranc MM (1978) Acute renal failure: association with administration of radiographic contrast material. JAMA 239:125–127
7. Lang EK, Foreman J, Schlegel JU, Leslie C, List A, McCormick P (1981) The incidence of contrast medium induced acute tubular necrosis following arteriography. Radiology 138:203–206
8. Milman N, Stage P (1974) High-dose urography in advanced renal failure. II. Influence on renal and hepatic function. Acta Radiol [Diagn] 15:104–112
9. Moreau JF, Kreis H, Barbanel C, Michel JR (1975) Effects des produits de contraste iodés sur la function des reins transplantés. Nouv Presse Med 4:2643–2646
10. Moreau JF, Droz D, Noel LH, Leibowitch J, Jungers P, Michel JR (1980) Tubular nephrotoxicity of water-soluble iodinated contrast media. Invest Radiol 15:S54–S60
11. Mudge GH (1980) Nephrotoxicity of urographic radiocontrast drugs. Kidney Int 18:540–552
12. Older RA, Korobkin M, Cleeve DM, Schaaf R, Thompson W (1980) Contrast-induced acute renal failure: persistent nephrogram as clue to early detection. AJR 134:339–342
13. Pengloan J, De Groc F, Moreau JF, Rouleau P, Perrier M, Bagros P (1980) Insuffisance rénale aiguë après urographie intraveineuse. Nouv Presse Med 9:2151–2154
14. Prinseau J, Jardin F, Sanchez A et al. (1977) Insuffisance rénale aiguë après U.I.V. chez le diabétique: fréquence de l'acidose lactique sous traitement par la metformine. Ann Med Interne (Paris) 128:173–177
15. Webb JAW, Reznek RH, Cattell WR, Kelsey Fry I (1981) Renal function after high dose urography in patients with renal failure. Br J Radiol 54:479–483

# The Urinary Concentration of Urographic Radiocontrast Drugs: The Role of Sodium Chloride Excretion and Free-Water-Production

G.H. Mudge

## Introduction

The urinary concentration (U) of the urographic radiocontrast drugs (Uro-RCD) has been of obvious importance in the development of urographic techniques. In addition urinary concentrations have often been considered a possible factor in the pathogenesis of nephrotoxic reactions. With these two clinical implications in mind we have investigated the physiological factors which determine the urinary concentration of Uro-RCD. The same drugs, often in slightly different formulations, are used for other purposes besides classical urography, particularly for angiography. The renal response is essentially the same regardless of the diagnostic intentions, with the exception of renal angiography during which high transient concentrations of Uro-RCD may be achieved in the renal circulation.

Historically the first urographic drugs were secreted by the renal tubule and thereby achieved high concentrations in the urine. Diodrast is probably the best known example. With the introduction of the triiodinated derivatives of benzoic acid, such as diatrizoate, tubular secretion was no longer of physiological importance since these compounds were simply filtered and not secreted. Since they were also not reabsorbed, it followed that the *amount* of Uro-RCD excreted in the urine depended simply on the amount filtered. While this conclusion is still valid tubular functions may be of great importance in determining the *concentration* of Uro-RCD in the urine. These functions include the mechanism by which the urine is either concentrated or diluted as well as the processes which regulate the reabsorption of the major solutes, particularly sodium chloride. The relationship between these several tubular functions and the excreted load of Uro-RCD is complex and the importance of each factor may fluctuate during the course of the urographic procedure itself [2].

## Methods

Details have been published [3, 4] and are briefly summarized. Dogs were deprived of water overnight and anesthetized. Urine was collected from ureteral catheters. For most experiments the contrast drug was diatrizoate; we have a few recent experiments with iopamidol and ioxaglate. Standard clearance techniques were used with measurements of all major urinary solutes including the contrast drug. Urine samples were collected at short intervals (often one-half minute) immediately after the bolus injection of the contrast drug and at longer intervals after the diuresis had started to subside. No radiographs were taken.

## Results

### Renal Response to Acute Diuresis

Under the conditions of these experiments there is a rapid transition from antidiuresis to diuresis. With a high dose of diatrizoate it was not unusual for urine flow to increase from 0.3 to 10 ml/min in less than 2 min. This is an osmotic diuresis which results from the filtration of a nonreabsorbable solute, i.e., diatrizoate and its attendant cation. Parenthetically the osmotic effect of the attendant cation is the same whether diatrizoate is administered (and excreted) as the sodium or meglumine salt.

Figure 1 shows the changes in concentration of urinary solutes. There is a sharp drop in total osmolality which gradually returns to controls within an hour. The major urinary solutes can be divided into (1) the contrast drug, here depicted as diatrizoate multiplied × 2 to account for the attendant cation, (2) urea, (3) chloride and its attendant cation, and (4) "other". The point to be emphasized is that the urinary concentrations of urea and "other" are quite predictable. During antidiuresis their concentrations may be high but these become negligible during the peak of diuresis and for at least 20 min after injection. On the other hand the concentration of chloride can vary over a wide range. In Fig. 1 the concentration was high in both experiments during the controls. In other protocols much lower values have been observed. In Fig. 1 note the difference between A and B regarding chloride concentrations after the injection of the Uro-RCD. These differences develop immediately and persist for at least an hour. In A urinary chloride is far lower than in B; the concentration diatrizoate is higher in A than B despite the fact that total osmolality is in the reverse order.

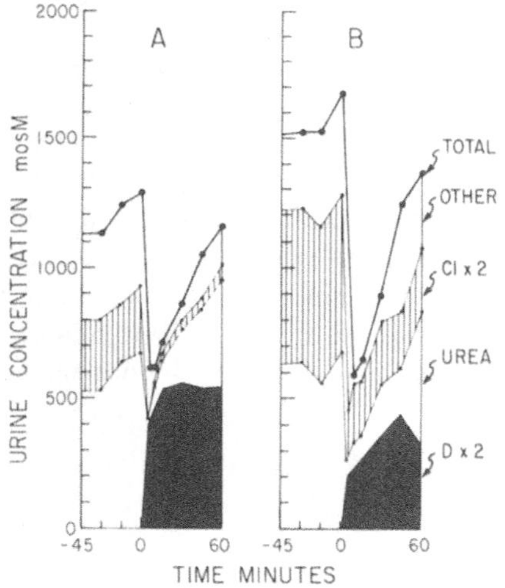


**Fig. 1.** Relation of urinary chloride (C1) to diatrizoate (D) concentration in urine. Bolus injection of sodium diatrizoate 1.2 mmol/kg at zero time; 62% and 55% of the injected dose were excreted within 60 min for A and B, respectively. Molar concentrations of Cl and D have been multiplied × 2 to account for osmotic effect of attendant cation. Concentration of "other" is calculated by difference between total osmolality and sum of measured components. Note the drop in total osmolality immediately after bolus injection with subsequent gradual rise

**Free-Water Formation**

Instead of simply describing the urine as either dilute or concentrated, when free-water formation is calculated one has a quantitative measurement of these processes as rates per unit time. Positive free-water = $V - C_{osm}$ (dilute urine); negative free-water = $C_{osm} - V$ (concentrated urine). In either instance free-water is operationally defined as the volume of distilled water which would have to be either added to or substracted from the urine actually formed over a given period of time (usually 1 min) in order to make that urine isosmotic to plasma. In the case of dilution of the urine, positive free-water is actually formed by the reabsorption of solute (principally sodium chloride) without water. In the case of concentrated urine, negative free-water is formed by the diffusion of water itself in the direction of reabsorption.

**Equation for Concentration**

We have previously [2] derived a mathematical expression which accurately predicts urinary diatrizoate concentration ($U_D$) under all conditions:

$$U'_D = K' \frac{U'_D V}{U'_D V + U_Z V \pm K' \text{ (free water)}}$$

in which $U'_D$ is the same as $U_D$ but corrected to osmotic terms for the obligatory attendant cations, $K'$ is plasma osmolality which under most conditions is almost constant, and $U_Z V$ refers to all osmotically active constituents of the urine other than $U'_D V$. During the sustained diuresis of urography $U_Z V$ consists principally of urea, "other solutes", and chloride plus its attendant cation. Of these, the first two are minor and vary but little from one experiment to another; the latter, i.e., chloride, varies over a wide range (Fig. 1). If other factors remain constant, it is evident from the equation that the lower the value for $U_Z V$, the higher that for $U'_D$. However, as discussed in detail elsewhere [2], the relationships are further complicated by the fact that the absolute value for free-water formation depends on total solute excretion ($U'_D V$ plus $U_Z V$) which varies over a wide range during urography. The sign as well as magnitude of free-water formation also depends on the action of vasopressin.

Several consequences may be summarized: (1) there is no necessary relationship between the rate of Uro-RCD excretion (UV) and its urinary concentration (U); (2) while U tends to vary with total osmolality, this relationship may be obscured by simultaneous changes in other solutes, particularly sodium chloride; and (3) from the dose of Uro-RCD it is not possible tp predict accurately the value for U either during urography or in the subsequent 24 h.

## Human Studies

To evaluate the applicability of these findings to man we studied 79 patients undergoing intravenous pyelography (IVP) with 60 ml of sodium and meglumine diatrizoate (Renograffin-60). We measured the composition of the urine obtained at the last voiding before

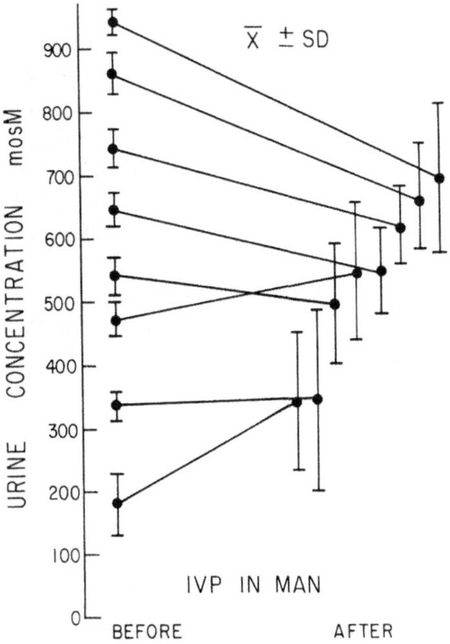


**Fig. 2.** Effect of IVP on urine osmolality. Summary of 79 patients. Values immediately prior to IVP have been subdivided into eight groups

the IVP and the first one after it. There was no special program of water intake prior to the procedure. Figure 2 shows the wide range of urine osmolalities in the control period. The administration of Uro-RCD lowered the osmolalities that were initially high and raised those that were initially low. Both responses are characteristic of osmotic diuresis and are the result of the relationship of solute excretion to water reabsorption. For the latter group of patients, the rise in osmolality may also have resulted from stimulation by the contrast drug of the posterior pituitary to release antidiuretic hormone.

Although osmolality was reasonably predictable, as described above, this did not apply to the urinary concentration of diatrizoate (Fig. 3). Data are shown for three groups of patients in whom the urine osmolality was low, intermediate, or high, and in whom the sums of chloride and diatrizoate were in a relatively narrow range for each group. Note the variations in the urinary diatrizoate concentrations throughout all groups.

## Iopamidol and Ioxaglate

We have done seven preliminary experiments in the antidiuretic anesthetized dog and injected doses that were equi-osmotic (not equal iodine) to our previous studies with diatrizoate. From a physiological point of view the osmotic diuresis induced by the newer agents is similar to that induced by diatrizoate as judged by the transient changes in filtration rate, free-water production, urea secretion, and the rate of excretion of the

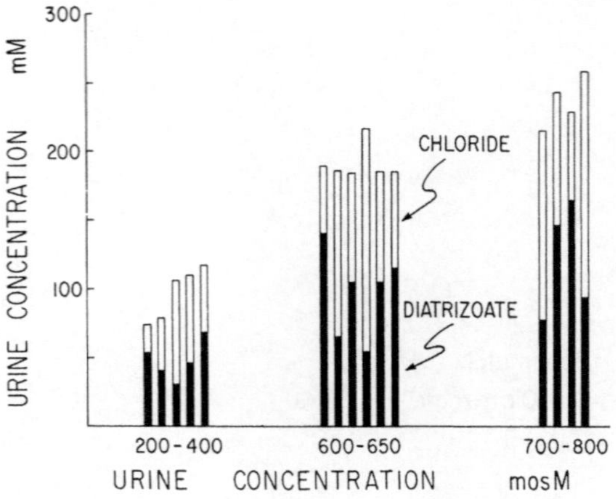


**Fig. 3.** Relationships of concentrations of chloride and diatrizoate to osmolality. Analysis of urine obtained at first voiding after IVP in patients selected as described in text. For comparison to radiological values, 100 mM diatrizoate equals 38 mg iodine per ml

Uro-RCD. As previously reported, changes in chloride excretion were unpredictable [1].

In this experimental model the newer agents appear to differ from diatrizoate in one respect. This is illustrated in Fig. 4 for iopamidol. The results with ioxaglate (Hexabrix) were similar. In the experiment of Fig. 4, two IVPs were done, the first with sodium diatrizoate, the second with iopamidol. The interval between the two was sufficiently long to permit excretion of most of the diatrizoate and also to allow the urine osmolality to ascend toward control levels. Note that after iopamidol the osmolality fell to lower values and that this persisted for a longer period of time. Because of the relationship between osmolality and the rate of solute excretion the data of Fig. 4 are difficult to interpret unless all factors are taken into account. For this purpose Fig. 5 summarizes the

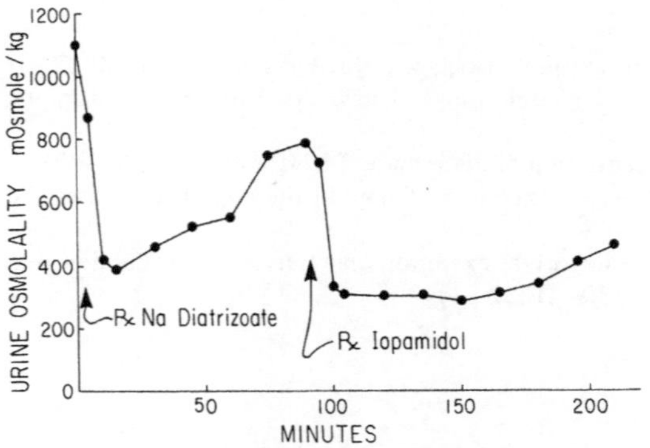


**Fig. 4.** Effect of diatrizoate and iopamidol on urine osmolality in the dog. Both urographic agents were given as a bolus, approximately over a period of 1 min, at dose calculated to be 4.8 mosmol/kg, which is the same as the intermediate dose of diatrizoate previously reported [2, 3, 4]

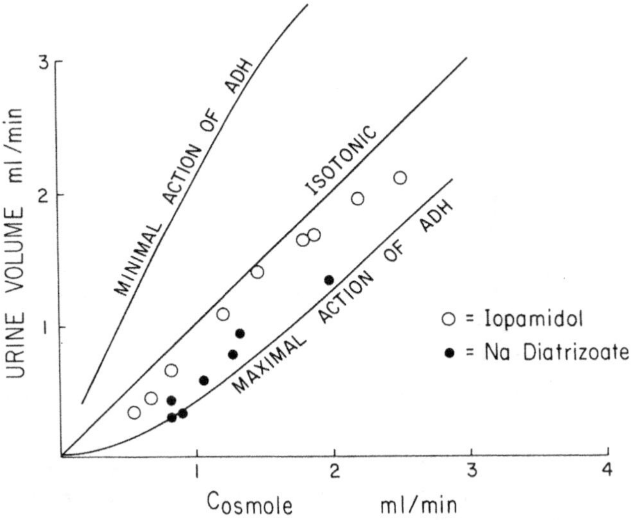


**Fig. 5.** Effect of diatrizoate and iopamidol on relationships of osmolar clearance ($C_{osmol}$) to rate of urine flow. Data from same experiment as Fig. 4. Values for minimal and maximal action of antidiuretic hormone (ADH) are taken from the literature

same data in a different plot. Note that at all rates of solute excretion, calculated as the clearance of osmoles, the data with iopamidol are consistently different from those with diatrizoate. During osmotic diuresis the urine is less concentrated with the newer agents than with diatrizoate. At present the physiological basis for such an action is not known.

*Acknowledgment.* The original investigations reported herein were supported by N.I.H. grants Am 16960 and AM 06818. We are indebted to Laboratoire Guerbet for a supply of Hexabrix and to Bracco Industria Clinica S.p.A. and E.R. Squibb and Sons for supplies of iopamidol.

## References


1. Mudge GH (1974) Renal function during intravenous urography. In: Wesson LG, Fanelli GM Jr (eds) Recent advances in renal physiology and pharmacology. University Park Press, Baltimore, pp 349–359
2. Mudge GH (1980) The maximal urinary concentration of diatrizoate. Invest Radiol 15:S67–S78
3. Mudge GH, Berndt WO, Cooke WJ (1974) Renal excretion of urea in the dog during onset and subsidence of diuresis. Am J Physiol 227:369–376
4. Mudge GH, Cooke WJ, Berndt WO (1975) Electrolyte excretion and free-water production during onset of acute diuresis. Am J Physiol 228:1304–1312

# Variations of Urinary Sodium Concentration After Contrast Media with Different Osmolality

J. Dupuy, J. Pengloan, P. Thienpont, J.L. Jourdan, H. Nivet, and Ph. Rouleau

The consequences of water-soluble contrast media (CM) on different renal functions are not well known. Their effect on sodium and water elimination has been compared to that of osmotic diuretics. Gruskin et al. [2] have shown that three-iodinated CM induce increased sodium elimination as prolonged as CM elimination. The experiments carried out by Ziegler et al. [3, 4] show that ionic CM inhibit active sodium transport. We have studied the evolution of urinary sodium concentration $[Na^+]$ u in man after CM with different osmolality.

## Method

Two CM were used on two groups of 60 intravenous urographies (IVU): sodium and methylglucamine diatrizoate (SMD) with an osmolality of 2100 mOsm/kg and sodium and methylglucamine ioxaglate (I) with an osmolality of 580 mOsm/kg. The amount of $Na^+$ and pH are comparable. Advanced renal failure (creatinine > 300 $\mu$mol/liter) was excluded from this study. There was no control made of the sodium supply during the days preceding the IVU. During the study no water intake was permitted. The amount of CM varied (50–100 cc) according to the diagnosis requirements. The urine passed before and throughout the 30 min following the CM injection was studied.

## Results

Age, sex ratio, amount of CM and injected iodine, urinary concentration of the electrolytes, and the urea were comparable in both groups. Only the amount of injected osmoles (mOsm/kg) varied statistically in the two groups (Tables 1, 2). SMD or I injections do not modify $[Na^+]$ u but there is a statistically significant decrease in the urinary concentration of $Cl^-$, $Ca^{++}$, and urea. This decrease is greater after SMD injection (Tables 3, 4). There remains a difference between $[Na^+]$ u observed in osmotic diuresis, between 50 and 70 mmol/liter [1] (Fig. 1) and a statistically significant difference can be seen between theoretical $[Na^+]$ u of 70 mmol/liter and the $[Na^+]$ u averages observed after SMD ($P < 10^{-3}$) and I ($P < 10^{-6}$). Estimated osmolality is comparable in the two groups before CM is injected and decreases after CM injection; the percentage decrease is 26% after SMD and 16% after I ($P < 10^{-4}$) (Table 5).

**Table 1.** Comparison between the two study groups

| | Age | ♂/♀ | Quantity CM (ml/kg) | Quantity iodine (g/kg) | Quantity osmoles (mOsm/kg) |
|---|---|---|---|---|---|
| SMD | 56.81 ± 19.00 | 33/27 | 0.84 ± 0.19 | 0.31 ± 0.07 | 1.77 ± 0.41 |
| Ioxaglate | 51.16 ± 18.61 | 38/22 | 0.99 ± 0.37 | 0.31 ± 0.12 | 0.57 ± 0.21 |
| Comparison among means | NS | NS | NS | NS | $P < 10^{-9}$ |

SMD, diatrizoate of Na and meglumine

**Table 2.** Comparison between urinary electrolytes and urea concentration before CM. Injection in the two study groups

| | $Na^+$ mmol/l | $Cl^-$ | $K^+$ | $Ca^{++}$ | Urea |
|---|---|---|---|---|---|
| SMD | 85.48 ± 55.32 | 107.50 ± 67.42 | 60.55 ± 34.94 | 2.02 ± 1.79 | 284.76 ± 102.60 |
| Ioxaglate | 102.45 ± 55.33 | 128.24 ± 77.25 | 60.30 ± 38.36 | 1.94 ± 1.50 | 272.20 ± 106.40 |
| Comparison among means | NS | NS | NS | NS | NS |

SMD, diatrizoate of Na and meglumine

**Table 3.** Variations of urinary electrolytes and urea concentration after diatrizoate

| | $Na^+$ mmol/l | $Cl^-$ | $K^+$ | $Ca^{++}$ | Urea |
|---|---|---|---|---|---|
| Before SMD | 85.48 ± 55.32 | 107.50 ± 67.42 | 60.55 ± 34.94 | 2.02 ± 1.79 | 284.76 ± 102.60 |
| After SMD | 88.80 ± 37.60 | 77.73 ± 37.75 | 40.93 ± 20.73 | 1.34 ± 0.89 | 166.54 ± 77.76 |
| Comparison among means | NS | $P < 0.01$ | $P < 10^{-3}$ | $P < 0.01$ | $P < 10^{-9}$ |
| Variance ratio $F$ | $P < 2$ ‰ | $P < 2$ ‰ | $P < 2$ ‰ | $P < 2$ ‰ | $P < 5\%$ |

SMD, diatrizoate of Na and meglumine

## Conclusion

Injection of the two CM studied does not cause any variation in $[Na^+]$ u, which remains superior to that observed in osmotic diuresis; urinary concentration in other electrolytes and urea decreases considerably. The results of our study suggest that ionic CM inhibit tubular reabsorption of sodium. This phenomenon is independent of CM osmolality.

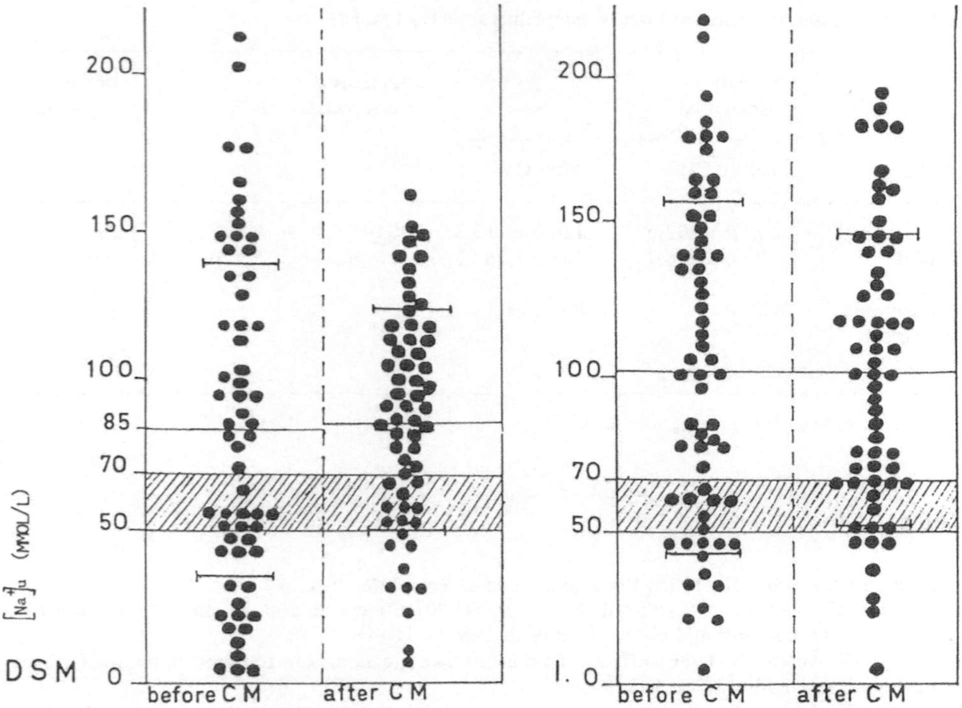


**Fig. 1.** Variations of $[Na^+]u$ after CM

**Table 4.** Variations of urinary electrolytes and urea concentration after ioxaglate

| | $Na^+$ mmol/l | $Cl^-$ | $K^+$ | $Ca^{++}$ | Urea |
|---|---|---|---|---|---|
| Before Ioxaglate | 102.45 ± 55.33 | 128.24 ± 77.25 | 60.30 ± 38.36 | 1.94 ± 1.50 | 272.20 ± 106.40 |
| After Ioxaglate | 101.73 ± 45.20 | 96.21 ± 54.64 | 50.95 ± 24.34 | 1.42 ± 1.11 | 201.30 ± 87.30 |
| Comparison among means | NS | $P < 0.01$ | NS | $P < 0.03$ | $P < 10^{-4}$ |
| Variance ratio $F$ | NS | $P < 2\%$ | $P < 2‰$ | $P < 5\%$ | NS |

**Table 5.** Variations of estimated urinary osmolality after the two CM

| mOsm/l | Urinary osmolality Before CM | After CM | Comparison among means | $F$ | % of decrease of osmolality |
|---|---|---|---|---|---|
| SMD | 577.9 ± 203.6 | 426.0 ± 113.3 | $P < 10^{-6}$ | $P < 2‰$ | −26% |
| Ioxaglate | 600.6 ± 206.7 | 505.3 ± 153.3 | $P < 0.01$ | $P < 5\%$ | −16% |
| Comparison among means | NS | $P < 0.01$ | | | |
| Comparison % | | | | | $P < 10^{-4}$ |

SMD, diatrizoate of Na and meglumine

## References


1. Gennari FJ, Kassirer JP (1974) Osmotic diuresis. N Engl J Med 291:714–720
2. Gruskin AB, Oetliker OH, Wolfish NM et al. (1970) Effects of angiography on renal function and histology in infants and piglets. Journal Pediatr 76:41–48
3. Ziegler TW, Olsen LS (1980) Effects of radio-contrast media on Ion transport in the toad urinary bladder. Invest Radiol 15:552–553
4. Ziegler TW, Ludens JH, Fanestil DD et al. (1975) Inhibition of active sodium transport by radiographic contrast media. Kidney Int 7:68–76

# Nephrotoxicity of Iodinated Contrast Media: A Preliminary Report on Five Compounds Used for Urography

A. Pinet, C. Vincent, J.P. Revillard, N. Pozet, and J. Bertrand

The nephrotoxicity of contrast media in common use today may be regarded as almost negligible. However, several reports on contrast medium-induced renal failure have been published and several risk factors have been identified as, for instance, pre-existing renal insufficiency and diabetes mellitus [1]. The relative nephrotoxicity of various contrast media has not been clearly assessed as yet.

The present study was designed to compare the nephrotoxicity of five different contrast media, three ionic products:
Na methyl glucamine ioxitalamate (Telebrix 38, 38 g I/100)
Meglumine ioxitalamate (Telebrix 30, Meglumine, 30 g I/100)
Monoacidic dimeric Na methylglucamine ioxaglate (Hexabrix, 32 g I/100)
and two nonionic products:
Iopamidol 370 (37 g I/100)
Iopamidol 300 (30 g I/100).

Several parameters of renal function were determined in two groups of patients undergoing intravenous pyelography, one with normal renal function, and the other with mild or moderate renal insufficiency.

## Patients and Methods

Forty patients were studied (21 males, 19 females, aged 17–74). Twenty-seven of them had a serum creatinine level below 123 μmol/liter and the 13 others had elevated serum creatinine.

Serum and urine samples were taken before injection and after 30 min and 24 h. Serum samples were immediately frozen at –40 °C. Urine samples were centrifuged for 10 min at 2000 g. pH was measured and adjusted to 7.0 if necessary. Part of the urine sample was used for enzymatic activity measurement; the remaining part was stored frozen. Creatinine concentration was measured on a technicon Auto-Analyzer (Technicon I N11b). β2 microglobulin was measured by a radioimmunoassay developed in our laboratory [6]. N-Acetyl-Glucosaminidase and β-Glucuronidase activity were determined according to the methods described by Marhund [4]. The amount of proteins in the urine was determined with the Biorad protein assay with albumin as reference (bio-rad laboratories).

Polyacrylamide gel electrophoresis in SDS was performed according to the method of Laemmli [3].

**Table 1.** Patients included in the study

| Contrast medium | *N* Patients | Normal renal function | Renal insufficiency |
|---|---|---|---|
| Iopamidol 370 | 5 | 3 | 3 |
| Iopamidol 300 | 8 | 4 | 4 |
| Telebrix 30 | 2 | 2 | 0 |
| Telebrix 38 | 13 | 9 | 4 |
| Hexabrix | 12 | 9 | 3 |

## Results and Discussion

### Serum Creatinine

Creatinine levels remained remarkably stable at 30 min and 24 h in the 27 patients with normal renal function. Conversely, a moderate increase in serum creatinine levels was observed at 30 min and 24 h in three out of four patients who received Telebrix 38, and only at 24 h in two out of four patients who received Iopamidol 300 and in two out of three patients who received Hexabrix. Mean serum creatinine was 589 μmol/liter before urography with Iopamidol 300, and 677 μmol/liter 24 h later.

### Serum β2 Microglobulin

Serum levels of β2 microglobulin remained within normal values in all patients with normal renal function. However, among the patients who received Hexabrix a moderate increase of serum β2 microglobulin was observed 24 h after the injection (mean values 1.65 mg/liter before urography, 1.81 mg/liter after urography; $0.02 < \mathbf{P} < 0.05$, **t** test on paired values). Among patients with renal insufficiency, a slight increase of serum β2 microglobulin occurred in one case with Iopamidol 370, one with Telebrix 38, and two with Hexabrix. The groups of patients are too small, however, to draw any firm conclusion from these changes.

### Urine pH

Whatever the contrast medium used, the urine pH rose at 30 min and returned to initial values at 24 h. This is likely to be attributed to an increase in urine output and urine dilution since opposite changes of urine creatinine concentration were regularly observed.

### Urine β2 Microglobulin

Individual values were found to be highly dispersed. Since the concentration of urine β2 microglobulin varies with urine dilution, only the ratios β2 microglobulin/creatinine were used for comparison. As shown in Table 2, the slight increase at 30 min did not reach statistical significance.

**Table 2.** Changes in the ratios of urinary concentration of β2 microglobulin/creatinine after injection of contrast media

| β2 microglobulin/ creatinine | Before | 30 min | 24 h |
|---|---|---|---|
| Iopamidol 370 | 0.0327 ± 0.0448 | 0.0429 ± 0.0642 | 0.0320 ± 0.0495 |
| Iopamidol 300 | 0.0835 ± 0.0953 | 0.1165 ± 0.1413 | 0.1036 ± 0.1261 |
| Telebrix 30 | N.D.[a] | N.D. | N.D. |
| Telebrix 38 | 0.0760 ± 0.0660 | 0.0997 ± 0.0630 | 0.0981 ± 0.0708 |
| Hexabrix | 0.0304 ± 0.0503 | 0.0354 ± 0.0627 | 0.0228 ± 0.0283 |

[a]N.D., not done

## Urine N-Acetylglucosaminidase and β-Glucuronidase

Enzymatic activities were also calculated with reference to urine creatinine. Despite the great heterogeneity of individual values, the changes in urinary enzymatic activities were clearly related to the type of contrast medium: no change was observed with Iopamidol 300 and 370, a mild elevation with Telebrix 30 and Hexabrix and a marked increase reaching 3 to 4 times the initial level with Telebrix 38. The elevation was less important at 24 h (Table 3).

**Table 3.** Changes in urinary enzymatic activity after injection of Telebrix 38

| | Before | 30 min | 24 h |
|---|---|---|---|
| *N*-Acetylglucosaminidase/ creatinine | 0.0179 ± 0.0165 | 0.0547 ± 0.1073 | 0.0301 ± 0.0343 |
| β-glucuronidase/creatinine | 0.0286 ± 0.0208 | 0.1214 ± 0.2118 | 0.0575 ± 0.0377 |

## Proteinuria

No quantitative change of proteinuria was observed with Iopamidol 300, Iopamidol 370, and Telebrix 30. Conversely in the 14 patients who received Telebrix 38 a marked increase in proteinuria could be demonstrated 30 min after the injection (about 10 times the initial levels) but it no longer persited at 24 h. Individual responses, however, were remarkably heterogeneous. Comparable changes were observed with Hexabrix, although the magnitude of the increase was smaller than with Telebrix 38. SDS polyacrylamide gel electrophoresis was performed in some patients only. Using this technique it is possible to define a tubular proteinuria made of fractions smaller than albumin and a glomerular proteinuria made of albumin and proteins of higher molecular weight. Because of the diversity of individual responses, it has not been possible as yet to define the electrophoretic pattern of each contrast medium. For instance in one patient with normal renal function and physiological proteinuria, injection of Telebrix 38 induced a marked glomerular proteinuria at 30 min. The pattern was again normal at 24 h. After injection of Iopamidol 300, a mixed pattern (glomerular and tubular) was observed at 30 min, with return to the initial state at 24 h. In one patient with interstitial nephritis and tubular proteinuria, the electrophoretic pattern was not changed after injection of Iopamidol 300.

## Conclusion

The tubular nephrotoxicity of contrast media has been documented by histological studies showing cytoplasmic vacuolisation of renal tubular cells. Cytoplasmic swelling was reported to occur after injection of low osmolar molecules such as metrizamide, Ioxaglate, and Iopamidol [5]. Our results indicate that tubular nephrotoxicity should be regarded as a negligible risk for the contrast media under study since no major change in $\beta 2$ microglobulin excretion nor in urine enzymatic activities were observed. Proteinuria is frequently recorded after injection of contrast media and it has been regarded as a good indicator of the effects of these compounds on kidney function both in clinical situations and in experimental studies [2]. In our study only two compounds, Telebrix 38 and, to a lesser extent, Hexabrix, were found to induce significant proteinuria. Electrophoretic studies, however, revealed in some cases the occurrence of a transient "glomerula proteinuria" which is likely to reflect the increase in vascular permeability. Owing to the great heterogenity of individual responses, further studies are needed to determine possible differences of effects among contrast media.

## References


1. Byrd L, Sherman R (1979) Radiocontrast-induced acute renal failure. A clinical and pathophysiologic review. Medicine 58:270–286
2. Golman S, Holtas S (1980) Proteinuria produced by urographic contrast media. Invest Radiol [Suppl] 15:S61–S66
3. Laemmli UK (1970) Cleavage of structural proteins during the assembly of the head of bacteriophage T4. Nature 227:680–685
4. Marhund D (1976) Rapid colorimetric assay of a $\beta$-galactosidase and N-Acetyl-$\beta$-Glucosaminidase in human urine. Clin Chim Acta 73:453–461
5. Moreau JF, Droz D, Noel LH, Leibowitch J, Jungers P, Michel JR (1980) Tubular nephrotoxicity of water-soluble iodinated contrast media. Invest Radiol [Suppl] 15:S54–S60
6. Vincent C, Revillard JP (1976) Comparison of radio-immunoassay and lymphocytotoxicity inhibition techniques for the determination of $\beta 2$ microglobulin. J Immunol Methods 10:253–259

# Acute Renal Failure Initiated by Contrast Media

K. Golman, Å. Aulie, C. Tørnquist, and T. Almén

## Introduction

About 1 year ago Dr. Mudge [1] concluded in an excellent review on the nephrotoxicity of urographic drugs: "The shortcomings of retrospective clinical case reports are all too obvious, particulary in dealing with incidence and mechanism and although the evidence is overwhelming that toxicity is real both the nature and the magnitude of the problem remain uncertain".

Different mechanisms of the acute renal failure after contrast media have been suggested and different animal models have been used to evaluate the possible mechanism.

One of the leads which might be found in the many clinical reports is the fact that relatively many of the patients where the contrast media produce acute renal failure are diabetic patients.

If the acute renal failure could be imitated in animals with diabetes it would be possible to study the causative factor.

We have recently reported [2] the possibility of producing acute renal failure in normal rabbits using slow infusion of extreme high doses of urographic contrast media. We therefore decided to repeat this technique in animals with experimental diabetes.

## Methods

A total of 100 female Wistar rats were used. Fifty of them were made diabetic by one or two intravenous injections of streptozotocin (50 mg/kg, Upjohn) 1 year before the contrast medium injection. The hyperglycemia was controlled by enzymatic determination of glucose blood level (Glox) 1 week and 1 month after the streptozotocin treatment and 1 day before the contrast medium injection.

The contrast media examined were metrizamide (Amipaque), diatrizoate (Urografin), and iohexol. All were injected at a concentration adjusted to an osmolality of 500 mmol/kg $H_2O$. The doses were 10 and 12 g I/kg and the infusion rate 60 mg I/min. Animals not injected with streptozotocin served as controls.

The degree of kidney damage was measured indirectly by blood urea level. The urea level was determined before and 1–3 days after the contrast medium injection by an enzymatic method (Boehringer). Rats which did not receive streptozotocin and with normal blood glucose level were used as controls. These control rats were injected with contrast media using the same procedure as in the diabetic rats.

An increase in urea level of more than 40% above the precontrast injection level was considered "status renal failure".

The Wilcoxon rank test was used for statistical evaluation of the results. $P < 0.05$ was considered significant.

## Results

Ten and 12 g I/kg were chosen as these were the highest possible doses for infusion of diatrizoate. Higher doses were only tolerated after injection of the nonionic media.

Table 1 shows the effect of the streptozotocin treatment. A significant increase in blood glucose level was obtained at least during the 1st month after the treatment. Blood glucose level returned to the preinjection level during the 1 year observation period, but the small vessel effects sustained during this period estimated from the colour change of the eyes of the rats.

**Table 1.** The effect of the streptozotocin treatment

| Contrast Medium | Dose g I/kg | Blood glucose (mM) mean ± SD | | |
|---|---|---|---|---|
| | | Before | After 1 month | After 1 year |
| Metrizamide | 10 | 7 ± 2 | 23 ± 5 | 9 ± 2 |
| | 12 | 9 ± 2 | 24 ± 8 | 8 ± 3 |
| Diatrizoate | 10 | 7 ± 2 | 24 ± 7 | 12 ± 6 |
| | 12 | 8 ± 1 | 29 ± 7 | 11 ± 7 |
| Iohexol | 12 | 8 ± 2 | 24 ± 10 | 8 ± 3 |

**Table 2.** Number of animals reacting with renal failure after injection of different contrast media

| Contrast medium | Dose g I/kg | Group | |
|---|---|---|---|
| Metrizamide | 10 | Diabetic | 1 of 10 |
| | 10 | Control | 3 of 10 |
| | 12 | Diabetic | 4 of 10 |
| | 12 | Control | 5 of 10 |
| Diatrizoate | 10 | Diabetic | 2 of 10 |
| | 10 | Control | 0 of 10 |
| | 12 | Diabetic | 1 of 10 |
| | 12 | Control | 6 of 10 |
| Iohexol | 12 | Diabetic | 2 of 10 |
| | 12 | Control | 0 of 10 |

After contrast medium injection ten animals in the diabetic and 14 animals in the control group had an increase in blood urea level. There were no significant differences between the diabetic and the normal rat.

Table 2 shows that there were no significant differences between the contrast media in the diabetic rats. In the control rats there were significantly less animals reacting with renal failure after injection of iohexol than after injection with diatrizoate or metrizamide.

## Discussion

Despite the fact that the diabetic rats have been troubled by the hyperglycemic condition for about half their life-span these rats were not affected more than the normal control rats. This might be explained by the recent finding by Hostetter et al. [3] indicating that the glomerular filtration rates in moderately hyperglycemic rats are increased above control level and that a decreased glomerular filtration rate is only found in severely hyperglycemic conditions.

The rats in our study were moderately hyperglyemic and as a support for the result of Hostetter it should be noted that in about 10% of the diabetic rats even a significant decrease in blood urea level was noted. After the contrast medium injections the decrease was sustained for 2–3 days. The frequency of rats reacting in the control group were considerably lower than what has been found previously in a similar study on rabbits [2]. A further increase in dose is not possible as an increase results in death of the rats from other causes than renal failure (the death occurred within a few hours after the injection).

## Conclusion

The kidneys of moderately hyperglycemic rats are not more affected by urographic contrast media than the kidneys of normals rats. The situation might be different in severely hyperglycemic rats.

*Acknowledgement.* The authors gratefully acknowledge the assistance of Britt-Marie Lilja, Kerstin Thyberg, and Birgit Persson.

## References

1. Mudge GH (1980) Nephrotoxicity of urographic drugs. Kidney Int 18:540–552
2. Golman K (1981) Acute renal failure after contrast medium injection. A method for early detection. XIV Int Congress of Radiology, Brussel
3. Hostetter TH, Troy JL, Brenner BM (1981) Glomerular hemodynamics in experimental diabetes mellitus. Kidney Int 19:410–415

# Summary of the Discussion

J. F. Moreau

Dr. Ansell mentioned the CM nephrotoxicity in patients with myoglobinuria and the differential diagnosis between nephrotoxic accidents and renal vein thrombosis.

Dr. Touraine posed a question about the actual rate of renal accidents, which is certainly higher than the 200 cases of anuria reported in the literature may suggest.

Dr. Moreau pointed out the lack of precision usually found in the clinical literature dealing with neprotoxic accidents, the lack of interest often shown from nephrologists teams who are not motivated enough in promoting CM nephrotoxicity studies and the possibility of preventing anuric accident in high-risk patients when the discussion of the urographic or angiographic procedures involves physicians and radiologists.

Dr. Brasch mentioned he found immune complex on the kidneys of rabbits he made allergic to CM according to a protocol experiment presented at the first session. The immune complex were found when the rabbits kidneys were sacrified at the end of the 1st month. The experiment is still continuing and the type of immunoglobuline has not yet been identified.

Dr. Lasser recalled that he formerly demonstrated a tubular reabsorption of the cation methylglucamine (10%–15%). Dr. Mudge and Dr. Benness did not confirm that data.

Several questions dealing with proteinuria induced by CM injections were posed, mainly by Dr. Charmes, Dr. Touraine, and Dr. Revillard. They pointed out the high rate of proteinuria observed during the 24 h following an angiography, even done with the new low osmolar agents. This proteinuria occurs even in living kidney donors who are considered as the archetype of normal kidneys. It is a global, nonspecific proteinuria which vanishes without renal functional sequelae. Proteinuria dos not result from an injury of the basal membrane of the glomerular vessels. Dr. A. Pinet thought that the proteinuria results from the vasoactive effect of intra-arterial CM injections, even when the CM is low osmolar. Dr. Charmes suggested that the proteinuria results from a change in the polarity of the basal membrane. Dr. Golman shared this opinion because he never found electron microscopic nephronic lesions certainly related to CM effects. Dr. Moreau recalled that proteinuria inconsistently follows an IVU and that it is an unreliable test of nephrotoxicity when the proteins are not specific.

Dr. Lasser was quite amazed to hear that diabetes mellitus does not increase the nephrotoxic risk when there is no preexisting renal failure nor underlying nephropathy. Dr. Moreau confirmed what he said during the conference, pointing out that (1) there is no truly good clinical literature dealing with this problem in humans and (2) he is not aware of renal accidents in nonazotemic diabetics except in a few cases of patients treated with metformine. However, his lack of wide experience leads him to introduce a statement.

Dr. Pengloan mentioned two cases of acute renal failure following angiographic procedure using Hexabrix injections. In both cases, oligoanuria developed in patients with preexisting renal insufficiency: both patients quickly recovered without added sequelae. Dr. Moreau mentioned he is worried about the risk of dissociation of the iodinated molecules which had been discussed the day before. Dr. Mudge reported that he transiently observed an unidentified yellow pigment in the urine output of the dogs submitted for injections of Hexabrix and Iopamidol.

# Section E:
# Various Topics

# The Effect of X-ray Contrast Media on the Endothelium of the Aorta and Vena Cava in Rats

Ch. Gospos, N. Freudenberg, J. Staubesand, and H. Koch

Using radiographic contrast media for aortography-, arteriography, and phlebography one must be aware of two complications due to contrast media: First, anaphylactoid reactions and second, local complications especially thrombosis. Endothelial damage produced by the contrast media is generally considered to be the primary cause of these complications [4]. The following factors contributing to the more harmful effects of contrast media on the endothelium are currently under discussion [5];

1. The chemical structure of the medium
2. The cation component used in the making up of the solution
3. Details of administration, such as the temperature of the medium and the rapidity of the injection
4. The physicochemical properties of the solution such as Pk value, protein-binding capacity, lipophilia, and osmolality

The hypertonicity of the contrast media particularly is considered by some investigators to be responsible for the endothelial damage following the intravascular injection of the contrast media [3]. In our study we tested the effect of the four contrast media diatrizoate, ioxitalamate, metrizamide, and ioxaglate on the endothelium of the aorta and vena cava of the rat. Furthermore, we examined the effect of a hypertonic solution, i.e., a 22% sorbit solution ($CH_2$ $(CHOH)_4$ · $CH_2OH$) with the same osmolality as that of diatrizoate. The control animals received physiological salt solution.

For our investigations we used standardized conditions: we injected 1 ml of each contrast medium with an iodine content of 300 mg through a catheter into the aorta and i.v. in the vena cava. To assess the endothelial alteration we used three investigation methods:

1. Scanning electron microscopy
2. Transmission electron microscopy
3. "*Häutchen* method"

In order to recognize early morphological alterations of the endothelial cells as caused by contrast media, we first investigated the ultrastructure of the aorta with scanning and transmission electron microscopy 12 h and again 10 days after contrast media injection. The morphological investigations were performed as a blind study. Using the "*Häutchen* preparation", the tritiated thymidine index of the endothelium of the aorta and vena cava was determined by autoradiography. The tritiated thymidine index corresponds to the regeneration rate of the endothelium. An increase of the tritiated thymidine index of the endothelium must therefore be considered as indicating a reactive reparation process following previous damage [1].

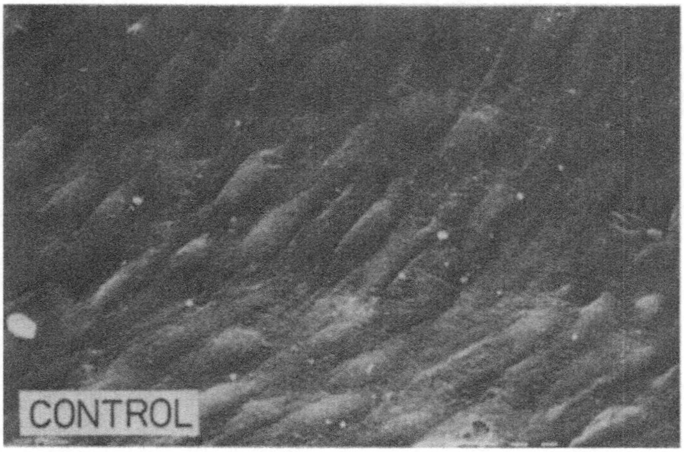


**Fig. 1.** Scanning electron micrograph of aorta. Endothelium with a smooth surface, well-developed marginal folds and nuclear crests. x 1000

## Results

The ultrastructural investigations on the aorta of the control animals with scanning electron microscopy showed a smooth endothelial surface, well-developed marginal folds, and nuclear crests (Fig. 1). After injection of ioxaglate, the aortic surface showed an intact endothelial coat. The endothelial cells appeared to be swollen, with prominent nuclear crests and with rather indistinct and partly irregular folds.

After sorbit injection, the endothelial surface was for the most part inconspicuous. The endothelial cells were flat and showed well-developed marginal folds. In comparison with the controls, only single cells showed a prominent nuclear crest. Twelve hours after the injection of diatrizoate, swollen endothelial cells could be seen without distinct marginal folds.

After injection of ioxitalamate one could see more distinct irregularities on the surface of several cells. Some endothelial cells were swollen and shrunken. In most instances the cellular outlines were irregular. After injection of metrizamide, the aortic surface was irregularly ruffled with focal accumulations of blood elements. Higher magnification demonstrated many crater-like endothelial defects of different sizes (Fig. 2). The endothelial outline could not be clearly distinguished. These crater-like structures were scattered throughout the whole aorta.

The ultrastructural investigations of the aorta with transmission electron microscopy showed single endothelial necroses 12 h after the injection of diatrizoate, ioxitalamate, and metrizamide, but not after administration of ioxaglate and sorbit solution. Ten days after injection of diatrizoate, ioxitalamate, and metrizamide, the ultrastructure of the aortic endothelium returned to normal. These ultrastructural investigations demonstrated different degrees of endothelial alteration, which were studied in their dynamic aspects with the "*Häutchen* method" to determine the endothelial proliferation kinetics. Three days after injection with diatrizoate, ioxitalamate, and metrizamide, the regeneration rate of the aortic endothelium (Fig. 3) was 3 times higher than the regeneration rate of the

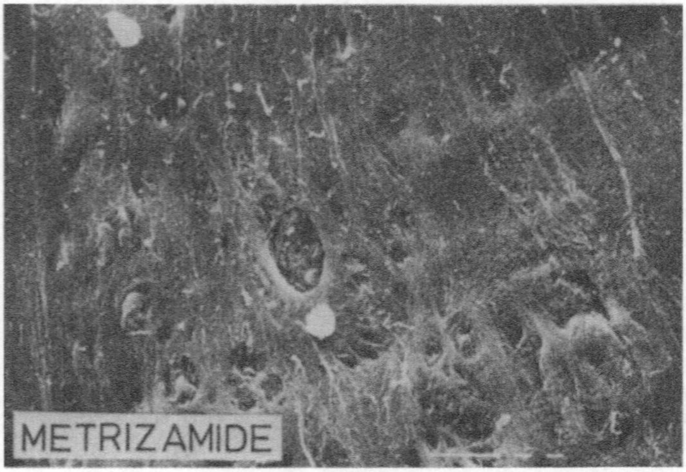


**Fig. 2.** Scanning electron micrograph of aorta 12 h after administration of metrizamide. Endothelium with many crater-like defects of different sizes and indistinct cellular marginal folds. x 700

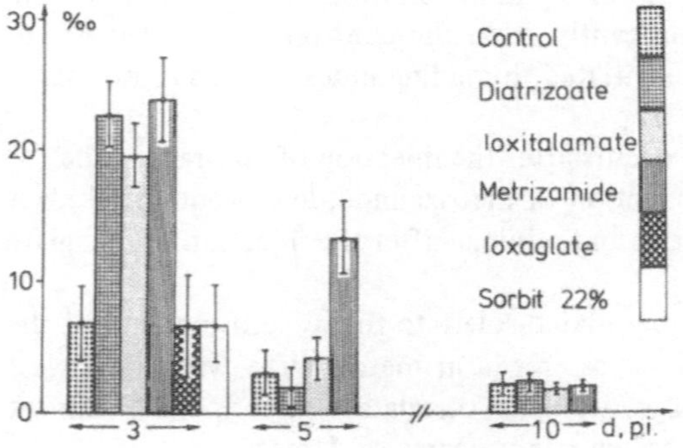


**Fig. 3.** $^{3}$H-thymidine indices (in‰) of aortic endothelial cells at different times (d, p.i., days after injection) of controls and after administration of diatrizoate, ioxitalamate, metrizamide, ioxaglate, and 22% sorbit solution

controls. At a similar time after the injection of ioxaglate and the 22% sorbit solution, there was no apparent change in the regeneration rate of the aortic endothelium in comparison with the controls. The endothelial proliferation returned to normal again on the 5th day after the injection of diatrizoate and ioxitalamate. After administration of metrizamide, however, the regeneration rate returned to its normal value after only 10 days.

Figure 4 shows the kinetics of DNA synthesis of the endothelium of the vena cava of the controls, and rats treated with the four contrast media and the 22% sorbit solution. Three days after administration of diatrizoate, ioxitalamate, and metrizamide, the tritiated thymidine index shows a tenfold increase, and after injection of ioxaglate a fivefold increase: a significant difference compared with the control animals. After injection of a

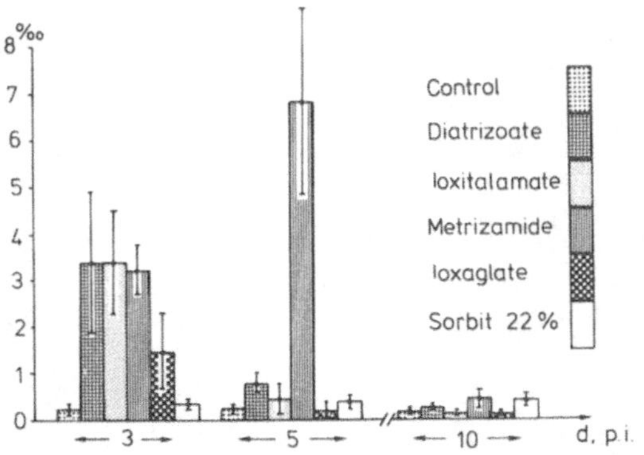


**Fig. 4.** $^3$H-thymidine indices (in ‰) of the endothelium of the vena cava at different times (d, p.i., days after injection) of controls and after administration of diatrizoate, ioxitalamate, metrizamide, ioxaglate, and 22% sorbit solution

22% sorbit solution, no significant difference of the tritiated thymidine index is observed. On the 5th day the DNA rate after injection of diatrizoate, ioxitalamate, and ioxaglate is again within the control range, whereas after administration of metrizamide, the tritiated thymidine index still differs significantly from the controls by a factor of 16. Ten days after injection of metrizamide the tritiated thymidine index returns to normal.

The following conclusions can be drawn:

1. Endothelial damage of different degrees occurs after the injection of contrast media.
2. This damage is most severe after the injection of metrizamide, less pronounced after the injection of diatrizoate and ioxitalamate, and minimal after the injection of ioxaglate and sorbit solution.
3. Obviously the damage observed cannot be related solely to the hyperosmolality of the contrast medium [2] because the X-ray contrast medium metrizamide with the lowest osmolality suffered the most severe damage, whereas ioxaglate with osmolality almost identical to that of metrizamide produced only a minor degree of damage.

## References


1. Freudenberg N, Riese K-H (1980) Standortunterschiede des normalen Gefäßendothels und Veränderungen durch Endotoxinschock. Arbeitstagung des Tübinger Arbeitskreises für Gefäßerkrankung e.V. Berchtesgaden am 13. und 14.6.1980
2. Gospos Ch, Freudenberg N, Mathias K, Hauenstein KH (in press) Hyperosmolalität von Röntgenkontrastmitteln – ein Faktor für die Endothelschädigung? Fortschr Röntgenstr 1981
3. Gottlob R, Zinner G (1965) Die Bestimmung der endothelschädigenden Wirkung injizierbarer Lösungen. Der Einfluß des osmotischen Druckes und des pH. Wien klin Wschr 77:149–157
4. Lasser EC Die Toxizität von Kontrastmitteln, Status 1977. Symposium der Fa. Schering, Berlin 1977. Hrsg.: Zeitler. In: Kontrastmittelzwischenfälle. Medizinisch-wissenschaftliche Buchreihe der Schering AG, Berlin Bergkamen
5. Schmid HW (1971) Untersuchungen der Toxizität der physikalisch-chemischen Eigenschaften und der hämolytischen Aktivität von trijodierten Röntgenkontrastmittelsalzen in wäßrigen Lösungen. Pharm Acta Helv 46:134–313

# Rapid Injection of a Cold Water-soluble Triiodide for Cardiovascular Investigation. Physicochemical Basis, Injection Technique, Tolerance, Prospects of Utilization

M. Ducos de Lahitte, C. Manelfe, A. Bonafe, and J. P. Marc-Vergnes

A rapid injection of a cold water-soluble triiodinated contrast medium for cardiovascular investigation is an original method of injection. We have developed and used it for intravenous angiography (IA) with the last 800 patients of our series (more than 1900 patients). Our concern to improve the quality of films, by using doses of contrast medium (CM) equal to or less than 1 cc/kg by injection, led us to modify our initial technique of injection. The injected mass is adapted to the investigation of every area from the pulmonary arterial tree to the arteries of lower limbs.

## Physical Basis

The use of a bolus of CM is necessary in IA. This bolus must be as compact as possible to avoid its dilution across the arterial pulmonary tree. It must be propelled at the same speed as the flow in big venous trunks; i.e., a strong flow and a low speed. With a peripheric venous route in order to obtain a compact bolus in the superior vena cava, a rapid peripheral injection followed by an immediate flushing out is necessary. This rapid injection involves a venous approach with a large diameter and a CM as viscous as possible to avoid dilution. The immediate flushing out necessitates a medium as viscous as possible to propel the bolus without diluting it. The sodium methylglucamine ioxitalamate solutions (with 38 g iodine/100 cc) have a viscosity varying with temperature (Table 1). The variation is from 6.1 cstokes for 38 °C to 29.3 cstokes for 5 °C. The very high viscosity of CM and the flushing out will allow the bolus to be propelled, to diminish the time length of venous parietal contact, and to effect its propulsion to the right

**Table 1.** Cinematic viscosity (centistokes)

| Temperature | Water | Macromolecules | Triiodinated |
|---|---|---|---|
| 38 °C | 0.69 | 1.1 | 6.1 |
| 30 °C | 0.80 | 2.1 | 8.5 |
| 20 °C | 1.00 | 3.7 | 12.8 |
| 10 °C | 1.30 | 6.6 | 20.5 |
| 5 °C | 1.52 | 11.5 | 29.3 |

Cinematic viscosity: dynamic viscosity / volumic mass
C.G.S. unit: stoke: $cm^2$ $5^{-1}$

auricle. This cardiac compartment is then saturated by a strong low speed flow. The CM cools without any effect (checking by laser diffusion down to 0 °C). But the macromolecules (M) are affected between 0 °C and 2 °C, when they change into a nonhomogeneous gel. Therefore we believe that cooling ought to be limited to 5 °C: bolus of 18 cc CM flushed out with 40 cc of M.

## Chemical Bases

A chemical hypothesis is being checked. The CM is a solution saturated with salts of ioxitalamate. The cooling lowers the ionization percentage of the solution and at the same time its hyperosmolality. The cooling reduces biochemical reactions between CM and venous membrane.

## Injection Technique

With a fasting patient, hydrated, without general anesthesia or premedication a Cathlon catheter was inserted (14-G) in the basilic or cephalic vein. We assessed the circulation time between the arm and tongue with dehydrocholate (varying from 10 to 30 s). With a pneumatic injector with two syringes we injected 1 cc/kg CM; approximate flow was from 20 to 25 cc/s and immediate flushing out with 40–50 cc M. In a standard examination we performed two successive injections; the film for masking was exposed 2 or 3 s before the beginning of the series.

## Tolerance

The tolerance to this rapid injection must be excellent as we use the substraction technique in order to visualize the arterial tree. We perform a local anesthesia of the tongue with viscous Xylocaine orally, after assessment of circulation time. This local anesthesia does not suppress the larynx reflex and allows a postexamination food intake. It totally suppresses the coughing reflex during the beginning of arterial opacification. The use of cooled CM significantly lowers teh burning sensation following rapid injection of triiodinated. The cooling, the increase in viscosity, the immediate flushing out, and the local anesthesia are now major factors of an excellent tolerance.

## Prospects of Utilization

The cineangiocardiography study of this injection technique has shown that the bolus moves with a speed near to physiological speed in right and pulmonary circulation. Thus we get a dilution as low as possible which afford several utilizations.

Total visualization of pulmonary arterial tree with 15–20 cc and with only one anterioposterior projection is possible (Fig. 1). It is nonaggressive and allows a screening. Doses of 20–25 cc with radiocinemra allow minimal kinetic study of right and left cardiac cavities.

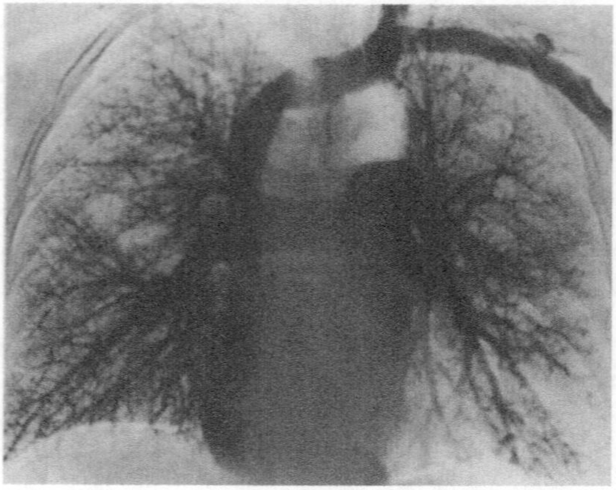

**Fig. 1.** Pulmonary arterial tree

A dose of 0.5–0.8 cc/kg allows the investigation of the left cavities and thoracic aortic arch with right posterior incidence.

Supra-aortic examination with 1 cc/kg visualizes from the aortic arch to the carotid siphons (Fig. 2).

At the abdominal level a dose of 1 cc/kg is sufficient to allow the investigation of the abdominal aorta, renal arteries, aortoiliac bifurcation (Fig. 3). Thus we can demonstrate the arteries of the lower limbs.

This injection method allows the examination of outpatients, as well as patients with heparinotherapy. It allows the supervision of known arterial lesions, the control of early

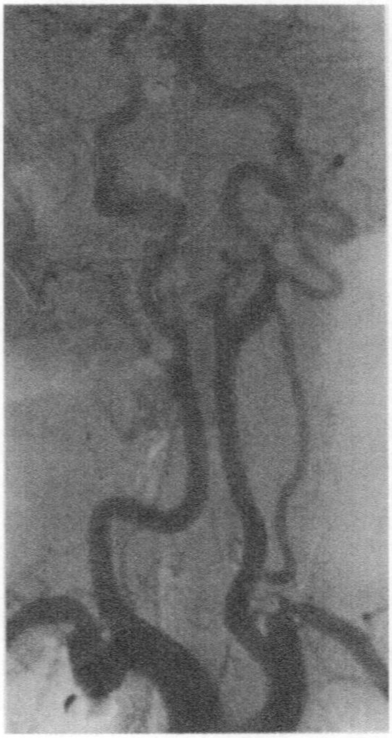

**Fig. 2.** Extracranial cerebral arteries

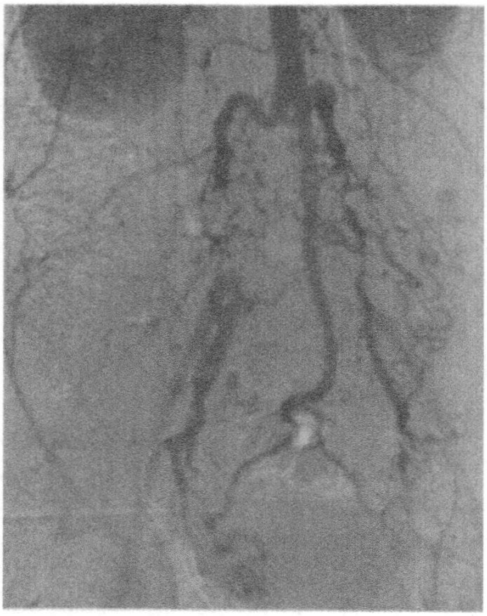

**Fig. 3.** Thrombosis of subrenal aorta and collateral circulation

postoperative patients, and the control of percutaneous transluminal angioplasties, as well as the detection of arterial stenosis or occlusion.

The rapid injection of cold CM is an easy, cheap solution with numerous clinical applications at a stage as early as the film substraction. We believe that this method is the first step before using digital angiography in real time.

*N.B.:* The figures presented here are classical substraction film of IA; their definition and contrast show the tolerance and interest of examination.

## References


1. Ducos de Lahitte M, Marc-Vergnes JP, Rascol A et al. (1980) Intravenous angiography of the extracranial cerebral arteries. Radiology 137:705–711
2. Viallet P, Sendra L, Chevrot L et al. (1959) Angiocardiopneumographie élargie. Méthode d'opacification vasculaire générale par voie veineuse. Masson, Paris

# Comparison of Hexabrix and Urografin in the Study of Postphlebographic Thrombotic Side Effects

A. Høfrup, B. Eliasen, A. Reimer-Jensen, and J. Praestholm

Many studies have shown a high incidence of phlebitis as a complication of phlebography, when using a high-osmolar contrast medium [1, 2, 5].

From January 1979 until December 1980 we performed a double-blind, prospective study of the postphlebographic thrombotic side effects, comparing the conventional contrast medium, Urografin 60%, with the low-osmolar contrast medium, Hexabrix, provided by Guerbet Laboratories.

Included in the investigation were all patients admitted to our department for phlebography of the lower limb, who consented to participate in the investigation.

Excluded from the investigation were primarily patients with:

1. A history of thrombophlebitis of the deep veins of the lower limb
2. Varicose ulcers
3. Inflammatory skin lesions
4. Active arthritis

Secondarily patients with signs of deep vein thrombosis on the phlebograms were excluded. The Fibrinogen Uptake Test [3, 4] was used to detect deep vain thrombosis after phlebography of the lower limb.

Investigative procedure was as follows: On the 1st day the patient was given an i.v. injection of 100 $\mu$Ci $^{125}$I-labeled Fibrinogen. The next day a Fibrinogen Uptake Test was performed, followed by phlebography. The following 3 days Fibrinogen Uptake Tests were carried out. The patient was interviewed and underwent a medical examination.

Phlebography of the lower limb was performed with the patient in semi-erect position and a torniquet round the ankle. Forty milliliters of contrast medium were injected through a dorsal foot vein. Film exposures were made, guided by fluoroscopy during injection, and after the injection the needle was flushed with a 0.9% saline solution. When the patient was back in the supine position, the leg was elevated and the calf was pressed in effort to remove all contrast medium. Every patient recieved two injections.

The material consisted of 35 patients, with 47 legs investigated. There were 22 females and 13 males. The youngest patient was 24 years old, and the oldest was 72 years old. Twenty-four legs received Hexabrix and 23 legs received Urografin.

The results concerning postphlebographic thromboses are as follows: In the Hexabrix group no signs of thrombophlebitis were found, using the Fibrinogen Uptake Test. In the Urografin group we found seven cases of deep vein thrombosis. The difference is significant using Fishers Exact Test at the 5% confidence level.

The more usual adverse reactions to i.v. injections of contrast media were distributed as follows between the two groups: five patients complained of pain during the injection in the Urografin group, whereas four patients in the Hexabrix group showed urticaria and two patients developed periorbital edema. The difference between the two contrast media is not significant.

One patient had to be excluded from the thrombosis study. She received only one injection, which was immediately followed by severe nausea and fall in blood pressure. Because of that the code was broken. After 2 days she was discharged in good condition. No other patients received any treatment because of adverse reactions.

The conclusion of this study is: We found an incidence of postphlebographic vein thrombosis of 30% using the conventional contrast medium Urografin 60%.

No cases of phlebitis were found after phlebography in an identical group of patients, using a low-osmolar contrast medium, Hexabrix.

We therefore suggest that the old hyperosmolar contrast media in phlebography are replaced by Hexabrix or other low-osmolar contrast media.

## References


1. Albrechtsson U, Olsson C-G (1976) Thrombotic side-effects of lower limb phlebography. Lancet 1:723–724
2. Bettmann MA, Paulin S (1977) Leg phlebography: the incidence, nature and modifications of undesirable side-effects. Radiology 122:101–104
3. Browse NL et al. (1971) Diagnosis of established deep vein thrombosis with the fibrinogen uptake test. Br Med J 4:325–328
4. Kakkar V (1972) The diagnosis of deep vein thrombosis using the $^{125}$I fibrinogen test. Arch Surg 104:152–159
5. Ritchie WGM et al. (1974) The effect of contrast media on normal and inflamed canine veins. Invest Radiol 9:444–455

# Effects of Contrast Material on Blood Volume

Y. Huet, E. Wirquin, H. Geschwind, and J. Loiret

Since angiocardiographic methods are extensively used to assess ventricular function and repeated injections of contrast medium are required in valvular, coronary, and congenital heart diseases, it is important to evaluate the hemodynamic changes that result from the introduction of a large quantity of contrast material into the vascular system.

These changes are thought to be the result of multiple factors such as the volume of contrast material injected its hypertonicity, the pharmacological effects of the iodine and sodium ions, and the myocardial toxicity of the agents [1].

Previous studies revealed a sharp rise in the serum osmolality with a similar sharp fall in the hematocrit, suggesting a marked dilutional effect [4]. The purpose of the present study was to evaluate the changes in both plasma and red cell volumes and to compare two different osmolarity contrast media.

## Material and Methods

The material consisted of 21 patients with valvular heart disease ranging from 25 to 70 years who underwent diagnostic cardiac catheterization. Biplane cineangiocardiography was performed in the left ventricle with a Gensini 8 F catheter using a pressure injector that was programmed to deliver the bolus of contrast medium of 1.2 ml/kg body weight in 3 s at a rate of 20 ml/s.

Twelve patients were injected with sodium and meglumine diatrizoate (2100 mosm/liter) (Radioselectan 76, Schering) and 11 patients with sodium and meglumine ioxaglate (600 mosm/liter) (Hexabrix, Guerbet). To evaluate the changes in both plasma volume and red cell volume, the concentration changes of $^{125}$I-labeled albumin and of $^{51}$Cr-labeled autologus erythrocytes were measured during control conditions and at 1, 5, 10, 20, 30, 40 min after the injection of contrast material [3]. Results are expressed as mean ± standard deviation. The paired *t* test or analysis of variance was used to compare data from control periods with those obtained after the injection of contrast medium and to compare the effects of the two contrast materials. A $P$ value $< 0.05$ was considered statistically significant.

## Results

The validity of measurements of both plasma and red cell volumes was corroborated by close correlation between measured and computed volumes since averaged values of

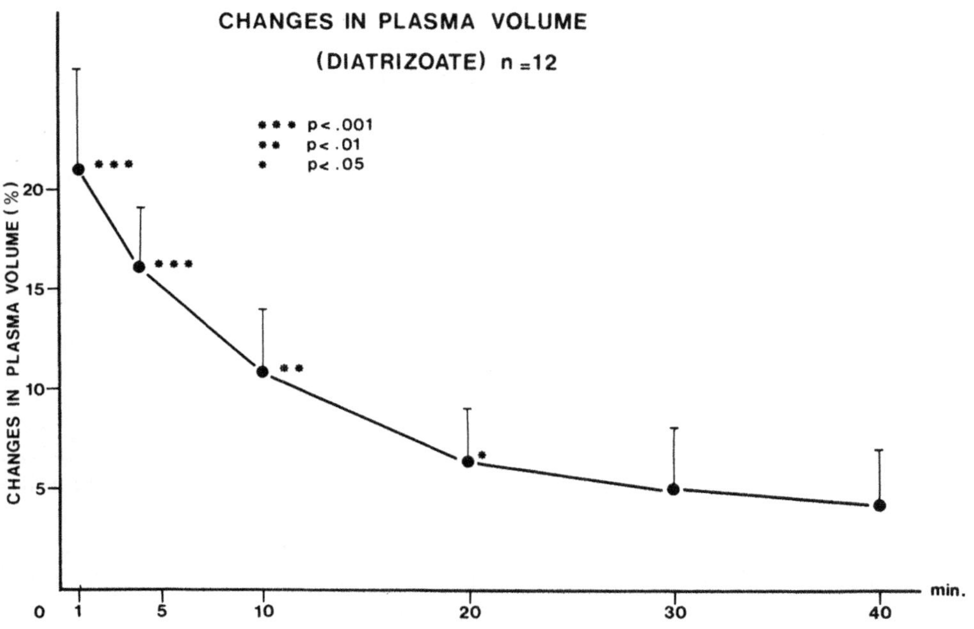


**Fig. 1.** Increase in plasma volume provided by the injection of diatrizoate

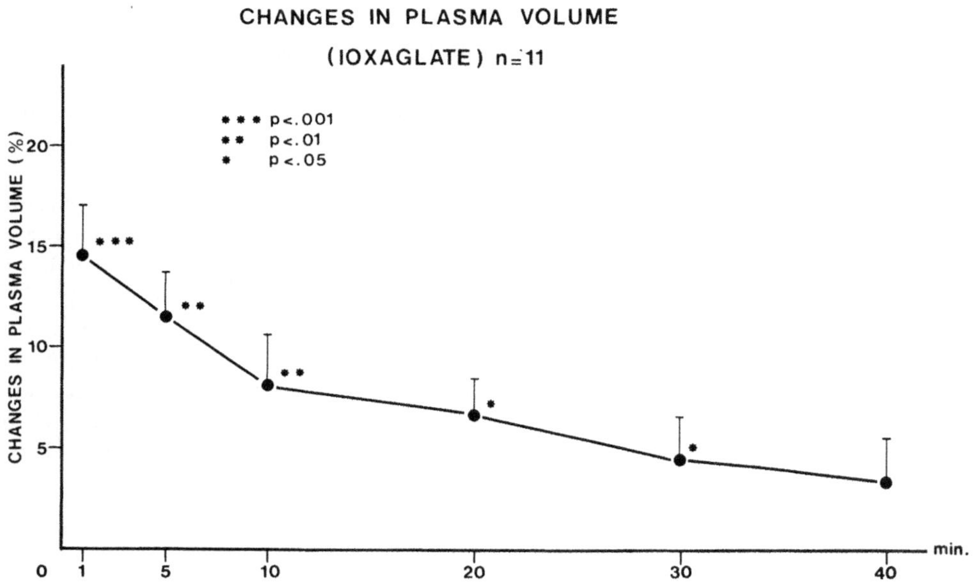


**Fig. 2.** Increase in plasma volume provided by the injection of ioxaglate

plasma volume were 2758 ± 149 ml and 2719 ± 185 ml, respectively. Averaged values of red cell volumes were 1760 ± 138 and 1780 ± 145 ml, respectively.

The introduction of contrast material into the vascular system resulted in a marked increase in plasma volume, whatever the contrast medium. Diatrizoate and ioxaglate resulted in a peak increase of 20.2% (from 41 ± 10 to 49 ± 11 ml/kg) (Fig. 1) and 14.6% (from 42 ± 7 to 48 ± 8 ml/kg) (Fig. 2) respectively. These changes were very significant ($P < 0.001$).

The peak increase occurred within the first minute after the angiography. Then plasma volume fell sharply. By 20 min, there was still a significant increase in plasma volume that reached 7% ($P < 0.05$). A return toward normal values was not observed until 40 min but the change was not significant by either 30 or 40 min. The same pattern of response was observed with ioxaglate.

In comparing the changes in blood plasma volume resulting from the injection of diatrizoate with those provided by ioxaglate (Fig. 3), it was evident that the same pattern of response was observed. However, the peak increase obtained with ioxaglate was significantly lower than that observed with diatrizoate (+20.2% and 14.5% respectively, $P < 0.01$). Even 5 min later, the difference was significant (15.7% vs 11% respectively, $P < 0.05$). However, later there was no significant difference between the two groups.

There were only slight changes in red cell volume. Both the injection of diatrizoate and ioxaglate resulted in a slight decrease in red cell volume within the first 10 min followed by a slight increase at 20 min. Although these changes were higher for diatrizoate than for ioxaglate, they did reach statistical significance.

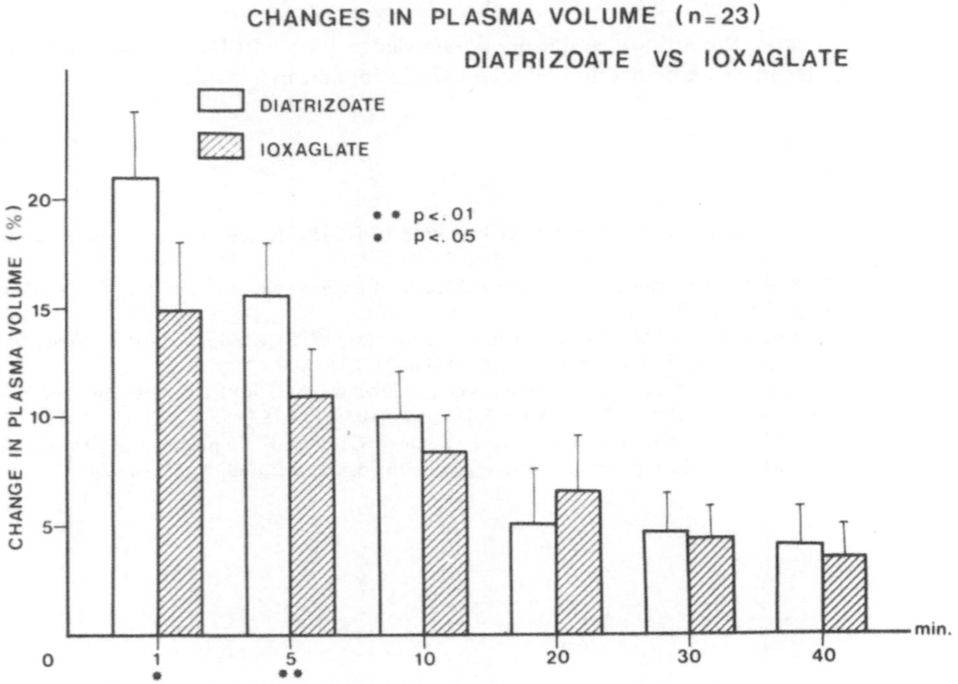


**Fig. 3.** Comparison between the increase in plasma volume provided by diatrizoate and ioxaglate

## Discussion

Intravascular injection of radiographic contrast material results in a complex series of potentially deleterious effects. Most of these effects have been attributed to the contrast material's hypertonicity [5]. The increase in osmolality is responsible for the direct negative inotropic effect [2]. The dilutional effect of contrast medium was documented previously by the fall in both electrolyte parameters and in the hematocrit [4]. This effect was attributed to transfer of fluid from the interstitial space to the intravascular compartment. Thus this study showed a significant increase in blood volume. In the present study, we demonstrated the increase in plasma volume without a change in red cell volume and showed the peak increase to occur almost immediately after the angiography. Moreover, the change in plasma volume may be related to the osmolality of contrast material since diatrizoate resulted in a significant higher peak increase in plasma volume than ioxaglate. The fall of the increase in plasma volume was similar for both contrast media, and control levels were not reached at 40 min.

## Clinical Implications

Thus, contrast media with low osmolality should be utilized to avoid the hemodynamic consequences of an increase in total blood volume. But whatever the contrast medium, 20 min should be managed between angiographies to allow fluid and electrolytes to return toward control levels so that hemodynamic and angiographic measurements could be achieved under basal conditions.

*Acknowledgments.* The authors gratefully acknowledge the contributions of Françoise Veyssiere for technical assistance and Mireille Labylle for editorial assistance.

## References

1. Friesinger GC, Schaffer J, Criley M, Gaertner RA, Ross RS (1965) Hemodynamic consequences of the injection of ratio opaque material. Circulation 31:730–736
2. Gootman N, Rudolph AM, Buckley NM (1970) Effects of angiographic contrast media on cardiac function. Am J Cardiol 25:59–65
3. International Comittee for Standardization in Heamatology (1980) Recommended methods for measurement of red cell and plasma volume. J Nucl Med 21:793–800
4. Levin AR, Grossman H, Schubert ET, Winchesier P, Gilladoga A (1969) Effect of angiocardiography on fluid and electrolyte balance. Am J Roentgenol 105:777–783
5. Thomson KR, Mracr C, Evill CA, Fritzsche J, Benness GT (1980) Comparison of iopamidol, ioxaglate and diatrizoate during coronary arteriography in dogs. Invest Radiol 15:234–241

# Labeling of Embolizing Substances with Contrast Agents

D. Novak

This report concerns the labeling of embolizing substances with water-soluble, oily and solid contrast agents. The aim of this study was to find out which contrast agent is the best suitable for labeling of clinically and experimentally used embolizing substances. Embolization procedure should be controlled fluoroscopically, and therefore an embolizing substance should be radiopaque [1–7].

## Materials and Methods

### Embolizing Substances

*Solid Substances.* Gelfoam (gelatine), Tachotop (collagen), Avitene (microfibrilar collagen), Fibrospum (fibrin).

*Liquid Substances.* (1) Cyanoacrylates: Histoacryl (butyl-2-cyanoacrylate), Sicomet (ethylcyanoacrylate), Eudragit (poly(meth)-cyanoacrylate). (2) Silicones: Silastic (silastic elastomer 382 and medical grade silicone fluid 360), Sil-Gel (Sil-Gel 604 A and 604 B), (3) Polyurethane (aliphatic polyetherpolyol and isocyanate).

### Contrast Agents

*Water-soluble Contrast Agents.* Hexabrix (meglumine ioxiglamate and sodium ioxaglate), Amipaque (metrizamide), Dimer-X (dimeglumine iocarmate), Angiografin (meglumine amidotrizoate), Telebrix (meglumine ioxitalamate and sodium ioxitalamate).

*Oily Contrast Agents.* Lipiodol (ethylester of monoiodo- and diiodostearic acid), Duroliopaque (9-iodine and 10-iodine ethylester of stearinic acid), Pantopaque (ethyliodophenyl undecoate).

*Solid Contrast Agents.* barium sulfate and zirconium dioxide.

### Labeling

Each of ten embolizing substances was systematically labeled with each of ten contrast agents (Fig. 1). The labeling was performed with the addition of 10%, 20%, 30%, 40% and 50% contrast agent (Fig. 2). The labeled substance was examined macroscopically and roentgenographically. In order to test the behavior of the labeled embolizing sub-

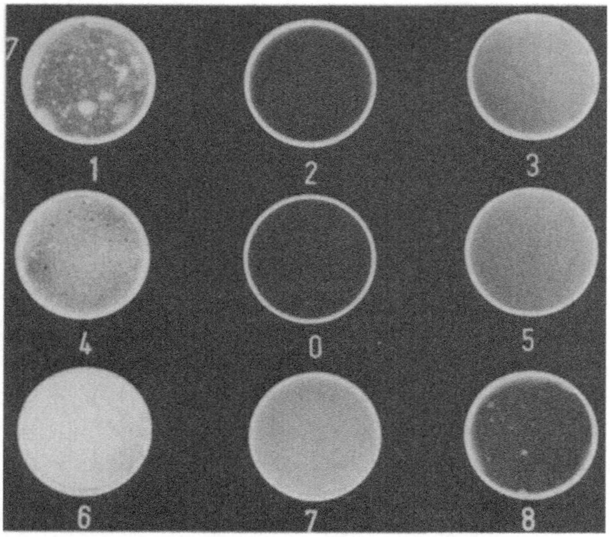


**Fig. 1.** Labeling of Silastic with different contrast agents. The best results are achieved with zirconium dioxide (6) and Pantopaque (7). Control (0)

stance in a biological environment experimental injections in "post mortem" as well as in "post nephrectomiam" kidneys were performed (Fig. 3). Kidney was used as a "tumor model" [6].

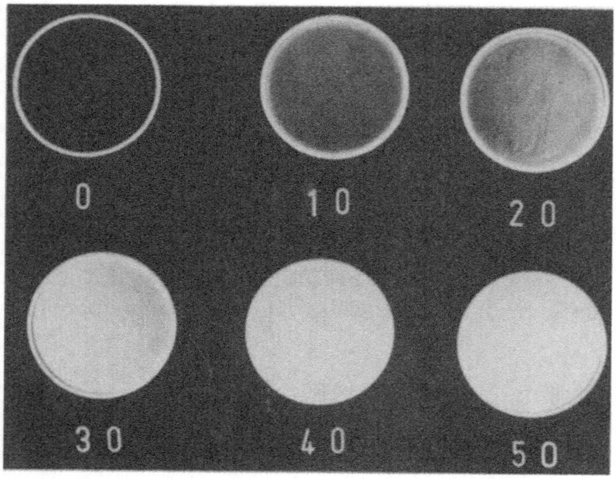


**Fig. 2.** Labeling of polyurethane with different concentrations (10%–50%) of zirconium dioxide. A homogenous mixture of high radiopacity was achieved with 30% of zirconium dioxide. Control (0)

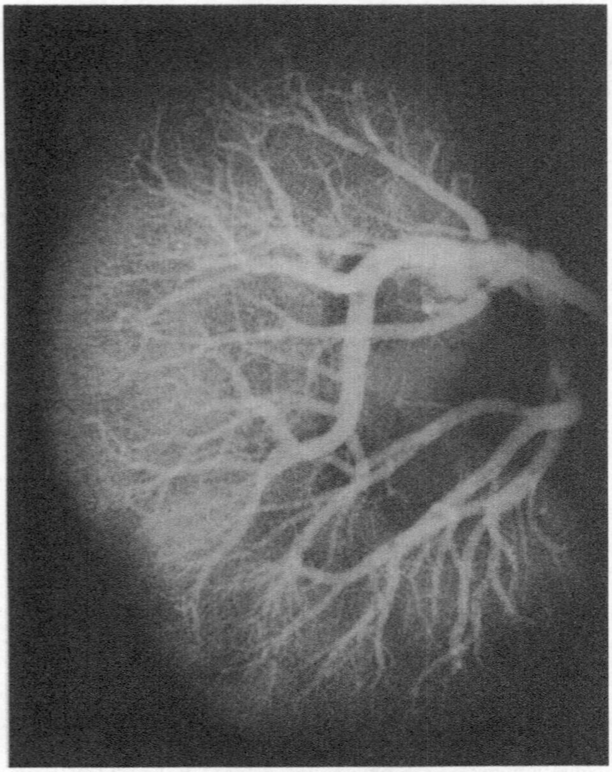

**Fig. 3.** Experimental embolization with ethylcyanoacrylate labeled with Pantopaque. A complete casting of renal vasculature was found

## Results and Discussion

The solid biological substances Gelfoam, Tachotop, Avitene, and Fibrospum were labeled most successfully with water-soluble contrast agents. Cyanoacrylates could be labeled with all oily contrast agents, but the most stabile solution was achieved with Pantopaque. A concentration of 20%–30% Pantopaque results in sufficient radiopacity of cyanoacrylates. Cyanoacrylates are visible under fluoroscopy during injection and in postembolization roentgenograms (Fig. 3).

Silicones are the best labeled with Pantopaque and Zirconium dioxide. In order to achieve sufficient radiopacity a concentration of contrast agent of 20%–30% was also needed. Polyurethane is also best labeled with Pantopaque and zirconium dioxide.

Embolizing substances are not radiopaque per se [3, 6, 7]. This disadvantage of embolizing substances could be very easily avoided by labeling the substance with contrast agents. Labeled, radiopaque embolizing substance is then injected more safely under fluoroscopic control. Postembolization follow-up could be performed using a plain film [4, 5]. Labeled embolizing substances casting tumor vessels remain radiopaque for a period of time up to 12 months [4, 5]. Due to the labeling of cyanoacrylates with oily contrast agents another favorable effect is achieved: oily contrast agents lead to prolongation of the polymerization time up to 30 s [1, 7]. It means that labeled cyanoacrylates could be injected more safely. Working in such a way the danger of overspilling or reflux is also minimized [1, 3, 6, 7].

## Conclusions

Labeling of solid embolizing substances with water-soluble contrast agents, and liquid cyanoacrylates with oily contrast agents, as well as silicones and polyurethane with pantopaque or zirconium dioxide diminishes the risk of embolization because the radiopaque embolizing substance could be injected under fluoroscopic control more safely. Also follow-up examination after embolization is simplified. Labeling of embolizing substances has become a prerequisite for a successful and complication-free transcatheter embolization.

## References


1. Cromwell LD, Kerber CW (1979) Modification of cyanoacrylate for therapeutic embolization: preliminary experience. Amer J Roentgenol 132:788–801
2. Greenfield AJ (1980) Transcatheter vessel occlusion: selection of methods and materials. Cardiovasc Intervent Radiol 3:222–228
3. Günther R, Schubert U, Georgi M, Marberger M (1977) Technik der therapeutischen Katheterembolisierung der Niere mit Histoacryl (Butyl-2-cyanoacrylat), aktuelle urol 8:299–303
4. Novak D (1980) Transkatheter-Embolisation von Nierentumoren. In: Loose KE, Loose DA (Hrsg) Gefäß-Patient-Therapie. Verlag Gerhard Witzstrock, Baden-Baden Köln New York, pp 232–236
5. Novak D (1980) Coaxial and balloon catheters in tumor embolization. Experimental results and follow-up studies. In: Veiga-Pires JA (ed) Intervention radiology. Excerpta Medica. Amsterdam Oxford Princeton, pp 302–308
6. Novak D, Weber J, Wieners H, Zabel G (1981) New liquid and semiliquid embolizing substances for tumor embolization. An experimental study. Ann Radiol 24:428–431
7. Pap J, Baratz M, Merimsky E (1981) Infarction of renal tumors using Isobutyl-2-cyanoacrylate and Lipiodol. Amer J Roentgenol 137:781–785

# Contrast Media in Arthrography. Experimental Study

G. Pallardy, R. Abelanet, G. Correas, B. Gerardin, and J. C. Zenny

## Purpose of the Study

Accuracy and efficiency of positive contrast arthrography depend on the delay between injection of contrast medium and occurence of cartilage absorption.

Six hundred knee arthrograms were reviewed in a previous study in order to compare several water-soluble contrast media. This revealed that cartilage absorption occurs later with ioxaglic acid than with triiodinated substances. With triiodinated substances, an overall 10-min delay is available to study the articular components. Beyond this, blurring of the edges of menisci and articular cartilage do not permit additional radiographs. If the examination is incomplete or an area is doubtful, complete resorption of contrast medium is necessary before a new injection may be carried on, i.e., more than 2 h after first injection or else the following day. With a hexa-iodinated substance, cartilage absorption occurs later, the delay being more than 20 min for menisci, and 30 min for articular cartilage. So, about ½ h is available to study the articular components.

We attempted to obtain a more delayed absorption, but dilution of contrast medium and variations of amount injected showed no significant modification. We therefore thought it worthwhile to complete this patient review by an experimental study on animals. This was done to compare absorption of contrast medium by the various articular components, and to assess how to modify it.

## Material

For articular study on animals, the rabbit is a good compromise (moderate cost and hind limbs of convenient size). In fact, a larger animal would have provided more facility for study of articular cartilage. But cost, positioning, and sacrifice brought too many problems for our modest resources. We systematically used the mid-articulation of the hind limb, which corresponds to the knee in man. This articulation has many common points with the human knee: supra patellar bursa, patella, menisci, posterior ossicles of fabella type. On the other hand, there is a major difference – communication between the articular cavity and a bursa of the extensor of the second digit.

We experimented on 22 rabbits. Arthrograms were performed with two contrast media, which we thought to have different properties: eight rabbits were studied with microcrystalline suspension (Dimer X), and 14 others with a hexa-iodinated substance (Hexabrix). In all 37 articulations were studied, 12 of them using Dimer X, and the other 25 Hexabrix; for technical reasons, both hind limbs of each rabbit were not available all the time (e.g., extra-articular injection, etc.).

## Methods

The same sequence was used for all animals: Premedication with Valium and atropine. General anesthesia by intravenous injection of sodium thiopental (Nesdonal), through the marginal vein of the ear. Articular puncture with a 21-gauge needle, and injection of 2.5 ml contrast medium under fluoroscopic control. In six cases, the contrast medium was mixed with fluorescein (four cases) or Terramycin (two cases). Frontal and lateral radiographs of each articulation using screenless films. Death of the animal was obtained by increasing the amount of anesthetic, rabbits being particularly sensible to overdosage. According to a predetermined sequence, rabbits were killed at various intervals, ranging from several minutes to 2 h following injection. Only one animal was killed 2 days later. The successfully opacified hind limbs were amputed at the hip level, lateral radiographs being then performed on screenless films. Each mid-articulation was carefully dissected, and radiographs of the various components are taken: femoral condyles, menisci, proximal portion of tibia. Dissection proved a difficult procedure: due to the fragility of the articular cartilage, care had to be taken not to damage it. Thin sagittal sections were cut through femoral and tibial epiphyses, parallel to the long axis of the bones, using an electrical saw. Slice radiographs are then performed with metallographic films (Structurix). In six cases, the sections were also studied with a fluorescence microscope.

This sequence has proved to be successful for the 12 articulations opacified by Dimer X, and for most of those performed with Hexabrix.

However, with Hexabrix, the fluorescence microscopic study of some femoral condyles proved unconclusive.

So we attempted unsuccessfully to add Terramycin. Then we tried to mix it with fluorescein, but the diffusion of the latter occurred so rapidly that it could be found widespread along the entire limb in tendon sheaths.

## Results

The first results, mainly radiological, can be thus summarized:

1. Destiny of intra-articular contrast medium after death: whatever the substance used, microcrystalline or water-soluble suspension, it remains in the articulation after death, until organism proliferation and putrefaction occur. To avoid the latter, refrigeration at under 0 °C is required.

But, in the living animal, the contrast medium has a rather fast resorption, totally disappearing after 1½–2 h. It seems that this phenomenon is stopped by death and the concentration of the substance depends only on the delay between injection and sacrifice (the densities are assessed on sequential radiographs using a Macbeth photographic densitometer, with adjacent bone as reference).

2. Even after death, there is no leakage of contrast medium through the capsule, and no extra-articular substance can be demonstrated on radiographs.

3. Similarly, neither radiological nor microscopic study shows subchondral issue of contrast medium.

4. The absorption of opaque substance by articular cartilage slowly increases, as long as the animal is alive. But here again, this is stopped by death, and the residual opacity depends upon the delay between injection and sacrifice, and then remains unchanged.

Given the small thickness of articular cartilage of the rabbit, we cannot say if the absorption is progressive from the articular edge or if it occurs suddenly. Our observations rather favor the second hypothesis, but this is too subjective to be assessed.

## Conclusion

Thirty-seven arthrograms were performed on 22 rabbits submitted to anesthesia and killed at sequential intervals. We found mainly that resorption of articular contrast medium, and absorption by cartilage, are biological phenomena which proceed when the animal is alive, but are stopped by death, as long as putrefaction has not occurred. This is not a common finding in the literature, since, until now, absorption and resorption have been regarded as mechanical processes.

We intend to carry out a more detailed study to determine factors able to delay cartilaginous absorption. The same sequence will be applied. The position of iodine molecules will be determined, either using isotopic iodine, or using an electron microscope with special procedures of fixation.

## References

No study concerning absorption of contrast medium by cartilage has been found in the literature.

*Acknowledgment.* This work was supported by INSERM grant ATP 78102.

# Iodinated Compound and Thyroid Status

A. Piffanelli, P. B. Romelli, G. Giovannini, A. Caputo, R. Rossi, D. Pelizzola, L. Ricci, G. Camerini, and A. Toti

Among the many exciting developments in the study of the behavior of contrast media [4], little attention has been paid to the suggested correlation of the iodinated agents with thyroid hormone physiology. To what extent could the accumulation of iodinated drugs influence the thyroid metabolism? Although some data indicate that minimal absorption of free iodine generally occurs [3], we have not yet elucidated the interrelationship of the absorption, distribution, binding, and biotransformation of the amount of iodide contained in an ordinary contrast media dose. During the recent past years few studies have reported certain changes in circulating iodo-thyronines in several groups of subjects given different contrast media [1, 5]. A better insight of hormonal status could be achieved with the measurements of free fractions of thyroid hormones. We therefore decided to carry out a prospective study of the hormonal trends during the 3 months after contrast media administration.

## Materials and Method

Fifty-three clinically euthyroid patients were studied; they had not been receiving iodine-containing drugs. All subjects, subdivided into four groups, were given a single dose of four different contrast agents according to the diagnostic examination performed (Fig. 1). Venous blood samples were obtained during a 24-h period and then once daily at 9 a.m. after the contrast media injection; additional samples were obtained once weekly for 3 months (Table 1). Sera were separated and the various specimens from individual patients were stored at $-20$ °C, until studied concurrently. Serum $T_3$, $T_4$, $rT_3$, TSH, $FT_3$, $FT_4$ were measured by RIAs described previously. Quality control tests according to the methods were carried out, to validate the overall accuracy.

## Results

The values of the six hormones at various time periods of study were statistically analyzed according to the methods summarized as follows:

1. Average ± S.E. of the standardized data
2. Two-way analysis of variance (A.N.O.V.A.) between individuals and times
3. Correlation index between hormones results

The baseline values of the overall subjects showed, for each hormone, slight differences from a gaussian distribution, in accordance with other results from a so-called

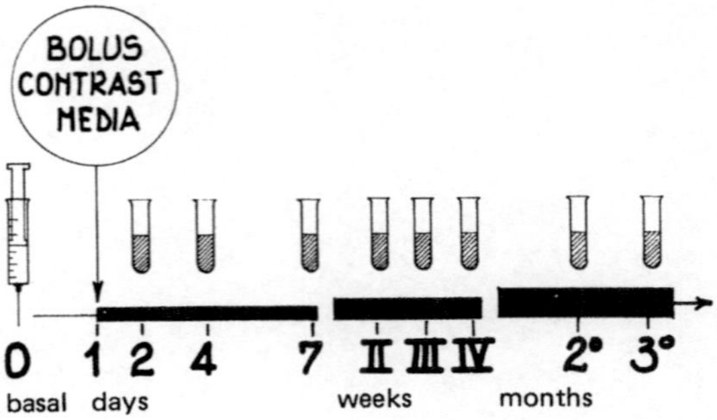


**Fig. 1.** Sample schedule

**Table 1.** Study material

| Materials | No. cases | | Total iodine concentration |
|---|---|---|---|
| Colangiography (iodoxanic acid i.v. ≅ 100 ml) | 12 | 10 ♀ / 2 ♂ | ≅ 45 g |
| Urography (sodium and methylglucamine diatrizoate i.v. ≅ 130 ml) | 18 | 10 ♀ / 8 ♂ | ≅ 38 g |
| Angiography (iodamid i.a. ≅ 100 ml) | 10 | 6 ♀ / 4 ♂ | ≅ 30 g |
| Angiography (iopamidol i.a. ≅ 80 ml) | 13 | 6 ♀ / 7 ♂ | ≅ 39 g |
| | 53 | | |

normal population (s. example in Fig. 2). Because of the high variability, either at different times from baseline, or among the subjects, the mean values of each parameter have been also expressed as the percentages of the changes from baseline (s. Figs. 3–7).

## Discussion

These changes were all within the so-called normal ranges for the various parameters evaluated. Is it possible to correlate the main results obtained to any characteristic mechanism of the thyroid physiology? The main regulatory influences on the thyroid function are summarized as follows:

1. Hypothalamic-pituitary-thyroid axis
2. Thyroid autoregulatory mechanism
3. Peripheral hormone deiodination processes
4. Effects of intrinsic and extrinsic variables

The mean TSH level at each time of investigation after contrast media administration was statistically indistinguishable from the mean baseline value. Therefore, the negative feed-back should be not involved. It is well known that various factors including drugs containing iodine, starvation etc., may drammatically influence the conversion of

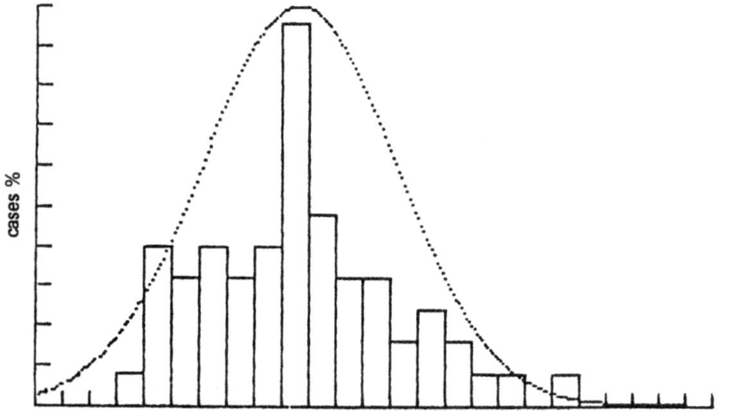


Fig. 2. Basal $TT_3$ distribution

$T_4$ to $T_3$ in peripheral tissue [5]. Other of our results, obtained in patients under chronic treatment of amiodarone, are complementary (increase of $rT_3$, decrease of $T_3$, etc.) to suggest that different mechanisms could be responsible for different features of so-called "low $T_3$ syndrome". This is undoubtedly an oversimplified view of the intrinsic mechanisms responsive to acute and chronic variations in the quantity of iodine excess [3]. Bound $T_4$ and $T_3$ are in rapid exchange equilibria with free fractions according of free fractions.

Perhaps for the people with a truly normal thyroid there is no level of iodine intake that cannot be accomodated by the variety of adaptive processes. Nevertheless, from

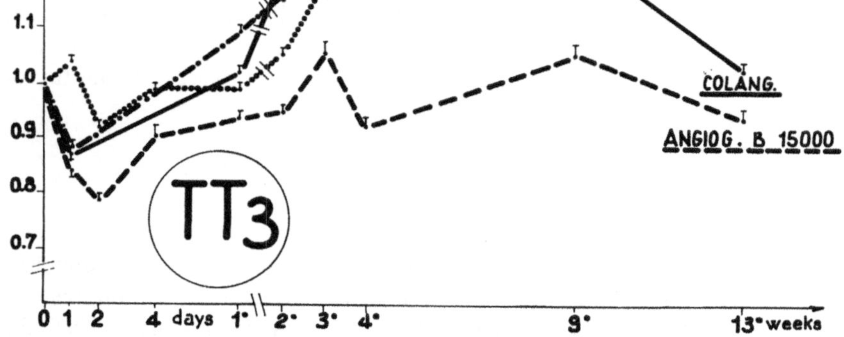


Fig. 3. Values of $TT_3$ expressed as percentages of changes from the baseline

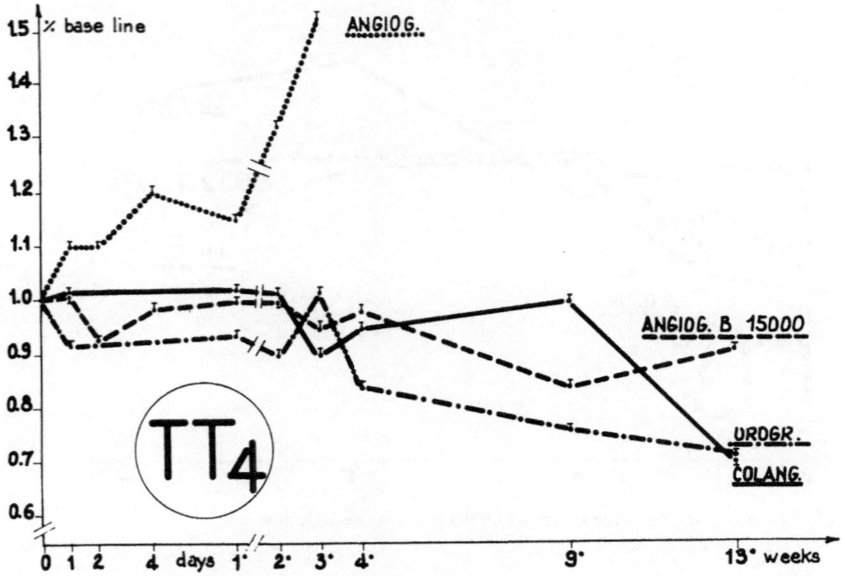


Fig. 4. Values of $TT_4$ expressed as percentages of changes from the baseline

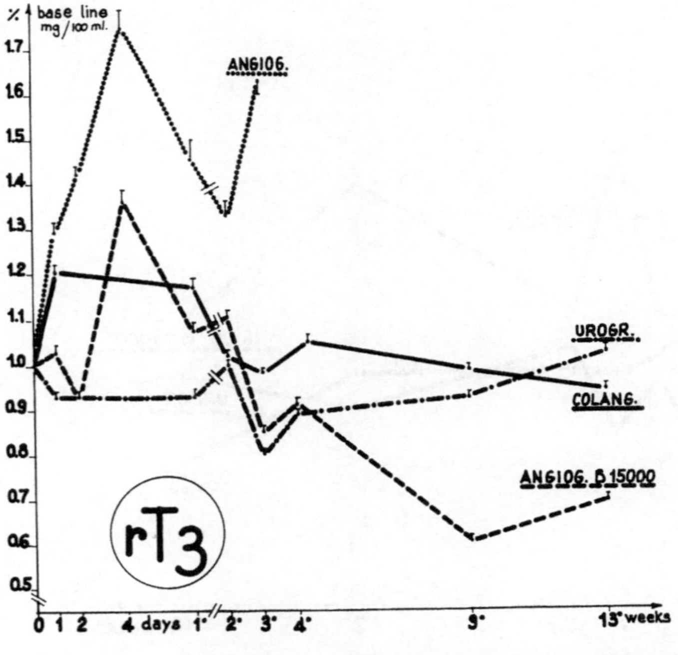


Fig. 5. Values of $rT_3$ expressed as percentages of changes from the baseline

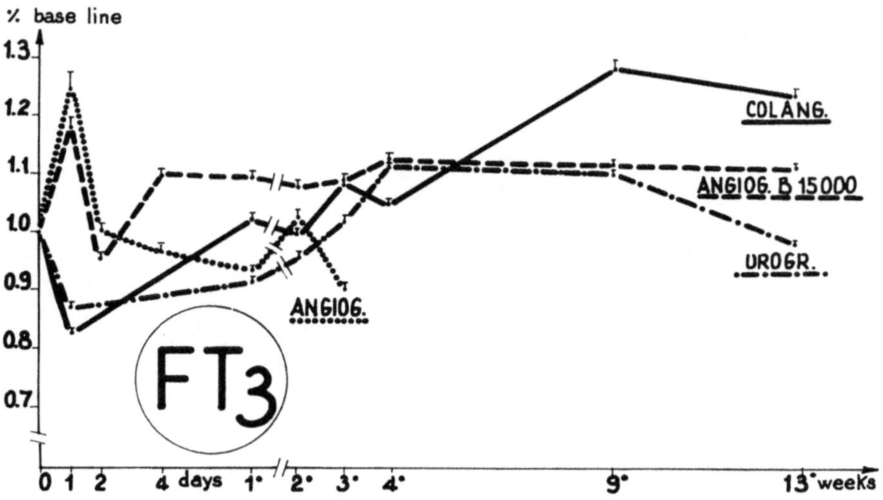


Fig. 6. Values of $FT_3$ expressed as percentages of changes from the baseline

the fact that exposure to additional iodine does sometimes result in frank thyroid disease (hyper- or hypo-), it is clear that an upper limit of normal or tolerable iodine intake should exist at least in some individuals, with underlying thyroid dysfunctions (autonomous nodules or previously treated thyrotoxicosis or thyroiditis, etc.).

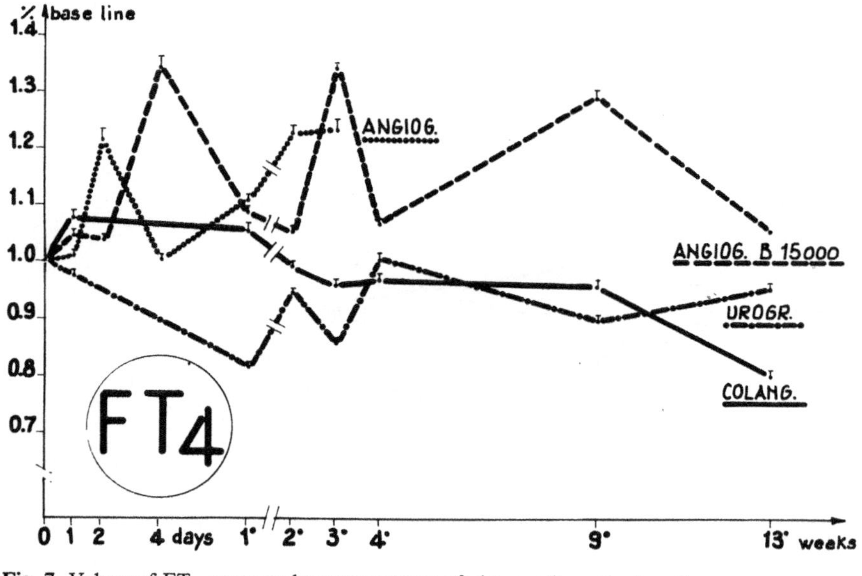


Fig. 7. Values of $FT_4$ expressed as percentages of changes from the baseline

Table 2. Angiography B 15 000

| $P < 0.5$ * <br> $P < 0.1$ ** <br> $P < 0.01$ *** | $TT_4$ | $rT_3$ | $FT_3$ | $FT_4$ |
|---|---|---|---|---|
| $TT_3$ | (0.57488) *** | n. s. | * | (−0.24666) ** |
| $TT_4$ | | (0.28170) *** | n. s. | n. s. |
| $rT_3$ | | | (−0.30027) *** | n. s. |
| $FT_3$ | | | | (0.16859) * |

## Conclusions

1. Administration of four different contrast media exerted slight but significant and prolonged effects on the hormonal thyroid status, in 53 euthyroid subjects (four subgroups), without any clinical expression of dysthyroidism.
2. Changes in serum $T_3$, $rT_3$, and $T_4$ demonstrated different trends for each iodinated compound, probably depending on the regolatory thyroid mechanisms, and CM pharmacokinetics (Figs. 3–5).
3. Plasma profiles of free fractions ($FT_3$, $FT_4$) slightly reflected consensual changes with circulating iodothyronines, at various time periods of study, demonstrating high correlation indexes with total fractions (Figs. 6, 7).
4. The five hormones profiles correlation study (s. example Table 2) suggests that different mechanism could be responsible for some features encountered of low $T_3$ syndrome.
5. These effects may be not only equivalent to giving various sources of iodide, but suggest more complex mechanisms (competition to steric binding to nuclear receptor, or others?).
6. It is apparent that man has a remarkable and possibly unique system of homeostatic thyroid hormone regulation.
7. Further correlations between time course hormone study and iodinated compounds pharmacokinetics are needed.

## References


1. Burgi H, Wimpfheimer C, Burger A, Zaunbauer W, Rosler H, Lemachand-Beraud T (1976) Changes of circulating tiroxine triiodotyronine and reverse triiodiothyronine after radiographic contrast agents. J Clin Endocrinol Metab 43:1203
2. De Groot LJ, Rue PA (1979) Roentgenografic contrast agent inhibit triiodothyronine binding to nuclear receptors "in vitro". J Clin Endocrinol Metab 49:4:538–542
3. Savoie JC, Massin JP, Thomopoulos P, Leger F (1975) Iodine induced thyrotoxicosis in apparently normal thyroid glands. JCE & M, vol 41, 4:685–691
4. Sternthal E, Lipworth L, Stanley B, Abreau C, Fang SL, Braverman LE (1980) Suppression of thyroid radioiodine uptake by various doses of stable iodide. The New England Journal of Medicine vol 303, 19:1083–1088
5. Yonckheer MH, Blockx P, Broeckaert I, Cornette C, Beckers C (1978) "Low $T_3$ Sindrome" in patients chronically treated with au yodine. Containing drug, amiodarone. Clinical Endorinology 9:27–35

# Binding of Contrast Media to Human Prealbumin: Another Cause of Thyroid Hormonal Disorder

J. Mathieu, Y. Looze, M. Deconinck, and R. Potvliege

## Introduction

It has already been shown that radiographic contrast media (RCM) can produce modifications of the thyroid metabolism. It is generally assumed that thyroid hormone secretion remains constant whatever the fluctuations in iodine supply. Hyperthyroidism when induced by RCM administration is accompanied by changes of the levels of circulating thyroid hormones [2].

Circulating thyroid hormones are found either free, or bound to serum globulin (thyroxin-binding globulin), prealbumin, and albumin in decreasing order of intensity [1].

Since it was found in a previous report [4] that RCM do have an affinity for prealbumin, it remained for us to investigate if RCM and the thyroid hormones did bind to the same site or not.

## Material and Methods

Prealbumin was isolated from the urine of a patient suffering from a nephrotic syndrome and purified using ammonium sulfate fractionation and ion-exchange chromatography on DEAE-Sephadex A-50 (Pharmacia). The preparation was found to be homogeneous using molecular filtration on Sephadex G-100 (Pharmacia), polyacrylamide gel electrophoresis in the presence of sodium dodecyl sulfate and isoelectric focusing experiment.

Fluorescence emission spectra were recorded at 25° using a Hitachi Perkin Elmer model MPF-2A spectrofluorometer equipped with an Osram XBO 150-W Xenon lamp and a RCA 1-P28 photomultiplier. Excitation and emission band widths were 5 nm each. A solution of L-tryptophan in water served as the standard.

The binding of 8-anilinonaphthalene sulfonic acid (ANS) to prealbumin was followed spectrofluorometrically [3]. Working conditions were chosen such that the measured fluorescence intensity was directly proportional to the quantity of ANS bound to the protein.

Prealbumin and ANS concentrations were determined spectrophotometrically (Zeiss spectrophotometer PMQ II) using appropriate molar extinction coefficients.

## Results

ANS fluorescence intensity when free in aqueous buffer is very low compared to its value when bound to proteins. From fluorescence studies as well as from other studies it has been concluded that two moles of ANS become bound to prealbumin [3].

The fluorescence intensity of prealbumin in the presence of saturating amounts of ANS decreased as increasing amounts of Biligrafin were added.

The results were interpreted using the Klotz equation:

$$1/r = 1/n + 1/n \cdot \mathrm{Ka} \cdot 1/[\mathrm{RCM\ free}]$$

where $r$ = [Biligrafin bound]/[prealbumin]

$n$ = number of binding sites of RCM to prealbumin

Ka = the binding constant

This analysis revealed that 0.82 mol of RCM bound prealbumin with a binding constant equal to 11.6 (Fig. 1).

## Discussion

The results clearly show that one out of the two ANS sites on prealbumin is thus susceptible to interact with RCM. The interaction is far to be strong but may be of physiological significance in view of the large amount of RCM used in clinical practice.

Previous work has shown prealbumin to possess common binding sites for ANS and thyroxine hormones.

It is thus suggested that RCM can displace one of the two thyroxine molecules from prealbumin, resulting in increasing amounts of free hormones in serum.

The reason some patients present high levels of circulating thyroxine after RCM administration has not yet been completely elucidated.

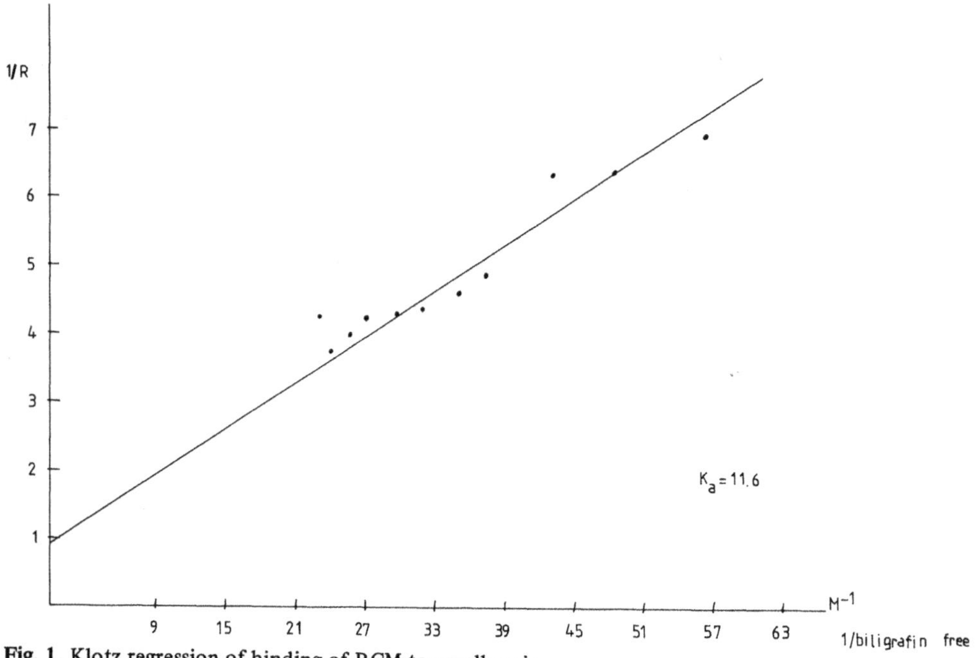


**Fig. 1.** Klotz regression of binding of RCM to prealbumin

## References


1. Burgi H, Wimpfheimer C, Burger A, Zaunbauer W, Rosler H, Lemarchand-Beraud T (1976) Changes of circulating thyroxine, triiodothyronine and reverse thiiodothyronine after radiographic contrast agents. J Clin Endocrinol Metab 43:1203
2. Brauman J, Brauman H, Van Camp B, Mathieu J (1976) Effect in vitro of ioglycamide on blood proteins and paraproteins. Acta Radiol [diagn] (Stockh) 18:715
3. Ferguson RN, Edelhoch H, Saroff HA, Robbins J (1975) Negative cooperativity in the binding of thyroxine to human serum prealbumin. Biochemistry 14:282
4. Wosilait WD (1977) A theorical analysis of the distribution of thyroxine among sites on thyroid binding globulin, thyroid binding prealbumin and serum albumin. Res Commun Chem Pathol Pharmacol 16:541

# Summary of the Discussion

J. F. Moreau

Dr. Eriksson recalled that his team demonstrated a relationship in rabbits between the vena cava endothelium damage severity and the CM concentration. This led them to contraindicate the injection of 76% CM for phlebographies. Dr. Bjork pointed out that the rate of venous complications in humans is low when the concentration of iodine is below 200 mg/ml.

Dr. Moreau posed a question about the most adequate CM for digitalized angiography. Dr. Ducos de la Hitte thought that digitalized angiography should lead to injection of 3 to 4 times smaller doses of CM and that Hexabrix is too fluid (even frozen) for taking the place of Telebrix in angiography of the peripheral vessels. Dr. Moreau asked the manufacturers why they do not make new media with a higher concentration of iodine; this should greatly improve the opacification of the peripheral vessels, which are poorly seen with a solution such as Hexabrix 32 g%. Mr. Lautrou answered that there is an exponential relationship between the concentration of iodine and CM viscosity; for instance, the viscosity of a 35-g iodine Hexabrix is raised to 15 centipoises: this would not be convenient for clinical use. Dr. Caille believed that angiography of the peripheral vessels should not be improved by i.v. injections of CM, in spite of digital imaging. Digitalized angiograms will continue to be obtained by intraarterial injections. But digitalization readily allows the doses required for intra-arterial carotidogram or aortogram to be divided 6 to 10 times.

Dr. X . . ., commenting on Geschwind's paper, thought that such large differences in the changes in plasma volumes obtained by two types of media, in spite of the similarity of the doses, the concentrations, and the injection rates, can be explained by a difference in osmolar doses only.

# Section F:
Various Topics

# Angiography in Lower Extremities with New Contrast Media: Review of Double-blind Studies

E. Zeitler, M. Georgi-Tönnesen, H. G. Hinski, H. Mader, and E.-I. Richter

Despite the considerable progress attributable to digital intravenous angiography (DIVA) [1, 3] contrast material now as before must be applied into the aorta and femoral arteries for total visualization of pelvic and leg arteries. The reason for this is the considerable extension of these body sections to be examined.

Exceptions are the examination after operation, fibrinolysis, PTA, and the diagnosis of tumors, where only one section must be analyzed angiographically [3]. In these cases, intravenous digital angiography is the method of choice in future.

With appropriate guidance of the patient and after premedication (Atosil, Atropin, Polamidon, Valium 5, Tranxilium 5) urographic contrast materials such as diatrizoate (Angiografin, Urografin) have been well tolerated so far for angiography of the lower legs without general anesthesia [5, 6]. Only sensations of pain and heat in the legs were uncomfortable for the patient. The severity of pain and heat varied individually.

Special pathologic findings were very often the reason for a local intensification of pain after contrast material application.

Patients with unilateral femoral artery occlusion reported a severe pain on the affected side in the thigh proximal to the occlusion. Patients with endangiitis or occlusions in various lower leg arteries or in the popliteal artery because of other reasons complained of increased pain in the leg proximal to the obliteration.

In normal arteries, however, patients reported a uniform distribution of pain, and, sometimes, the pain is felt to be severest in the feet. Unlike these patients, others with aortic artery occlusion or occlusions in both pelvic arteries report sensation of heat but not of pain.

**Table 1.** Contrast media

| | Generic name | Iodine content (mg/ml) | Osmolarity mOsmol/kg) |
|---|---|---|---|
| Ionic contrast medium Rayvist 300 | Meglumine ioglicinate | 300 | 1790 |
| Ionic contrast medium of low osmolarity Hexabrix | Ioxaglate | 320 | 600 |
| Nonionic contrast medium Solutrast 300 | Iopamidol | 300 | 620 |

Radiological Center, Nürnberg

**Table 2.** Randomized double-blind crossover trial

| I (*n* = 30) | | II (*n* = 48) | |
|---|---|---|---|
| A Solutrast 300<br>B Rayvist 300 | *n* = 15 | A Solutrast 300<br>B Hexabrix | *n* = 24 |
| B Rayvist 300<br>A Solutrast 300 | *n* = 15 | B Hexabrix<br>A Solutrast 300 | *n* = 24 |

Radiological Center, Nürnberg

The development of new contrast materials with reduced osmolarity such as Amipaque, Solutrast 300, Iopromide, and Hexabrix has made angiography in the legs less painful.

To objectify the grade of the sensation of pain and heat the patient complains of during leg angiography, we carried out two randomized double-blind crossover trials. We tested (Tables 1, 2) the water-soluble nonionic contrast material Solutrast 300 with the ionic contrast material Rayvist 300 and the ionic Hexabrix with low osmolarity. Another randomized double-blind study between Hexabrix and Iopromide has not yet been concluded.

To quantify the sensation of pain and heat the patient feels, we used the visual analogous scale method (Fig. 1) (dolorimeter, calorimeter) first used for the control of contrast media sensations by Tillmann et al. in 1979 [4]. On the scale from 0 to 100 the graduation 0 means: no pain or no heat, and 100 on the scale means: unbearable sensation of heat or pain. The patients were asked to note the degree of pain or heat felt following every injection by marking the visual analogous scale with a pencil.

## Material

Fifteen patients in collective I first received an injection of 80 ml Solutrast and then 80 ml Rayvist (AB) with a flow rate of 22 ml/s into the aorta 4 ± 3 cm proximal the aortic bifurcation. The second injection followed 10 ± 5 min later.

In an additional 15 patients the same injections were carried out but in retrograde order (BA). None of the patients was given an analgesic premedication. The Seldinger technique was used, and a catheter introduced from the groin under local anesthesia with 1% Xylocaine.

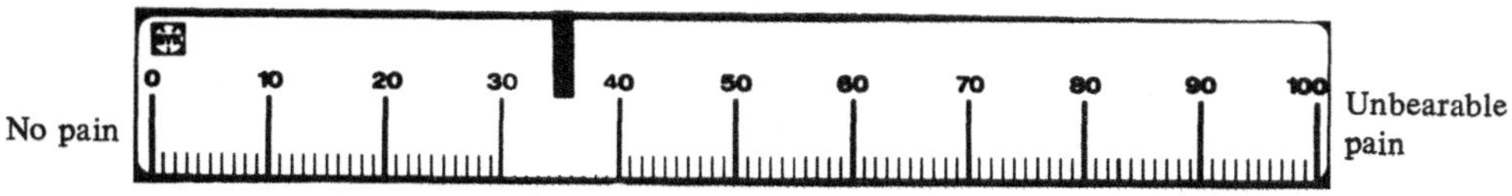


**Fig. 1.** Dolorimeter, Calorimeter. The visual analogous scale

In the double-blind crossover trial in collective II 24 patients were first administered Solutrast 300 and then Hexabrix (AB). An additional 24 patients were first administered Hexabrix and then Solutrast (BA).

## Results

Collective I (Solutrast 300/Rayvist 300)

There were no significant differences in the makeup of the patient groups to be compared as to age, sex, clinical indication for angiography and the ascertained obliteration forms and locations (Tables 3–5).

**Table 3.** Collective I ($n$ = 30)

| AB | | Sex / Age | | BA |
|---|---|---|---|---|
| | 46.7% | Male | 80% | |
| | 53.3% | Female | 20% | |
| 67 | | Mean age (y) | | 64 |
| | 37 | Youngest | 40 | |
| | 85 | Oldest | 84 | |

A, Solutrast 300; B, Rayvist 300
Radiological Center, Nürnberg

**Table 4.** Collective I ($n$, 30)

| AB | Indication | BA |
|---|---|---|
| 5 | Claudication | 5 |
| 3 | Rest pain | 5 |
| 6 | Gangrene | 4 |
| 0 | Embolic occlusion | 2 |
| 1 | Functional disorders | 0 |
| 1 | Postop. control | 2 |

A, Solutrast 300; B, Rayvist 300
Radiological Center, Nürnberg

**Table 5.** Collective I ($n$ = 30)

| AB | Angiographic diagnosis | BA |
|---|---|---|
| 11 | Occlusion | 13 |
| 6 | Stenosis | 6 |
| 2 | Normal | 1 |
| 2 | Postoperative | – |

A, Solutrast 300; B, Rayvist 300
Radiological Center, Nürnberg

When comparing leg pain after Solutrast 300 with Rayvist 300 injection in the series A : B, a significant difference of $P < 0.01$ was found in the sequence AB, and of $P < 0.001$ in the sequence BA (Fig. 2).

The crossover statistical analysis [2] regarding the difference in sequence and period was not significant, a difference resulting from this of $P < 0.001$ between the preparations related to the sensation of pain during leg angiography.

The same analysis was made concerning the feeling of heat. The tests were made under the same conditions, and the result was a significant value of $P > 0.05$ only when

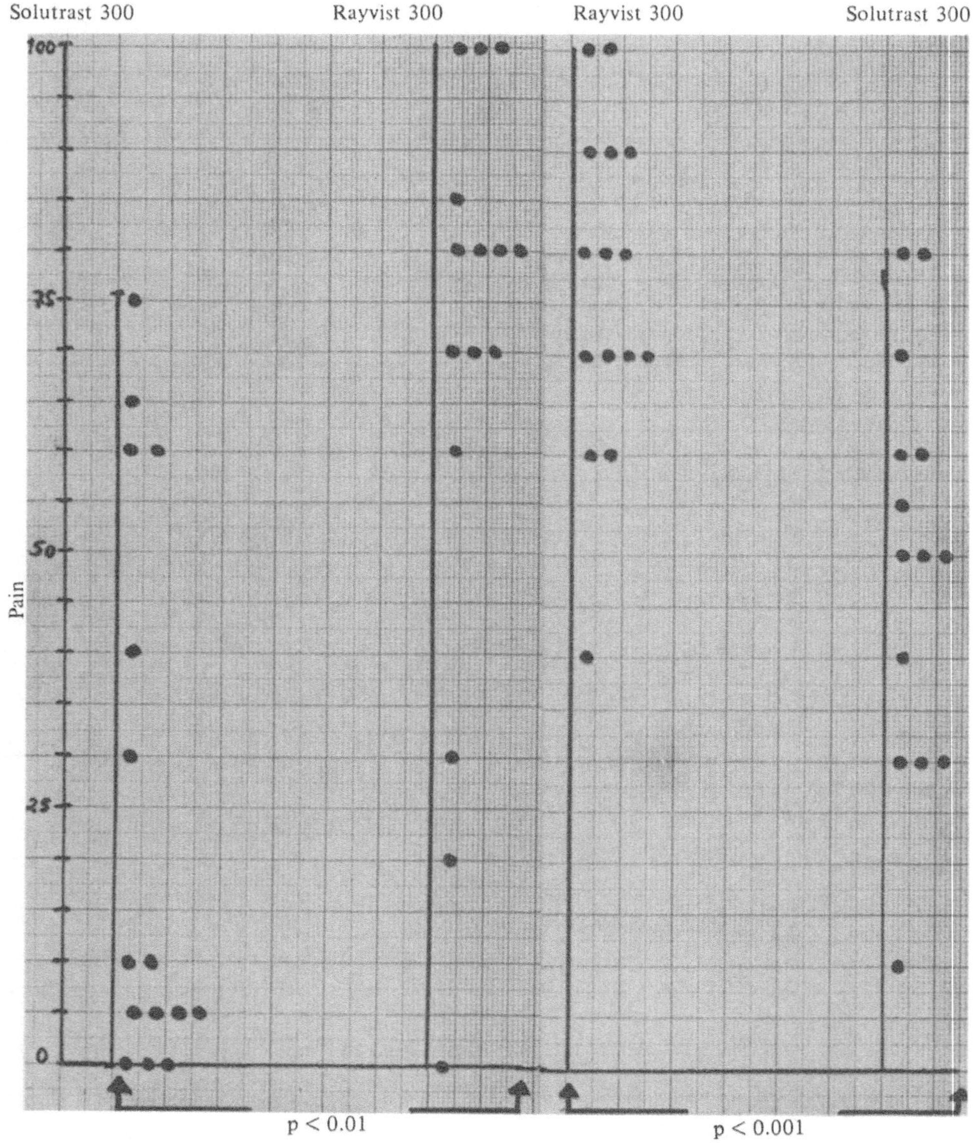


**Fig. 2.** Comparison of Solutrast 300 and Rayvist 300 in the sequence AB and in the sequence BA

**Table 6.** Collective II ($n$ = 48)

| AB | Sex/Age | BA |
|---|---|---|
| 62.5% | Male | 66.7% |
| 37.5% | Female | 33.4% |
| 60 | Mean age (y) | 61 |
| 34 | Youngest | 38 |
| 81 | Oldest | 84 |

A, Solutrast 300; B, Hexabrix
Radiological Center, Nürnberg

**Table 7.** Collective II ($n$ = 48)

| AB | Indication | BA |
|---|---|---|
| 10 | Claudication | 13 |
| 2 | Rest pain | 2 |
| 8 | Gangrene | 7 |
| 5 | Embolic occlusion | 1 |
| 1 | Functional disorders | 2 |
| | Postop. control | 3 |

A, Solutrast 300; B, Hexabrix
Radiological Center, Nürnberg

**Table 8.** Collective II ($n$ = 48)

| AB | Angiographic diagnosis | BA |
|---|---|---|
| 15 | Occlusion | 12 |
| 10 | Stenosis | 6 |
| 2 | Normal | 4 |
| – | Postoperative | 2 |
| 6 | Art. sclerot. lesion | 6 |

A, Solutrast 300; B, Hexabrix
Radiological Center, Nürnberg

Solutrast was used for the first contrast injection. If Rayvist was injected first, no statistical significance was found.

General side effects on both contrast materials were noted in 3.3%.

## Collective II (Solutrast 300/Hexabrix)

No difference existed in the characteristics of both groups, and no significant difference was found with regard to the parameters pain and sensation of heat (Tables 6–8). Hence it follows that the two contrast materials caused an equally low feeling of heat and pain (Fig. 3).

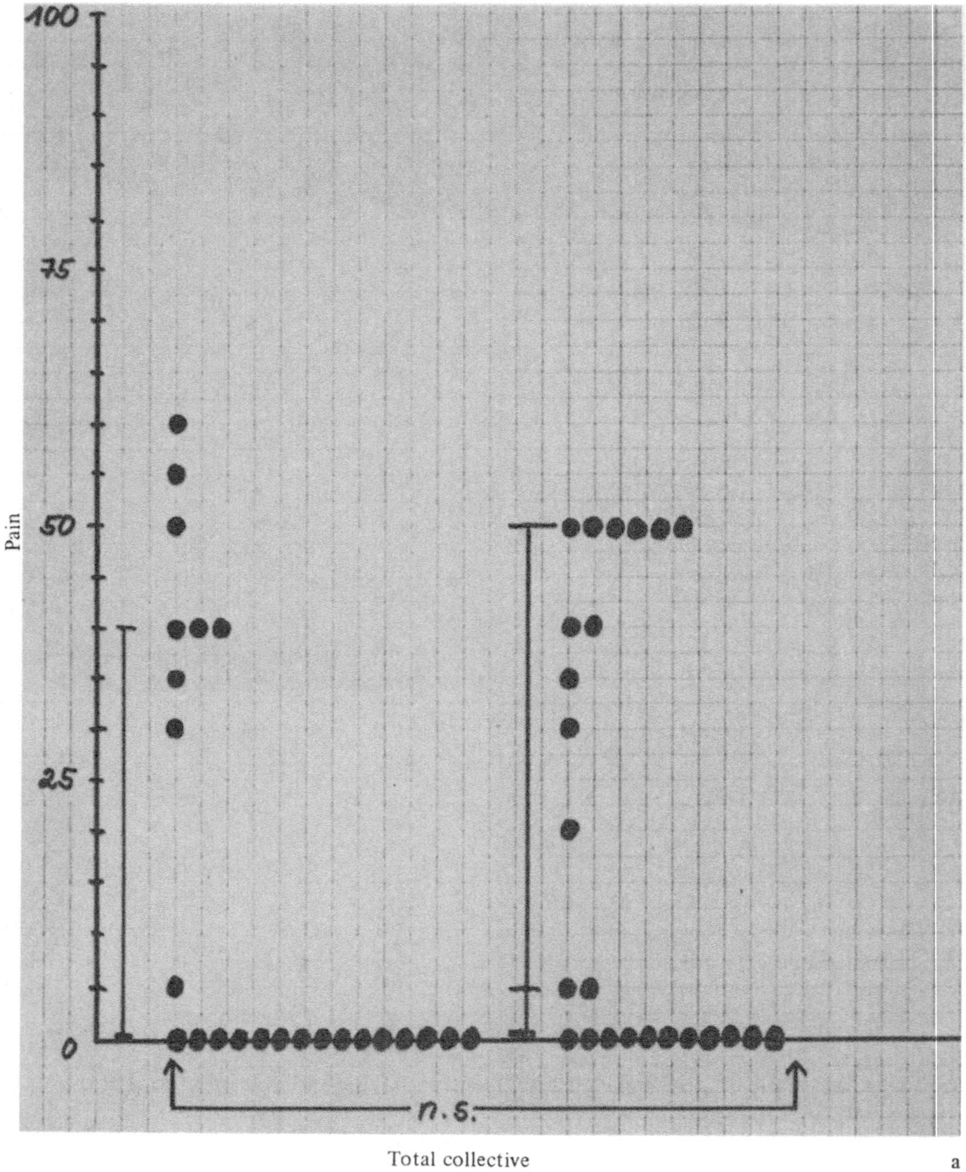


**Fig. 3a, b.** Comparison of Solutrast 300 with Hexabrix in the sequence AB (a) and in the sequence BA (b)

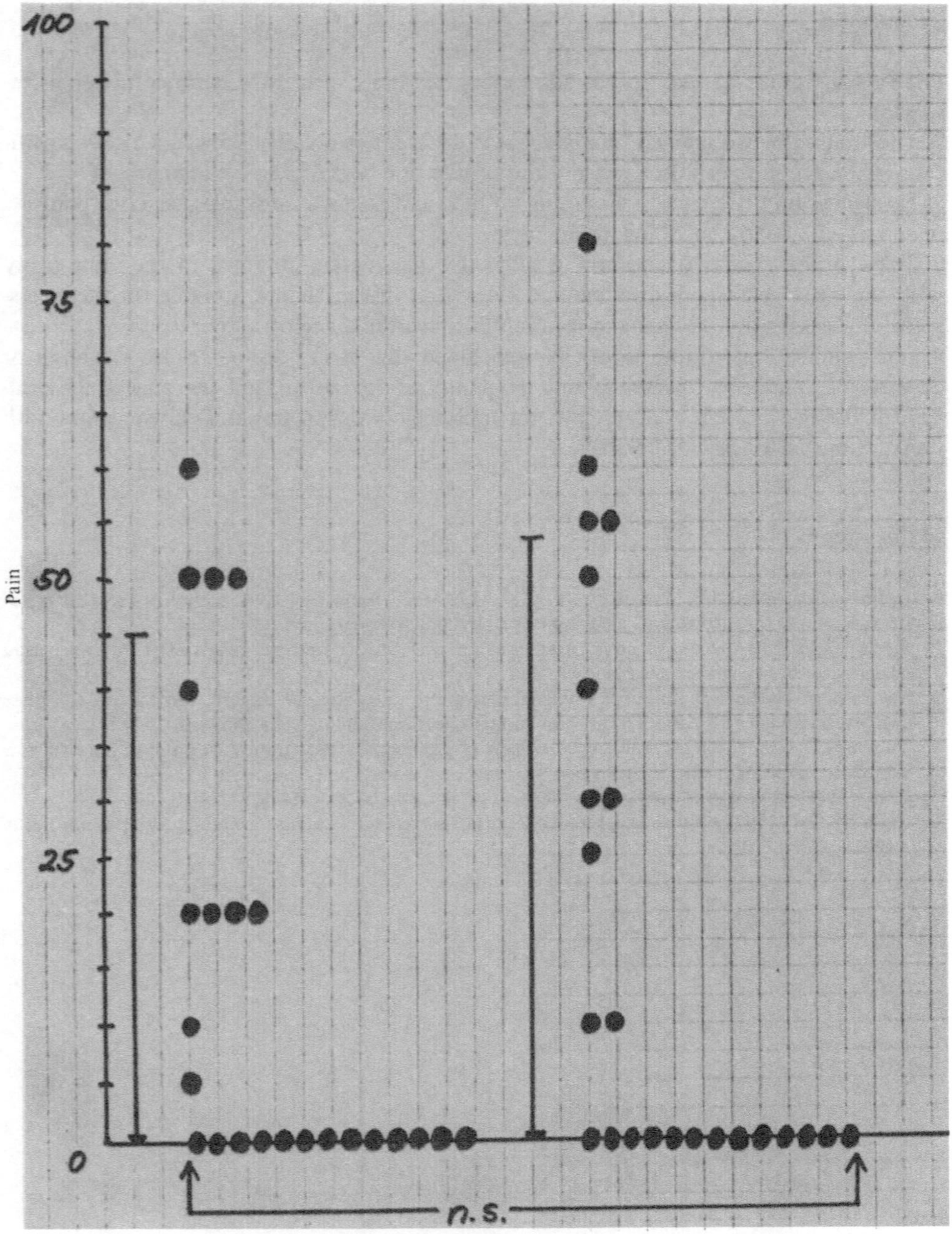


Total collective A:B (n.s.)

b

## Discussion

The varying results of two double-blind crossover trials with three contrast materials revealed:

1. The trial with two contrast materials with different osmolarity showed a highly significant difference in the subjective sensation of pain and heat during leg angiography.
2. No significant difference in the feeling of heat and pain was provable using two contrast materials with nearly equal low osmolarity.
3. These differing results concerning subjective parameters obtained in the same study with the visual analogous scale method show that this method is suitable for the assessment of the sensation of heat and pain felt during arterial angiography.
4. For practical application it can be concluded that it is possible to use Hexabrix or Solutrast as equivalent water-soluble preparations for pelvic and leg angiography, although the one is a ionic and the other a nonionic contrast material. Decisive is that both preparations have a low osmolarity.

## References


1. Crummy AB, Strother CM, Sackett JF et al. (1980) Computerized fluoroscopy, a digital subtraction technique for intravenous angiocardiography and arteriography. AJR 135:6
2. Koch GG (1972) The use of none-parametric methods in the statistical analysis of the two-period change-over design. Biometrics 28:577–584
3. Seyferth W, Marhoff P, Zeitler E (1982) Transvenöse und arterielle digitale Angiographie – Erste Erfahrungen nach 120 Patientenuntersuchungen. Fortschr Roentgenstr 136, 3:301–309
4. Tillmann U, Adler R, Fuchs WA (1979) Pain in peripheral arteriography. A comparison of a low osmolality contrast medium with a conventional compound. Br J Radiol 52:102–104
5. Zeitler E (1978) Risks of artiography under local anesthesia. Ann Radiol 21:491–492
6. Zeitler E (ed) (1977) Neue Aspekte des Kontrastmittelzwischenfalls. Schering, Symposium Berlin 1977

# Patient Reactions During Hexabrix, Iopamidol and Conray Angiography

R.G. Grainger

Conventional ionic radiographic contrast media (CIRCM) cause a variable degree of warmth and even pain on arteriography in the conscious patient. The discomfort may be sufficiently distressing to cause the patient to cry out or move during the procedure. The cause of the warmth and feeling of heat is the peripheral vasodilatation caused by CIRCM, but the cause of the pain is not known. The pain sensation, however, correlates well with the heat sensation and they may have the same or similar pathogenesis. Probably vascular endothelial damage caused by CIRCM is responsible for at least some of the pain sensation.

It has been well established by ourselves and others [1, 2, 3] that both the pain and the warm sensation are related to the marked hyperosmolality of CIRCM.

We have shown that Hexabrix (ioxaglate salts), Iopamidol and Amipaque (metrizamide) when injected at 280 mg I/ml produce the same degree of peripheral vasodilatation in the anaesthetised dog on experimental femoral arteriography [3]. Maximal vasodilatation occurred 30–40 s after injection and peaked at x 1.3 above base line blood flow. Conray 280 (meglumine iothalamate) when injected at identical iodine concentration, volume and flow rates, caused vasodilatation peaking at x 2 base-line blood flow, and maximal at 30–40 s. The three new contrast media – Hexabrix, Iopamidol and Amipaque – all have the same osmolality which is about one-third that of CIRCM solutions of equivalent iodine concentrations. The equal vasodilatatory response to these three media suggests, therefore, that osmolality is of major influence in its causation.

Each of the three new low osmolality media (Hexabrix, Iopamidol, Amipaque) would therefore be expected to produce the same degree of vasodilatation in clinical peripheral arteriography, which can be anticipated to cause much less warmth and pain than CIRCM (e.g., Conray 280) injections.

We have therefore compared subjective patient reactions in conscious patients with no or minimum pre-medication, to Conray 280 (280 Img I/ml), Hexabrix 320 (320 mg I/ml) and Iopamidol (300 mg I/ml) in cerebral, aortic and ilio-femoral arteriography.

All injections were delivered via a trans-femoral percutaneous arterial catheter at the same volume and same flow rate for each contrast medium. At first we designed a double blind cross-over trial, but as patient numbers increased this was discontinued. Most patients received injections of two of the contrast media and did not know which was being injected.

A nurse who did not know which contrast medium was being injected asked the patient immediately after each injection, how he would grade the discomfort both of warmth and pain.

The grading was: No symptom = 0; slight symptom = 1; moderate symptom = 2; severe symptom = 3.

We found that this grading system was much simpler, easier to explain to the patient and more reliable than scoring on a linear 100-mm scale from 0 to 100.

## Results

### Cerebral Arteriograms

Injections of 8 ml made either into the termination of the common carotid artery or origin of the internal carotid artery at 6 ml/s.

**Table 1.** Reactions to Hexabrix 320 and Conray 280 on cerebral arteriography

| | Reactions | Nil | Mild | Moderate | Severe | No. of Injections | No. of Patients |
|---|---|---|---|---|---|---|---|
| *Pain* | Hexabrix 320 | 141 | 11 | 2 | 0 | 152 | 36 |
| | Conray 280 | 33 | 15 | 11 | 4 | 63 | 35 |
| *Heat* | Hexabrix 320 | 7 | 136 | 81 | 8 | 232 | 69 |
| | Conray 280 | 2 | 9 | 29 | 19 | 141 | 68 |

### Abdominal Aortography

Injections of 30–40 ml at 12 ml/s. Equal volumes of different contrast media injected in same patient at same aortic site.

**Table 2.** Reactions to Hexabrix 320 and Conray 280 on abdominal aortography

| | Reactions | Nil | Mild | Moderate | Severe | No. of Injections | No. of Patients |
|---|---|---|---|---|---|---|---|
| *Pain* | Hexabrix 320 | 44 | 0 | 0 | 0 | 44 | 15 |
| | Conray 280 | 9 | 4 | 0 | 7 | 20 | 15 |
| *Heat* | Hexabrix 320 | 10 | 12 | 17 | 5 | 44 | 15 |
| | Conray 280 | 5 | 1 | 4 | 10 | 20 | 15 |

### Ilio-Femoral Arteriography

Injections of 20 ml at 10 ml/s. Different contrast media injected with catheter at same arterial site.

### Comparison Between Intra-arterial Injections of Hexabrix 320 and Conray 280

Hexabrix 320 very rarely caused any pain on injection into the common carotid, internal carotid, iliac or femoral arteries or into the abdominal aorta. Of these territories, cerebral

**Table 3.** Reactions to Hexabrix 320 and Conray 280 on ilio-femoral arteriography

| | Reactions | Nil | Mild | Moderate | Severe | No. of Injections | No. of Patients |
|---|---|---|---|---|---|---|---|
| *Pain* | Hexabrix 320 | 56 | 4 | 0 | 0 | 60 | 24 |
| | Conray 280 | 9 | 5 | 13 | 8 | 35 | 24 |
| *Heat* | Hexabrix 320 | 1 | 28 | 27 | 4 | 60 | 24 |
| | Conray 280 | 0 | 3 | 10 | 22 | 35 | 23 |

arteriography with Hexabrix produced slightly more pain than in other territories, but only 11 carotid injections caused "mild" pain and only two caused "moderate" pain in 152 Hexabrix injections into the carotid artery. All the other 139 Hexabrix carotid injections were called "painless" by the patient.

Conray 280 injected into the same vascular territories caused frequent pain often graded "moderate" or "severe".

Heat sensation was also considerably reduced during the Hexabrix injections compared to the Conray 280 injections and was frequently described as "moderate" in severity compared to "severe" with the Conray injections.

We then extended the clinical trial to include Iopamidol 300 and the total results are presented in Table 4.

**Table 4.** Total results of the clinical trial

| | Conray 280 | Hexabrix 320 | Iopamidol 300 |
|---|---|---|---|
| Abdominal aorta (No. of injections) | (20) | (44) | (89) |
| Pain | 1.25 | 0.0 | 0.16 |
| Heat | 1.95 | 1.39 | 1.39 |
| Ilio-femoral arteries (No. of injections) | (37) | (60) | (40) |
| Pain | 1.65 | 0.07 | 0.3 |
| Heat | 2.41 | 1.56 | 1.52 |
| Carotid artery (No. of injections) | (68) | (156) | (169) |
| Pain | 0.76 | 0.10 | 0.08 |
| Heat | 2.60 | 1.38 | 1.50 |

Each score represents the average score of patient reaction to each injection. The higher the number, the more the patient reaction. Scoring system: 0, no reaction; 1, mild reaction; 2, moderate reaction; 3, severe reaction

## Conclusions

1. As anticipated from their iodine content, Hexabrix 320 and Iopamidol 300 produce angiographic results at least as good as Conray 280 in carotid, ilio-femoral arteriography or abdominal aortography.
2. Hexabrix 320 and Iopamidol 300 very rarely cause pain of even "mild" severity in any of the above arteriographic procedures.
3. Hexabrix 320 and Iopamidol 300 often cause a moderate degree of warmth in the above arteriographic procedures.
4. Conray 280 causes much more heat and pain despite having the least iodine content when compared with Hexabrix 320 and Iopamidol 300.
5. The following recommendations are made:
a) For arteriographic procedures known to be very painful (e.g. external carotid, brachial) a new low osmolar contrast medium, e.g. Hexabrix, Iopamidol (or probably also Iohexol and Amipaque) should be used throughout the procedure.
b) For all other angiographies under local anesthesia, the first injection may reasonably be a conventional ionic one (e.g. Conray, Urografin, Triosil). If this causes patient distress, then subsequent injections of a new low osmolar contrast medium should be used.
c) For patients under general anesthesia, unconscious or very heavily sedated, a conventional ionic contrast medium will probably be acceptable.
d) The above method of usage will enable the most cost-effective use to be made of the improved but expensive new low osmolar contrast media.
e) The virtually identical patient scores for heat and pain sensation for Hexabrix 320 and Iopamidol 300 injections (Table 4) into the carotid, ilio-femoral and aortic territories strongly suggest that it is the osmolality of contrast media which is responsible for these adverse subjective reactions.

## References


1. Grainger RG (1979) A clinical trial of a new low osmolality contrast medium. Sodium and meglumine ioxaglate (Hexabrix) compared with meglumine iothalamate (Conray) for carotid arteriography. Br J Radiol 52:781–786
2. Hilal SK (1966) Hemodynamic changes associated with the intra-arterial injection of contrast media. Radiology 86:615–633
3. Steiner RM, Grainger RG, Memon N, Weiss D, Kanofsky PB, Menduke H (1980) The effect of contrast media of low osmolality on the peripheral arterial blood flow in the dog. Clin Radiol 31:621–627

# Experience of Cerebral Arteriography with Iopamidol: Clinical Data

P. Dettori

A contrast medium which is completely inert and atoxic on the nervous system has not yet been found. However, hydrosoluble, nonionic, and low osmolality contrast media seem to be better tolerated. On account of this and on the basis of the good results obtained in myelographic investigations, we have used Iopamidol (nonionic contrast medium of Bracco, Milan) also in cerebral angiography [1, 2, 3, 4, 5].

## Material and Method

Randomized, double-blind, research was performed on 85 patients (Table 1), 38 males and 47 women aged between 1 and 72.

The contents of the vials, containing Iopamidol 300 (300 mg I/ml) and Conray 60 (methylglucamine salt 280 mg I/ml) were only known after a complete analysis of the material. The surgical technique and the investigated region are summarized in Table 2. Eighty-six angiographies of the internal or common carotid artery and seven of the external carotid, all by direct puncture, were performed. Fourteen angiographies (four carotid and ten vertebral artery) were carried out by a catheter via the femoral artery. Only one investigation was performed via the brachial artery.

The injected amount and the flow rate are indicated in Table 3. Conray was injected in 43 patients and Iopamidol in 42. Simultaneous technique was employed in 61 cases (frontal and lateral views were obtained with an injection of 10 ml contrast medium). In 24 cases some additional injections were made because of clinical problems. Only in these later cases did the amount of the contrast medium rise above 10 ml.

**Table 1.** Material: 85 cases

| M | F | Age (decades) | Cases |
|---|---|---|---|
| | | 1–10 | 7 |
| | | 10–20 | 11 |
| | | 20–30 | 6 |
| 38 | 47 | 30–40 | 7 |
| | | 40–50 | 19 |
| | | 50–60 | 16 |
| | | 60–70 | 19 |

**Table 2.** Technique 1: 108 examinations

| Artery | Direct puncture | Catheter by femoral artery | Brachial puncture | Conray | Iopamidol |
|---|---|---|---|---|---|
| ICA/CCA (90) | 86 | 4 | | 46 | 44 |
| ECA (7) | 7 | | | 2 | 5 |
| Vertebral (11) | | 10 | 1 | 5 | 6 |
| Total | 93 | 14 | 1 | 53 | 55 |

ICA, Internal carotid; CCA, common carotid; ECA, external carotid

**Table 3.** Technique 2: 85 cases

| Artery | Injected quantity (ml) | Flow rate (ml/s) | No cases | Conray | Iopamidol |
|---|---|---|---|---|---|
| Unilateral ICA/CCA | 10 | 4 | 45 | 24 | 21 |
| Bilateral ICA/CCA + oblique projection | 20 + 30 | 4 | 14 | 7 | 7 |
| Unilateral ICA/CCA + additional projection | 20 | 4 | 9 | 6 | 3 |
| ICA + ECA | 10 + 7 | 4 + 3 | 5 | – | 5 |
| ECA | 7 | 3 | 2 | 2 | – |
| Vertebral | 8 | Manually | 8 | 3 | 5 |
| ICA + Vertebral | 10 + 8 | 4 + Manually | 1 | – | 1 |
| ICA + brachial | 10 + 35 | 4 + 16 | 1 | 1 | – |
| Total Cases | | | 85 | 43 | 42 |

## Anesthesia

Local anesthesia was employed in 38 patients, analgesia in 25, neuroleptoanalgesia in 9, and general anaesthesia in 12. The quality of the contrast medium seems to be independent of the choice of the various kinds of anesthesia.

## Diagnosis

Final diagnosis of the patients with normal angiographic pictures is indicated in Table 4 and pathological angiographic findings are represented in Table 5. No difference was found by using either one of the contrast medium. The material was evaluated from two standpoints: (1) radiological results and (2) adverse effects.

**Table 4.** Normal pictures: 20 cases

| Diagnosis | No cases | Conray | Iopamidol |
|---|---|---|---|
| Pituitary adenoma | 4 | 2 | 2 |
| Cranial trauma | 2 | 1 | 1 |
| Ischemic attack | 5 | 2 | 3 |
| Epilepsy | 3 | 1 | 2 |
| Intracranial hypertension | 3 | 2 | 1 |
| Eosinophilic granuloma | 1 | – | 1 |
| Orbitary venous angioma | 1 | 1 | – |
| Occipital angioma | 1 | – | 1 |
| Total | 20 | 9 | 11 |

## Radiological Results (Table 6)

Only carotid angiographic examinations have been considered, as they represent the most homogeneous group of investigations from the technical point of view. Results were excellent in 44 cases, good in 32, and adequate in 14. No examination had to be repeated. No differences were noticed between the use of Conray and Iopamidol, but better results were obtained, of course, when the internal carotid was selectively injected.

## Adverse Effects

Neither during nor after the examinations were adverse effects observed, except for the habitual ones seen in all cerebral angiographic investigations. In 23 patients studied with local anesthesia, the EEG performed before and 6 h after the injection of contrast media (10 Conray and 13 Iopamidol), remained unchanged. On the basis of what the patients reported, it might seem that the sense of rash is decreased during the injection of Iopamidol into the external carotid artery.

## Conclusions

1. Iopamidol 300 can be considered a good contrast medium in cerebral angiography, with regard to radiological and diagnostic results.
2. Iopamidol is well tolerated at the employed doses; in particular no clinical or subclinical (EEG) signs of epileptic activity have been observed.
3. The injection of Iopamidol into the external carotid artery seems to be less painful than other contrast media.

**Table 5.** Pathological findings: 65 cases

| | Diagnosis | No cases | Conray | Iopamidol |
|---|---|---|---|---|
| Tumors (26) | Meningioma | 5 | 2 | 3 |
| | Glioma | 6 | 2 | 4 |
| | Metastasis | 5 | 4 | 1 |
| | Sella turcica tumor | 9 | 3 | 6 |
| | Orbitary tumor | 1 | | 1 |
| | Total | 26 | 11 | 15 |
| Vascular diseases (33) | Aneurisma | 10 | 4 | 6 |
| | Angioma | 4 | 3 | 1 |
| | Ischemic lesion | 15 | 8 | 7 |
| | Intracerebral hematoma | 4 | 2 | 2 |
| | Total | 33 | 17 | 16 |
| Cranial trauma (6) | Carotid-cavern. Fistula | 2 | 1 | 1 |
| | Subdural Hematoma | 2 | 1 | 1 |
| | Cerebral contusion | 2 | – | 2 |
| | Total | 6 | 2 | 4 |
| | Total | 65 | 30 | 35 |

**Table 6.** Radiological results: 90 investigations

| | Excellent | | Good | | Adequate | |
|---|---|---|---|---|---|---|
| | ICA | CCA | ICA | CCA | ICA | CCA |
| Conray | 15 | 5 | 8 | 8 | 2 | 6 |
| Iopamidol | 21 | 3 | 10 | 6 | 1 | 5 |
| Total | 36 | 8 | 18 | 14 | 3 | 11 |

## References


1. Dettori P (1979) Iopamidol in myeloradiculography. In: Congr Dtsch Ges Neuroradiol May 10–12, 1979
2. Hammer B, Lackner W (1980) Iopamidol, a new non-ionic hydrosoluble contrast medium for neuroradiology. Neuroradiology 19:119–121
3. Nuzzo G, Malaguti C, Mavilla L, Fagioli L, Trevisan C (1980) Mielografia cervicale con mezzi di contrasto radio-opachi idrosolubili non ionici (Metrizamide e Iopamidolo). – Radiol Med (Torino) 66:211–214
4. Signorini E, Ciorba E, Pellicioli GP, Caputo M, Piccinin GL (1979) First experiences with the clinical use of a new Hydrosoluble non-ionic contrast medium (Iopamidol) in the study of the subarachnoid space. Rays 4:47–68
5. Smaltino F, Ciccarelli R, Cirillo S et al. (1980) Mielografia con B 15 000, un nuovo mezzo di contrasto idrosolubile non ionico. Radiol Med (Torino) 66:203–205

# Painless Angiography with Newer Contrast Media

K. Mathias, P. Billmann, and E. Schmiedel

Since the early days of radiology the efforts to improve contrast media have played a major role in angiography. The contrast agent with which Haschek and Lindenthal performed the first angiogram in 1896 was composed of cinnabar, chalk, and petroleum, a mixture suited only for postmortem examinations.

For many years pain was the most unpleasant effect of contrast media in peripheral angiography. General anesthesia or preinjection of local anesthetics was required to prevent intractable pain. Now substances are available with a decreased osmolality of about 480–620 mosmol/kg. In two double-blind studies we tested iopamidol against ioglicinate and ioxaglinate.

The indications for angiography were chronic occlusive vessel disease in 78% of the cases and in the remaining patients acute arterial thrombosis, angiodysplasia, Raynaud disease, and control angiography after vascular surgery. Every patient was informed about the two contrast medium injections for intraindividual testing. About 70% of the patients gave their written consent to the study.

All patients received the same premedication, with 10 mg triflupromazine and a local anesthesia at the groin with 5–10 ml mepivacain. The bottles with the contrast agents were coded and the code was unknown to the examiner. The flow rate depended on the degree of vessel obstruction and varied between 10 and 16 ml/s. After each contrast medium injection the patient indicated the degree of pain on a dolorimeter. The dolorimeter is a ruler with 100 scale lines, where "0" signifies "no pain at all" and "100" "intractable pain." The data were evaluated by the Wilcoxon-Pratt and the nonparametric crossover test. We looked for differences in the heat- and pain-producing effects of the various contrast agents, and the influence of the first and second injection on the pain degree.

The first group consisted of 30 patients. In one case with vomitus after the first injection we canceled the second contrast medium application. Twenty-nine patients received iopamidol and ioglicinate in a randomized sequence. Iopamidol caused impressively less pain than ioglicinate. When iopamidol was given as the first substance the difference was highly significant ($P < 0.001$). The difference was less distinct ($P < 0.05$) when iopamidol was applied as second injection. The heat sensation was somewhat less after iopamidol, but the difference was not statistically significant.

In the second group, in which the patients received iopamidol and ioxaglinic acid, 28 of the 30 cases could be evaluated statistically. Mean age and indications for angiography were comparable to the first group. Heat and pain sensations differed nonsignificantly after these contrast agents. The pain degree for the same contrast medium was always higher ($P < 0.05$) when it was given as second injection.

Iopamidol caused no side effects in 57 applications. Three of 29 patients (11%) showed contrast medium reactions after ioglicinate and 4 of 28 after ioxaglinate (14%). The difference in the frequency of side effects between the two substances is not significant. The patients developed nausea (5), vomitus (1), hypotension (1), and urticaria (1).

After ioglicinate all patients complained of heat and pain sensations. This is the reason why this substance is not used any more in our department. Iopamidol and ioxaglinic acid have similar favorable qualities in peripheral angiography. With regard to these contrast agents it is better not to speak of "painless angiography", but of "angiography with less pain". This opinion is supported by the phenomenon that the second contrast medium injection always produced significantly more pain than the first one. Hyperosmolality and chemical structure of the available contrast agents are responsible for this effect probably caused by the damage of the vessel wall, the increased permeability of the endothelial cells, and the disturbed microcirculation. Further endeavors are necessary to develop isosmolar, highly compatible contrast media. Meanwhile we prefer ioxaglinate for peripheral angiography, because it is about 10% cheaper than iopamidol. But iopamidol may be of advantage in cerebral angiography because of its low neurotoxicity [1].

## Reference


1. Hammer B, Lackner W (1980) Iopamidol, a new nonionic hydrosoluble contrast medium for neuroradiology. Neuroradiology 19:119

# Hemodynamic Changes During Aortic Arch Angiography. A Comparative Study Using Two Contrast Media: Telebrix 30 (Ioxitalamate) and Hexabrix (Ioxaglate)

J. M. Caillé, A. M. Bidabé, P. Floras, and F. Guibert-Tranier

The development of area generations of contrast media prompted us to study their side effects and to compare them with classical products during 47 aortic arch examinations. Telebrix 30, the most commonly used, is a 66% solution of meglumine of ioxitalamic acid, which contains 30% iodine. Its osmolality is 1490 mosmol/kg $H_2O$. It was compared with Hexabrix, a mixture of 28.8% sodium salts and 28.8 meglumine salts of ioxaglic acid. This new product is unusual in its weak osmolality (580 mosmol/kg $H_2O$) when compared with classical products, through its iodine content (32%) is the same. It is a monoacid dimer, that is, a structure which can carry double the quantity of iodine carried by the ion in solution.

## Material and Methods

A first series of patients (19) underwent the examination under general anesthesia. The contrast used was Telebrix 30. A second group of patients (28) underwent the same angiographic exploration with intravenous premedication given 10 min before the examination. The substance used was Hexabrix. There was no statistically significant difference between the two series for age, sex, or pathological history.

Seldinger's technique was used. Seventy milliliters of contrast were injected in 3 s by an automatic injector (angioject 2 C.G.R.). A rapid film changer of large frame size was used. This enabled many pictures to be taken at an adjustable speed. Two injections were given to obtain the right anterior oblique and left anterior oblique views.

Hemodynamic measurements – heart rate and blood pressure – were measured at different times during the examination.

t0, Control measurement, before any drug administration
t1, Immediately after induction of anesthesia or premedication
t2, During a stable period 10 min after drug administration
t3, At the end of the first series of X-rays
t4, During the stable period 5 min after injection of contrast
t5, At the end of the second set of X-rays
t6, During the stable period 5-min after the second injection of contrast
t7, At the end of a third set of X-rays
t8, During the stable period at the end of the examination

**Table 1.** Hemodynamic measurements at different times during the examination

| | Heart rate | | | | Blood pressure | | | |
|---|---|---|---|---|---|---|---|---|
| | Telebrix | | Hexabrix | | Telebrix | | Hexabrix | |
| | Mean | *P* | Mean | *P* | Mean | *P* | Mean | *P* |
| t1 | 12.5 | | 8.8 | | 19.2 | | 10.1 | |
| t2 | 13.1 | n.s | 8.1 | n.s | 15 | n.s | 9.6 | n.s |
| t3 | 20.2 | <0.01 | 14.0 | <0.05 | 42.2 | <0.001 | 9.5 | n.s |
| t4 | 10.5 | n.s | 9.2 | n.s | 16.5 | n.s | 8.9 | n.s |
| t5 | 24.1 | <0.01 | 12.3 | n.s | 38.1 | <0.01 | 10.3 | n.s |
| t6 | 16.8 | n.s | 10.3 | n.s | 8.5 | n.s | 6.3 | n.s |
| t7 | 27 | n.s | 8.6 | n.s | 35 | <0.01 | 6.5 | n.s |
| t8 | 18.8 | <0.05 | 11.8 | n.s | 10 | n.s | 8.2 | n.s |

## Results

These are shown in Table 1. Variations in heart rate and blood pressure were expressed as a percentage of the value observed before anesthesia (t0). The values for each time were compared with the value at time t1, that is at the end of induction. Student's $t$ test was used and $P < 0.05$ was considered significant. Injection of Telebrix induces a fall in blood pressure of 42%, followed by return to the original value in the minute following injection. Each injection leads to a fall in blood pressure which is immediately reversible. A change in heart rate is seen at each injection. No significant change in blood pressure was seen after injection of Hexabrix. A just significant change in heart rate was seen only at the time of the first injection. No difference was found when images were compared. Hexabrix like Telebrix gives good visualization of vessels at all measurement times.

## Discussion

All contrast media depress myocardial activity, and cause direct or indirect vasodilatation due to hypovolemia. Change in heart rate and reduced blood pressure are, therefore, the hemodynamic changes seen. There is real depression of the myocardium due to the high osmolality of the substance [5]. However, Chahine et al. [2] draw attention to the ancillary role of direct myocardial depression. Bradycardia and hypotension, which could be related to the toxic action of contrast on the myocardium, are the same when contrast is injected far from the heart. There is, therefore, a second mechanism. Vasodilatation caused by the contrast substance seems to be the most important factor causing the fall in blood pressure. This direct action may be local or generalized [4]. Local dilatation of the peripheral vascular is a direct response to the osmolality of the substance injected.

There is generalized vasodilatation when large quantities of hypertonic substances are injected. There is a fall in peripheral vascular resistance, an increased cardiac flow, and a fall in systemic blood pressure. This generalized vasodilatation produces feelings of heat and pain.

There is also indirect vasodilatation due to hemodilution. Injection into the blood of a strongly hypertonic substance stimulates influx of water from the extravascular compartment to the vascular system, the blood volume increases by the Frank Starling effect and vascular dilatation occures [3]. Hypervolemia increases the work of the left ventricle and creates a hemodynamic state in which bradycardia is the result of blood pressure regulation. This explains why some authors have considered the bradycardia which follows injection of contrast as an indicator of toxicity of the substance.

## Conclusion

The hemodynamic side effects of angiography can be attenuated when a less hypertonic substance is used [1]. Ioxaglate, whose vasodilating action is weak, produces fewer hemodynamic side effects than a classical product such as Telebrix 30.

## References


1. Almen T, Aspelin P, Levin B (1975) Effect of ionic and nonionic contrast medium on aortic and pulmonary arterial pressure. An angiocardiographic study in rabbits. Invest Radiol 10:519–528
2. Chahine RA, Raizner AE (1976) The mechanism of hypotension following angiography. Invest Radiol 11:472–478
3. Cheymol G, Mouille P, Grasland D (1977) Pharmacological investigation of cardiovascular and hemodynamic effects of salts of ioxitalamic acid in anaesthetized dogs. Arzneim Forsch 27:393–397
4. Grainger RG (1980) Osmolality of intravascular radiological contrast media. Br J Radiol 53:739–746
5. Tragardh B, Lynch PR (1980) Cardiac function during left coronary arteriography in canines with Ioxaglate, nonionic compounds and Diatrizoate. Invest Radiol 15:449–451

# B 15 000: A Nonionic Contrast Medium in Peripheral Angiography

P. Falappa, M. Rossi, A.R. Cotroneo, F.M. Danza, and R.F. Baici

A new contrast medium (CM) B 15 000 (Iopamidol), was tested, in double-blind, on 60 patients with peripheral vascular diseases, for angiographic evaluation. This nonionic CM has many interesting chemical properties: high solubility in water; complete stability (control of solution after 24 months); highly concentrated solutions are performable (over 400 mg I/cc); its osmolarity and viscosity are fairly low. Furthermore, Bracco in order to various clinical applications, furnishes solutions with different concentrations: 200, 300, 370, and 400 mg I/cc. Intermediate concentrations (adding distilled water) are easily performable. In all our patients, hematological parameters, hepatic and renal functions, before and after angiographic examination, were tested. Transfemoral aortic catheterization or a simple femoral artery puncture, were the utilized methods. The amount of CM injected varied between 50 cc (femoral injection) and 80 cc (aortic injection). A small dose of 10 cc for positioning the catheter or the needle was always injected. The pharmacological treatment (local anesthesia) was the same for all patients. Examining our results, this new CM shows many clinical and technical interesting properties. The whole arterial network is well visualized, up to distal vessels, using the same technical data of angiography carried out with ionic CM (400 m.A., 0.08 s, 95–85 Kv). No toxic reactions were noted. Usually the injection of ionic CM causes a very severe pain, especially when distal vessels are compromised and collateral circulation is developed. The pain results from a direct interaction of ionic contrast media on arterial receptors. The nonionic structure of B 15 000, may explain the complete absence of pain (only a light heat sensation) during its administration. Therefore it is possible to carry out, where necessary, multiple injections in oblique views, without any trouble or risk for patients. In conclusion: absence of pain and toxic effects, together with a satisfactory opacification, make B 15 000 the choice CM in peripheral angiography.

# First Part: Discussion

E. Zeitler

## Conclusion

Conventional ionic contrast media cause a variable degree of warm discomfort and even pain on arteriography if the procedure is done without general anesthesia.

The double-blind studies demonstrated between different contrast media have shown that the pain at the time of leg arteriography is mainly due to the hyperosmolarity of the contrast agents. The mostly prospective double-blind trials give us the possibility of summarizing all results as follows:

1. Trials between contrast materials with different osmolarity showed a highly significant difference in the sensation of pain and also a quantitatively different feeling of heat during leg angiography.
2. The trials between different contrast materials with the same low osmolarity – non-ionic and dimers – have shown no significant difference in the sensation of pain and heat.
3. The visual analogous scale method is very useful for objectifying differences in subjective parameters if they are of interest to control contrast media in angiography.
4. For practical application in leg angiography it can be concluded that contrast media with low osmolarity can be used. Pain sensations are minimal and seldom even without general anesthesia and analgetic drugs.
5. Intravenous digital angiography will considerably influence the indication for arteriography.

Intra-arterial contrast material application for control angiographies after therapeutic intervention will become superfluous in future.

Nevertheless, pretherapeutic angiography in pelvic and leg arteries now, as before, is an inevitable procedure at the present state of development, as not only the pathologic changes but also the inflow and outflow arteries must optimally be demonstrated prior to each treatment procedure. Digital intravenous angiography, which is also applicable during intra-arterial contrast material injection, can provide information of the same quality, however, at reduced contrast material quantities. The improvement in contrast material and technology clearly shows that angiography without general anesthesia involves no discomfort for the patient. The allergic reaction is the only risk which must be considered now as well as in future.

# Compared Effects on Various Blood Parameters of Iopamidol and Iodamide in Man During Infusion Urography

G. Cittadini, G.A. Gambaro, G.A. Rollandi, and F. Romanzi

Water-soluble ionic organo-iodinated uroangiographic contrast media give rise to highly hypertonic solutions. In clinical use this results in the induction of hematic hyperosmolarity with all the well-known consequences on various organs. The extent of these effects depends on injection velocity and volume of solution introduced. Some of the side effects of contrast media (CM) depend on increased permeability of the brain-blood barrier, negative effect on cardiac inotropism, possible induction of nephrosis, all mechanisms in which hematic hyperosmolarity plays an important role.

In this report we wanted to verify if and to what extent a nonionic CM, the iopamidol, differed from a traditional ionic CM, the iodamide.

## Materials and Methods

Forty-two patients (25 women and 17 men, ages ranging from 20 to 83 years) who had normal preliminary renal function were randomly divided into two groups. The first group was submitted to urographic examination with iodamide (Uromiro, Bracco, Milan, Italy); the second was examined with iopamidol (Iopamiro, Bracco, Milan, Italy). Both CM were administered with infusion technique (100 ml in 7 min; 300 mg I/ml).

Venous blood samples were drawn from each patient immediately before, at the end of infusion, and 30 and 60 min later. To keep the needle open a 5% glucose solution was run at a velocity of 0.5 ml/min immediately after the second blood drawing.

The following blood tests were carried out: osmolarity, hematocrit, BUN, creatinine, sodium, potassium, calcium, chloride, and triglycerides.

## Results and Conclusions

The results for osmolarity and hematocrit measurements, which reached levels of significance in each comparison, are reported in graph form in Figs. 1 and 2. The pairs of average values refer to the percent variations with respect to the basal value, at the end of infusion, after 30 and 60 min. Factorial analysis of variance (two CM, three postinfusional blood samples) is reported in Tables 1 and 2.

Osmolarity increased an average of 8.5% for iodamide and 5.7% for iopamidol at the end of the infusion, returning to basal values after 60 min. The difference between "times of sample drawing" was highly significant ($P = 0.01$), that between CM significant ($P = 0.05$).

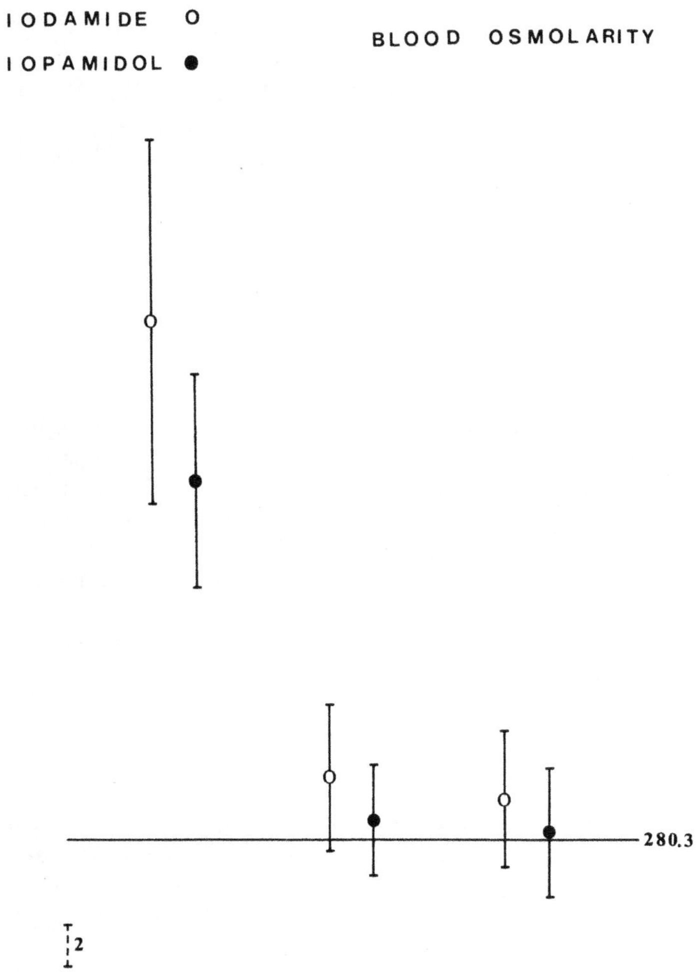


**Fig. 1.** Blood osmolarity in iodamide and iopamidol groups

**Table 1.** Iopamidol vs iodamide – blood osmolarity – factorial analysis of variance

| | D. of F. | $s^2$ | $F$ |
|---|---|---|---|
| Total | 125 | | |
| Between groups | 5 | 280.253 | 20.179** |
| Error | 120 | 13.888 | |
| Between CM | 1 | 59.451 | 4.280* |
| Between times | 2 | 655.505 | 47.198** |
| Interaction | 2 | 15.402 | 1.109 |

*, $P = 0.05$; **, $P = 0.01$

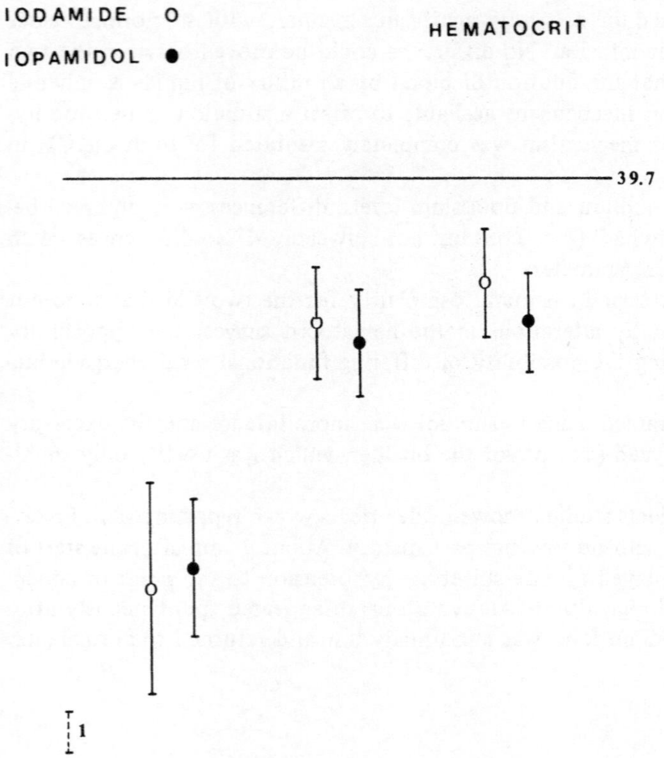


**Fig. 2.** Hematocrit in iodamide and iopamidol groups

**Table 2.** Iopamidol vs iodamide – hematocrit – factorial analysis of variance

| | D. of F. | $s^2$ | $P$ |
|---|---|---|---|
| Total | 125 | | |
| Between groups | 5 | 1607.766 | 30.109** |
| Error | 120 | 53.397 | |
| Between CM | 1 | 2.681 | 0.050 |
| Between times | 2 | 3914.499 | 73.308** |
| Interaction | 2 | 103.576 | 1.939 |

*, $P = 0.05$; **, $P = 0.01$

The hematocrit decreased in a highly significant manner, with subnormal values persisting up to 60 min after infusion. No difference could be proved between the two CM. This seem to indicate that the dilution of blood by an influx of liquids is only one of the possible compensation mechanisms available to offset a situation of hematic hyperosmolarity. However, this mechanism was completely saturated for both the CM in our experimental conditions.

For what concerns the sodium and potassium levels, differences were observed between "times of samples drawing" ($P = 0.05$) but not between CM. No differences worth noting were seen for the other parameters.

The different variations seen in hematic osmolarity for the two CM that were not completely compensated for by alterations in the hematocrit suggest the opportunity of experimentally investigating the possibility of differing functional renal charge induced by the two contrast media.

Urographic pictures obtained using iopamidol were more intense and the excretory tracts were more easily analyzed (except for the bladder, which was usually only slightly distended).

Only one of the 42 subjects studied showed side effects worth reporting. This involved a 42-year-old outpatient with no unusual past history. About 1 min after the start of the infusion the subject displayed intense shivering, hypotension to the point of collapse, nystagmus with signs of convulsion. All symptoms disappeared spontaneously after a few minutes. The basal sodium level was abnormally low and returned to normal later in the study.

## References


1. Bonati F, Felder E, Tirone P (1980) Iopamidol: new preclinical and clinical data. Invest Radiol 15 [Suppl] 310–316
2. Felder E, Pitrè D, Tirone P (1977) Radiopaque contrast media. XLIV-preclinical studies with a new non-ionic contrast agent. Farmaco [Sci] 32:835–839

# Conventional Versus Low Osmolality Nonionic and Dimeric Intravenous Contrast Media: Noninvasive Evaluation of Hemodynamic Effects

P. Vock and W.A. Fuchs

New types of contrast agents have been introduced that differ from conventional tri-iodinated substituted benzoic acids primarily by a lowered osmolality of less than twice the physiological value instead of 5–7 times [1]. Although the mechanisms of adverse reactions to contrast media are still incompletely understood, it is true to say that cardiovascular reactions – directly or indirectly – play an important part in contrast medium toxicity. It was the aim of the present study to compare noninvasively some of the parameters reflecting heart and circulatory function following i.v. application of different compounds. Impedance cardiography [2], having proved to be sufficiently exact for measuring relative, percentage changes of stroke volume, was chosen as principle testing method.

## Materials and Methods

Sodium-meglumine ioxaglate (580 mosm/kg, 320 mg I/ml) as a representative of mono-acid dimers and metrizamide (512 mosm/kg, 320 mg I/ml) as a nonionic compound were selected for study in addition to conventional sodium-meglumine diatrizoate. Inferior cavography with two individual 60-ml bolus injections in anteroposterior and oblique projection permitted two compounds to be tested. Thus two groups of 12 subjects each were exposed to diatrizoate and ioxaglate or ioxoglate and metrizamide respectively, the sequence of the compounds having been determined by randomization. Measurements were taken immediately before the injection as basic values and then during and after bolus application for 15 min. The same procedure was repeated for the second agent 20 min after the first injection. Statistical evaluation was done using the Wilcoxon test.

## Results

Neither for image quality and clinical parameters nor for ECG changes could there be found any significant differences among the compounds tested, though low osmolality products were preferred subjectively. The heart rate tended to decrease slightly within the first 10 s, increasing then for about 3 min with a peak at 30–60 s (105%–115% of basic value). Diatrizoate raised the cardiac rate significantly more than ioxaglate. The stroke volume too was lowered initially for 10–20 s (to 86%–99%), with a significantly stronger effect using metrizamide than ioxaglate. This phase again was followed by an increase of stroke volume less noticeable with metrizamide (103%), but more marked and

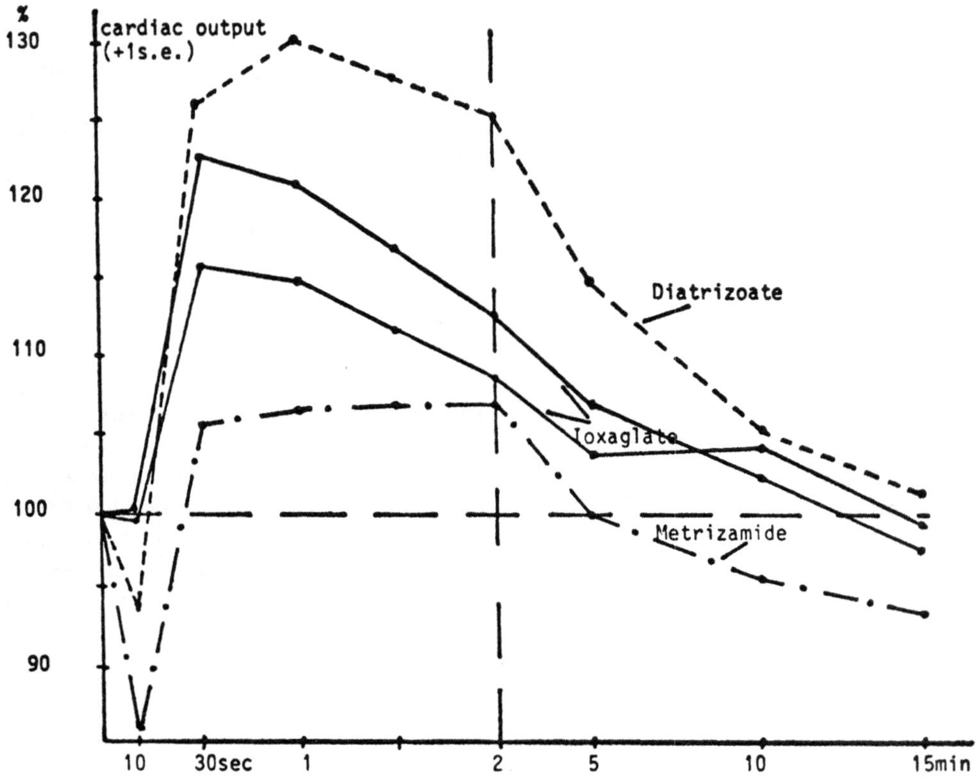


**Fig. 1.** Cardiac output after administration of three contrast media

persistent using diatrizoate (126%) in comparison to ioxaglate (115%/114%). The *cardiac output* consequently was also characterized by an initial decrease and a subsequent increase, the latter significantly higher using diatrizoate (Fig. 1).

## Discussion

Several mechanisms are involved in cardiovascular responses to contrast medium injection [1, 3, 4, 5] such as (1) direct effects on cardiac and vascular muscle cells and parasympathetic nerve system, (2) indirect release of mediators (i.e., histamine), and (3) osmolality-induced sludge of red blood cells and hemodilution, all these resulting in changes of pulmonary and systemic pressure and secondary reactive adaptations of circulation. Interpreting our results, we realize the influence of two patient groups making impossible direct comparison of metrizamide and diatrizoate, and we are conscious that timing and contribution of a particular mechanism may differ much in intracoronary, peripheral intra-arterial, and intravenous application of contrast agents. We conclude that the initial cardiodepressory phase, being slightly more expressed concerning stroke volume after the nonionic compound, is not related to osmolality. Similar to results of other investigations

[1, 4, 5], the consecutive increase of the three parameters is significantly more important with the conventional compound and thus caused primarily by hyperosmolality.

Although no severe adverse reaction has occurred, our experiments using noninvasive measurement suggest that compounds of lower osmolality might reduce the potential risk of cardiovascular side effects in routine intravenous injection of contrast media. In view of the financial aspect we think they should be preferred above all in cardiac failure and in the geriatric and pediatric age groups. In addition to better tolerance, by slower diffusion out of the vascular compartment, they offer better visualization of vessels in computed tomography and intravenous digital angiography.

## References


1. Grainger RG (1981) Formulation and clinical introduction of low osmolality contrast media. Radiologe 21:261–267
2. Kubicek WG, Kottke FJ, Ramos MU et al. (1974) The Minnesota impedance cardiograph: theory and applications. Biomed Eng (Berl) 9:410–416
3. Newell JD, Higgins CB, Kelley MJ, Green CE, Schmidt WS, Haigler F (1980) The influence of hyperosmolality on left ventricular contractile state: disparate effects of nonionic and ionic solutions. Invest Radiol 15:363–370
4. Petitier H, Crochet D, Bizais Y, Delumeau J, De Languerenne J, Le Douarin L (1978) Etude des effects hemodynamiques d'un nouveau produit de contraste a structure dimere monoacide. Ann Radiol 21:297–300
5. Trägardh B, Lynch PR (1980) Cardiac function during left coronary arteriography in canines with ioxaglate, nonionic compounds, and diatrizoate. Invest Radiol 15:449–451

# Comparative Study of the Effects to Two Contrast Media of Different Osmolarity on Pulmonary Hemodynamics and Lung Function

J.P. Senac, Ch. Prefaut, M. Adda, F.B. Michel, J. Lautrou, and V. Laporte

The aim of this study was to specify the modifications on pulmonary hemodynamics and lung function produced by ioxitalamate (Telebrix) (osmolarity = 2100 mosm/kg) and ioxaglate (Hexabrix) (osmolarity = 580 mosm/kg).

## Materials and Methods

The study was conducted during pulmonary angiographies carried out on 20 patients: 10 were given ioxitalamate and 10 ioxaglate (double-blind method). None of the patients presented cardiac, respiratory, or renal failure. Systemic arterial pressure and cardiac output (Qc) (thermodilution method) were measured every 5 min; mean pulmonary arterial pressure (Pap) and electrocardiogram were recorded continuously. The $O_2$ alveolar gradient ($D(A\text{-}a)O_2$) was also measured, both before and 10 and 25 min after the injection. The contrast media was injected into the pulmonary artery, the amount depending on body surface (35 cc/m$^2$). Injection flow was function of Pap: From 25 cc/s to 30 cc/s.

## Results

Results are shown in Tables 1, and 2. Our main observations were:
A significant increase in cardiac frequency with both media. However, Telebrix produced a sharp frequency drop in two patients, which influences the mean results.

**Table 1.** Means and standard deviations (in brackets) of the studied parameters before and after injection of ioxitalamate

| | Before | 5 min | 10 min | 15 min | 20 min | 25 min |
|---|---|---|---|---|---|---|
| Cardiac frequency (c/min) | 70.8 | 69.4 | 77.4 | 76.4 | 72.8 | 76.3 |
| | (12.3) | (15.7) | (13.5) | (12.2) | 13.8) | (14.8) |
| Cardiac output (l/min) | 5 | 6.1 | 6.3 | 5.7 | 5.7 | 5.6 |
| | (0.9) | (1.5) | (1.1) | (1) | (1) | (1.3) |
| Stroke volume (ml) | 73 | 91.1 | 83 | 76 | 80.9 | 74.5 |
| | (19.5) | (24.3) | (16.6) | (16) | (20) | (16.8) |
| Mean pulmonary artery pressure | 14.6 | 21.4 | 18.25 | 18.25 | 17.8 | 17.25 |
| (mmHg) | (5) | (6) | (5) | (5.6) | (6) | (5.9) |
| Alveolo-arterial oxygen gradient | 35.35 | | 40.6 | / | / | 39.5 |
| (mmHg) | (9.9) | | (11.8) | | | (10) |

**Table 2.** Mean and standard deviation (in brackets) of the studied parameters before and after injection of ioxaglate

| | Before | 5 min | 10 min | 15 min | 20 min | 25 min |
|---|---|---|---|---|---|---|
| Cardiac frequency (c/min) | 76.7 | 82.1 | 91.7 | 87.4 | 88.7 | 88.4 |
| | (13.8) | (14.8) | (12.2) | (12.7) | (16.7) | (14.3) |
| Cardiac output (l/min) | 4.85 | 5.8 | 5.8 | 5.97 | 6 | 5.6 |
| | (1) | (1.55) | (1.55) | (1.8) | (1.7) | (1.1) |
| Stroke volume (ml) | 65.1 | 71.7 | 64.1 | 69.1 | 68.4 | 64.2 |
| | (18.6) | (17.2) | (17.8) | (21.8) | (18.6) | (15.5) |
| Mean pulmonary artery pressure | 20.2 | 22.15 | 19.65 | 19.9 | 19.4 | 19.55 |
| (mmHg) | (8.3) | (7.9) | (6.25) | (6.5) | (6.3) | (6.3) |
| Alveolo-arterial oxygen gradient | 34.5 | / | 45.8 | / | / | 43.5 |
| (mmHg) | (6.5) | | (7.2) | | | (8.8) |

A significant increase in cardiac output with no apparent difference between the two media. But, when stroke volume is calculated by dividing cardiac output by cardiac frequency, a significant difference appears: ioxitalamate increases stroke volume significantly ($P < 0.01$), while ioxaglate does not.

With ioxitalamate, Pap increased significantly ($P < 0.001$) after 5 min, and 30 min later, the increase was still significant ($P < 0.01$), while with ioxaglate there was no significant increase.

With both media a significant increase in D (A-a) $O_2$ was observed after 10 and 25 min. Surprisingly, the effect was more pronounced with ioxaglate than with ioxitalamate.

## Discussion

The main hemodynamic observations of this study are that with the low osmolarity medium there is no significant modification in stroke volume or in mean pulmonary arterial pressure, whereas with the high osmolarity medium these modifications are very significant.

These results can be explained in the following way: The high osmolarity medium increases the medium fluid volume in pulmonary vessels. This in turn leads to an increase in stroke volume, which will increase cardiac output and pulmonary arterial pressure. The higher Pap can also be a result of red blood cell rheology, as described by Almen et al. [1]. These undesirable effects are not observed with ioxaglate, because its osmolarity is lower.

The alveolo-arterial gradient increases with both media, indicating that both cause hypoxia. This is hard to explain. At least two mechanisms can be involved. Shunt can be increased, either by an increase in the distribution of perfusion (a higher Pap) – this possibility exists only with the medium of high osmolarity – or by a decrease in ventilation: This possibility is consistent with the bronchoconstriction observed by Julien and Gamsu [2]. We can also speculate that contrast media induce lung edema, possibly through direct toxic effects.

In conclusion, although the medium of low osmolarity produces some hypoxia, it seems evident that the absence of significant hemodynamic effects makes it more usable during pulmonary angiography than the high osmolarity medium.

## References


1. Almen T, Aspelin P, Nilsson P (1980) Aortic and pulmonary arterial pressure after injection of contrast media into the right atrium of the rabbit. Acta Radiologica [Suppl] 362
2. Julien PJ, Gamsu G (1979) The effects of pulmonary angiography on bronchomotor tone. Invest Radiol 9:297–308

# Synergism of Radiographic Contrast Media and X-Irradiation

D. Carr, A.C. Walker, and R.G. White

The effect of large doses of abdominal X-irradiation and intravenous meglumine ioglycamate, individually and in combination, has been investigated in rabbits.

At the doses used, radiographic contrast medium alone caused no deaths. The X-irradiation alone caused only one death out of 15 animals. However, when radiographic contrast medium was administered 2 h after abdominal X-irradiation, there was a 60% and 70% mortality, using 750 and 400 rads respectively. Histology revealed pulmonary edema and necrotic hepatic and/or splenic foci in some of the fatal experiments.

A mechanism mediated via the kinin and clotting systems is postulated.

If the results can be extrapolated to humans, caution is advised in the administration of biliary radiographic contrast medium to patients undergoing a course of radiotherapy.

*Acknowledgment.* This work was supported by a grant from the Biomedical Research Committee of the Scottish Home and Health Department.

# Design and Synthesis of New Compounds for Hepatobiliary Imaging

C.A. Evill, M.J. Thompson, P. Habel, and G.T. Benness

Most radiologists are now well aware of the importance of the osmolality of contrast media and are familiar with the effects of osmotic diuresis on urinary iodine concentration. It has been shown that the less osmotic "dimeric" contrast media are more highly concentrated in urine than monomers. Experiments were carried out with monomer and dimer biliary molecules (iopodate and iopidamide) [1] to see if the osmotic differences would be seen in bile. It was found that iopodate and iodipamide reached almost identical iodine concentrations in bile. Results obtained by Berk [2] showed that the "monomeric" iopanoic acid also reached similar maximum iodine concentration in bile when excretion was adequate.

Excretion of all biliary contrast media causes an increase in bile flow rate; however, dimeric compounds are much more choleretic than the monomers. The excretion of 1 mmol iopidamide results in the excretion of about 25 ml bile, whereas the excretion of 1 mmol iopodate results in the excretion of only 9 ml bile.

It was suggested that micelle formation might explain the difference between the oral and intravenous agents. Iopodate and iopanoate are both excreted as the glucuronide conjugates. This conjugation produces a molecule with one highly water-soluble end and one more lipid soluble end. Such properties could enhance the incorporation of conjugated contrast molecules into bile salt micelles. In addition, it seems likely that glucuronide conjugation reduces reabsorption from the GI tract and this limits enterohepatic recirculation.

With these facts in mind it was proposed to design a conjugatable molecule carrying six, rather than three, iodine atoms in the hope that such a molecule might reach similar molar concentration to iopodate and thus have double the iodine concentration.

It was observed [3] that iopodate and iopanoate were excreted principally in conjugated form, while compounds such as iodipamide and ioglycamide, along with all the urographic agents, did not undergo significant metabolism. This is presumably due to the carboxylic acid groups of the former pair being further from the benzene ring, while in the latter compounds it is directly adjacent to the ring and thus may not be accessible to enzyme action.

For micelle formation a molecule with detergent-like properties and similar size to bile salt molecules seemed desirable. Such a compound would have to have one lipid soluble end and one water-soluble end.

With these considerations in mind a molecule with the general structure shown in Fig. 1 emerged.

Several compounds of the type shown have been produced and tested for biliary excretion in rats. So far no fully substituted compounds have been made. The testing was

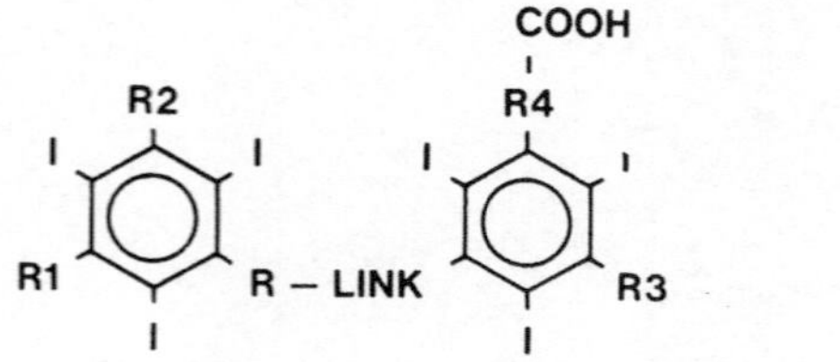


**Fig. 1.** Desirable structure of contrast medium molecule

carried out by administering 150 mg compound/kg to male hooded rats intravenously over 15 min. Some compounds were also tested via the intraduodenal route.

Figure 2 shows the bile flow rate obtained following administration of iodipamide, one of the new six-iodine compounds, and a three-iodine compound, shown on the left in Fig. 1. There is a rapid increase in bile flow following iodipamide, little change following the three-iodine compound, while the six-iodine compound appears to suppress bile flow. This result is consistent for all the six-iodine compounds so far tested.

Figure 3 shows the biliary iodine concentration reached with one of the new compounds following intravenous and intraduodenal administration. It can be seen that the new compound undergoes significant GI absorption. This is a desirable property as it would be preferable if the new molecules could be administered orally.

Figure 4 shows the iodine concentration reached with best of the new molecules compared with the maximum concentration reached with iopodate. This does not seem so impressive until the concentrations are compared at equal iodine excretion rates. Table 1 shows that at equivalent excretion rates the new compound reaches double the concentration of iodipamide and iopodate.

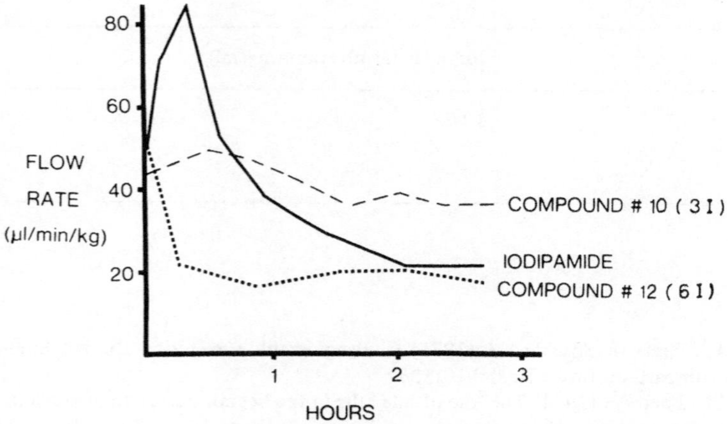


**Fig. 2.** Bile flow rates obtained following administration of iodipamide, compound # 10, and compound # 12

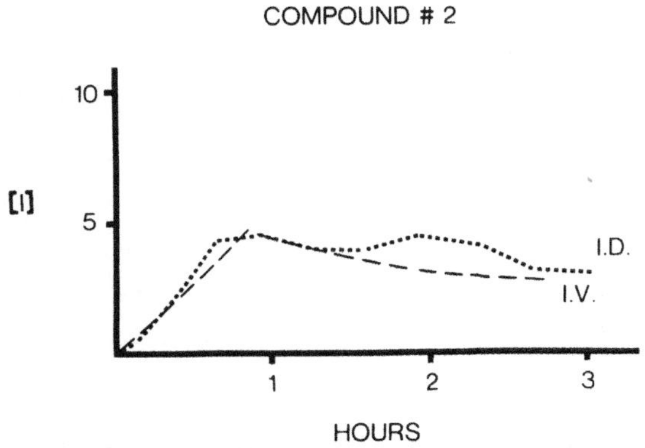


**Fig. 3.** Biliary iodine concentration with one of the new compounds following i.v. and i.d. administration

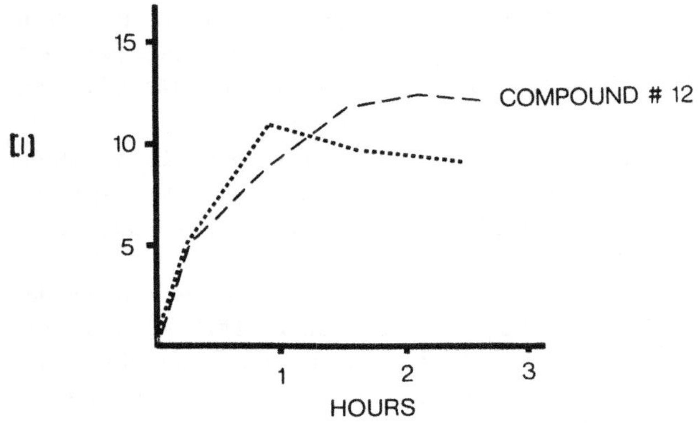


**Fig. 4.** Iodine concentrations reached with compound 12 and iopodate

**Table 1.** Iodine concentrations of three contrast media at an excretion rate of 200 mg I/kg/min

| | Iodine concentration (mg/ml) |
|---|---|
| Compound # 12 | 12 |
| Iopodate | 6 |
| Iodipamide | 6 |

## References


1. Benness GT, Evill CA, Varga D, Soschko M (1975) Cholangiographic excretion studies. Solu-Biloptin and Biligrafin comparison. Invest Radiol 10:526
2. Berk RN, Goldberger LE, Loeb PM (1974) The role of bile salts in the hepatic excretion of iopanoic acid. Invest Radiol 9:7
3. Goldberg HI, Lin SK, Thoeni R, Moss AA, Brito A (1977) Recirculation of iopanoic acid after conjugation in the liver. Invest Radiol 12:537

# Comparative Double-blind Study of Three Different Oral Contrast Media in Cholecystography

D. Doyon, A. Spira, F. Kunstlinger, H. Farah, Ch. Sassoon, A. Roche, and B. Ducot

## Introduction

In France, more than 90% of all oral cholecystograms are done using iopanoic acid (Telepaque), calcium iopadate (Solubiloptine), and bunamiodyl (Orabilix). A comparative double-blind study was carried out to determine the best oral contrast medium, their tolerance and the image quality obtained with these products in comparison with the literature on this subject [1, 2, 3, 4, 5, 6, 7].

## Material and Method

The patients in this study, performed from January 1980 to July 1981, for whom an oral cholecystogram was prescribed, were hospitalized (232) or outpatients (106). According to the status of the patient, the three contrast media were randomly allocated. The interpretation of the cholecystographic study was done by a radiologist who ignored which contrast medium was used for the examination. Before the radiographic study, the patients were asked if there was any prior jaundice, typical pain in the right upper quadrant, if they had had previous contrast medium studies and their actual bilirubin level, the type of meal they had the night before, hour of ingestion of the oral contrast medium, and finally if they experienced any secondary reactions after the ingestion of that product. The patients who had had a cholecystectomy or a biliary digestive anastomosis and those with a bilirubin level of more than 20 mg/liter were excluded from the study. The protocol for the radiologic examination was as follows:

a) A plain film of the abdomen in the few days preceding the examination. In few cases, a plain film dating less than 4 months was used.

b) The contrast medium was ingested after the meal the night before the examination (after a normal meal or a low-fat meal in 44% of the cases). The dose used for Telepaque was: six pills for 60 kg, seven pills for 61–70 kg, and eight pills for 71–80 kg. For Solubiloptine, it was 1 envelope dose. For Orabilix four pills were given for less than 60 kg, five pills for 61–70 kg, and six pills for over 70 kg.

c) Cholecystography was performed 1 day after the ingestion of contrast medium and effected in two steps:

A morphological study during which films were centered in the right upper quadrant in upright and decubitus positions with and without compression.

A functional study after a fatty meal (Bladex). The films were done at 5, 10, 15, and finally at 30 min.

Complementary films (tomography or standard) were used to determine or to confirm a pathologic process. If the gallbladder was nonvisualized a plain film of the whole abdomen and tomographic cuts of the right upper quadrant were taken. Sixty-six percent of all cone-down views were done below 70–80 Kvp. The technical quality, the quality of the gallbladder opacification, and biliary tree opacification, the quality of opacification after Bladex, the presence or absence of non-absorbed contrast medium in the digestive tract, and the radiologic diagnosis were mentioned on the cholecystographic report. This work was also associated with a prospective comparative cholecysto-echographic study, which is not included in this presentation. After verification of the comparability between groups for age, sex, height, weight, previous medical history, and symptomatology, this work analyzed the tolerance, the absorption, the opacification quality of gallbladder and biliary tree. The number of films used was also included. The statistical analysis used the CHI-2 and the variance analysis.

## Results

The 338 patients were divided into three groups. Group I: patients studied with Telepaque (111 cases); group II: patients studied with Solubiloptine (119 cases); group III: patients studied with Orabilix (108 cases). The medical history of one patient in four pointed toward a gallbladder pathology. Jaundice was noted in 17% of group I, 17% of group II, and 15% of group III (non significant difference). Numerous patients (54%) were taking medication at the time of examination. All medications including laxatives, oral contraceptives, barbiturates, and antibiotics were noted. There was no difference between groups concerning clinical or demographical characteristics.

*Tolerance.* The tolerance of the three products was judged according to the secondary effects reported by the patients. The tolerance was the worst in group I (Telepaque, secondary effects: 28%); this was due to a great number of patients complaining of diarrhea (14% for Telepaque, 1% for Orabilix, and 1% for Solubiloptine). For the other signs of intolerance, there was no difference between the three groups.

*Presence of Nonabsorbed Contrast Medium in the Digestive Tract.* This was observed more often in group I (68%) than in groups II and III (51% and 52%: $P < 0.05$).

*Gallbladder Opacification.* The greatest number of opacified gallbladders were observed with Solubiloptine (Solubiloptine, Orabilix, and Telepaque: 87%, 83%, 79% respectively). This difference is not significant. The quality of opacification was also non significantly different between the three groups.

*Visualization of the Main Bile Duct.* The opacification of the biliary tree prior to the fatty meal was observed in 28% with Telepaque, 30% with Solubiloptine, and 28% with Orabilix; after Bladex, it was 75%, 83%, and 68% respectively. There is a significant difference in these results, the opacification being obtained more often with Solubiloptine and less often with Orabilix.

*Relation Between Diarrhea and Quality of Gallbladder Opacification* shows that the quality of gallbladder opacification is independent of the diarrhea.

*Relation Between Nonabsorbed Contrast Medium and Quality of Gallbladder Opacification.* The quantity of residual nonabsorbed contrast medium is probably not related to the quality of gallbladder opacification ($P < 0.07$). The relation of renal opacification was never observed during this study. Lastly, the average number of films used does not differ significantly for the three groups (6.1, 6.6, and 6.7 respectively).

## Discussion

The comparative study of the three contrast media for oral cholecystogram showed the good tolerance of these products. The secondary effects, all without clinical importance, were observed in approximately 20% of cases.

*Relation Between Echographic Diagnosis and Nonopacification of Gallbladder for Each Product.* It was noted that the 20 nonopacified gallbladders with Telepaque were all abnormal at the echographic study. Of the 14 nonopacified gallbladders using Solubiloptine and Orabilix, five and three echographic studies were normal. This number is, however, insufficient to allow any conclusion, but it does emphasize the significantly greater incidence of diarrhea with Telepaque (14%). The other secondary effects such as vomiting, biliary pain, headache are rare and comparable for the three products.

The presence of nonabsorbed contrast medium retained in digestive tract is not rare. It is more often observed with Telepaque. This may, however, prevent other radiologic studies, particularly in hospitalized patients.

The quality of gallbladder and main bile duct opacification is the same for the three products. We have not found such a study in the literature comparing the three most popular oral contrast media for cholecystography (more than 90% of.the French market). The administration of oral contrast medium for cholecystography varies from one medical center to another [2, 4], but double dose oral cholecystography seems to have some risks [1]. In case of inadequate or nonvisualization, the interest of tomographic cuts is again noted. There is no relation between the provoked diarrhea and the quality of gallbladder opacification, neither between the presence of nonabsorbed contrast medium in the digestive tract and quality of gallbladder opacification. It seems interesting to note that in all cases in which gallbladder was not opacified with Telepaque, the echography was pathological. In the case of nonvisualized gallbladder using the two other products, the echographic study was not always abnormal. This suggests that some normal gallbladders may not be opacified when using Orabilix and Solubiloptine. However, the number of studies is insufficient to conclude definitely on this point.

## Conclusion

The comparison between three contrast media used in oral cholecystography is reported and permits us to conclude that the tolerance is the worst with Telepaque, essentially due to the frequent diarrhea associated with this product. Residual nonabsorbed contrast medium in digestive tract is also more frequent with Telepaque; however, diarrhea and presence of nonabsorbed contrast medium do not modify the quality of opacification, which is comparable for the three products studied.

*Acknowledgment.* Research undertaken with Inserm, financed by Cnamts (No. 79.1.394.8) and grant UER-Bicetre No. 80-808.

## References


1. Bismuth V, Jourde AM, Pouliot Ph (1975) Incidents et accidents de la biligraphie orale. Feuill Electroradiol XV:245–249
2. Burhenne HJ, Morris DC, Graeb DA (1981) Single-visit oral cholecystography for inpatients. Radiology 140:505–506
3. Farrell TE, Weldon WV (1961) A comparative study of Bunamiodyl (Orabilex) and iopanoic acid. (Telepaque): a clinical report on 200 cases. South Med J 54:54–56
4. Felson B (1976) Roentgenology of the gallbladder and biliary tract. A seminars in roentgenology reprint, July and October 1976. Harcourt Brace Jovanovich, New York
5. Pilbrow WJ (1980) Tomography of the biliary tract during oral cholecystography: a review of 200 cases. Clin Radiol 31:189–193
6. Tatelman M, Steel WB (1961) Comparative evaluation of oral cholecystographic media. Reprinted from J Mich State Med Soc 60:357–360
7. Whitehouse WM, Fink HE (1959) A controlled comparative statistical study of Orabilex and Telepaque in cholecystography. Univ Mich Med Bull XXV:238–242

# Can We Improve Cholecystography? A Multiple Factor Experiment

G. Cittadini, S. Cantoni, G.A. Gambaro, F. Romanzi

The diagnostic possibilities of echotomography in the study of gallbladder diseases have induced a revision of the role of oral cholecystography as the first instance examination of the cholecystopathic patient. Oral cholecystography has a fundamental role in the selection of patients suffering from gallstones who can be cured by medical treatment with biliary acids. This role is only fulfilled if the technique is as accurate as possible.

The percent of nondiagnostic cholecystographies is 19% in our patient population, dropping to 13% after immediate complement with a second dose of contrast medium (CM). The factors that influence these values are: the diet before the examination; the type of contrast medium; the modalities of administration.

On the basis of some reports in the literature [2, 3], it may be hypothesized that an interaction may exist between the pre-examination diet and type of CM used. It also seems important to give, immediately before administration of CM, a cholecystokinetic meal, which is able to induce a preliminary emptying of gallbladder.

In this study we investigated the effect on the quality of the cholecystographic picture of two different CM (iopanoic adic, Cistobil, Bracco, Milan, Italy; iocetamic acid, Colebrin, Schering, Milan, Italy) as related to the type of precholecystographic diet (fat-free diet; unrestricted diet; unrestricted diet with pre-evacuation of gallbladder).

## Materials and Methods

Two hundred and forty-nine patients were randomly divided into six groups, representing each of the six possible combinations of the three different diets and two types of CM employed.

Gallbladder pre-evacuation was obtained by administering a cholecystokinetic preparation (Byk Gulden Italia, Milan, Italy) immediately after supper. In all groups the CM was administered 30 min after the evening meal, subdividing the total dose (six tablets of 0.5 g each of iopanoic acid or iocetamic acid) within 15 min;

The cholecystogram, obtained 12–16 h after administration of CM, were classified into five groups on the basis of the degree of opacification of the gallbladder: 0 = no opacification; 1, 2 or 3 = degree of opacification inferior, equal, or superior to the 12th rib; 4 = equal or superior to the peduncle of the adjacent vertebral body. The intestinal residues of CM were evaluated with respect to their qualitative aspect [1].

For the single groups, a division was made between cholecystograms with opacification inferior to the median value of the entire series and those with opacification superior or equal to the median value. This resulted in a 2 × 2 × 3 contingency table (Table 1)

**Table 1.** Contingency table for two contrast media and three diets

Opacification inferior to median value

| | F-L D | FD | FD+KM | Total |
|---|---|---|---|---|
| Iopanoic acid | 13 | 26 | 30 | 69 |
| Iocetamic acid | 30 | 23 | 24 | 77 |
| Total | 43 | 49 | 54 | 146 |

Opacification equal or superior to median value

| | F-L D | FD | FD+KM | Total |
|---|---|---|---|---|
| Iopanoic acid | 29 | 20 | 11 | 60 |
| Iocetamic acid | 13 | 13 | 17 | 43 |
| Total | 42 | 33 | 28 | 103 |

based on the subdivision by median liable to statistical analysis with a distribution-free test of analysis of variance hypothesis [4].

## Results and Conclusions

In an overall evaluation (Table 2), the difference between the two CM was not significant ($P = 0.10$), nor was that between the three types of diet ($P = 0.20$). However, the interaction between CM and type of diet was highly significant ($P = 0.01$).

Analyzing the data in Table 1 allows us to conclude that:

1. Each contrast medium requires the appropriate diet, or viceversa each diet requires the appropriate contrast medium.
2. The appropriate diet to be followed with the use of iopanoic acid is an unrestricted diet with gallbladder pre-evacuation.
3. The appropriate diet to be followed with the use of iocetamic acid is a fat-free diet.

**Table 2.** Overall evaluation

| | $\chi^2$ | D. of f. | $P$ |
|---|---|---|---|
| Total | 19.533 | 5 | < 0.01** |
| Contrast media | 2.923 | 1 | 0.10 |
| Diet regimens | 4.073 | 2 | 0.20 |
| Interaction | 12.537 | 2 | < 0.01** |

## References


1. Evens RG, Schroer C, Koehler PR (1971) The importance of contrast absorption in the evaluation of the nonvisualized gallbladder. Radiology 98:365–398
2. Parkin GJS (1974) Dietary preparation for oral cholecystography. A critical reappraisal. Br J Radiol 47:452–453
3. Stanley RJ, Leland Melson G, Cubillo E, Hesker AE (1974) A comparison of three cholecystographic agents. A double-blind study with and without a prior fatty meal. Radiology 112:513–517
4. Wilson KV (1956) A distribution-free test of analysis of variance hypotheses. Psychol Bull 53:96–101

# Choice of Radiologic Contrast Medium: The Medico-legal Point of View

D. Fierro and M. Canale

The radiologist's responsibility in the case of contrast medium adverse reaction may be also a problem of correct choice. This seems especially true when comparing new nonionic contrast media to ionic ones. Many factors may influence the criteria of choice, but basic principles must be related to the protection of patients.

The introduction in radiodiagnostics of nonionic contrast media, with chemicophysical and toxicopharmacological characteristics capable of increasing their tolerance and therefore reducing their danger, emphasizes the importance of the radiologist's choice between ionic or nonionic contrast media.

Experimental radiology and its clinical applications of nonionic components which are now normally used in accordance with preliminary theoretical statements, allow a higher tolerance of the body and tissues or organs with which the opaque substance is in contact to be noticed, even if there are some differences arising from the instruments. Let us now briefly consider the essential data for choosing them in preference to any other.

Nonionic contrast media form a new class of molecular substances which, through three highly hydrophilic substitutes linked to the triiodobenzoic nucleus, greatly reduce the chemical toxicity, as they are not subject to an ionic scission in solution. Osmolarity, which is one of the basic parameters of tolerance, is reduced to 50%, with the same quantity of iodine. Salificate components and viscosity are also reduced. The nonionic components which are nearly completely eliminated through renal function are not metabolized. Stability in solution for iopamidol is total.

The study of clinical experiments of iopamidol of which Caresano has recently given a survey of literature together with a limited list of cases of Galliera Hospital, Genoa, reports a neurotoxic effect in the examination of cerebrospinal spaces inferior to that of lipo- and hydrosoluble ionic media, shown from a higher clinical tolerance.

Up to now, there have been no fatal complications; even immediate secondary effects are, comparatively, not very important as to frequency and seriousness. Ionographic results take advantage of a slower diffusion in liquor of nonionic media, compared with the salificate ones.

In angiography, the clinical tolerance is higher than the tolerance of salificate media, with a better collaboration of the patient, in an investigation described as "painless angiography"; there is also a lower incidence as to immediate reactions. The iconographic result can be laid upon the one obtained with ionic contrasts. Also for urography, there is a better clinical and biological tolerance and opacity appears to be darker from that contrast, in a preliminary phase, as a function of its low osmolarity.

Following these directions, it is possible to draw up a priority list of indications for the use of nonionic contrast media. The first progressive order of indications according to tolerance parameters can be modified, when there will be more precise valuations in regard to the progressive increase of cases.

## Priority List of Indications for Using Nonionic Contrast Media

1. Study on cerebrospinal liquor spaces
2. Angiographic procedures on patients presenting vascular pathology or in cardiovascular use
3. Angiographic procedures in the conscious patients
4. Other indications on the basis of theoretical premises and clinical experiments that must be confirmed:

High-risk patients (nontolerance to ionic media; impossibility to do anamnesis; patients with sickle cell anemia, etc.)
Patients under hemodialytic treatment
Patients in the infant period or infants with congenital heart disease

If the comparative assessment of risk is still the fundamental principle for making a choice between ionic and nonionic media, it is impossible to ignore that, in some cases, there are also economic problems which may influence the choice of contrast media. In fact, the present cost gives a ratio of 1 to 10, between ionic and nonionic media.

In the cases where the indication is nearly absolute (in our list, the study of cerebrospinal liquor spaces), there is no problem; in the same way it can be absolute when the contrast quantity is very low, for instance in the pediatric branch. In other cases, it is a problem of health policy or personal choice in the private branch.

When it has been asserted statistically that there is a minor danger using nonionic media, the radiologist must, nevertheless, point out to the Health Authority that it is necessary to choose the less dangerous contrast media.

In conclusion, from the medicolegal point of view, the problem of choice must be evaluated case by case, taking into account that there is the risk of severe reactions and that the problem will become less and less important as we reach a nonsignificant incidence.

## References


1. Almen T, Tragardh B (1973) Effects of non-ionic contrast media on the blood flow through the feloral artery of the dog. Acta Radiol [Suppl] (Stockh) 335:197–203
2. Caresano A (1980) Iopamiro in clinical trials: a review of the literature. Rays [Suppl] 6:1–31
3. Granger RG (1980) The osmolarity of intravascular contrast media. Br J Radiol 53:739–746
4. Hammer B, Lackner W (1980) Iopamidol, a new nonionic hydrosoluble contrast medium for neuroradiology. Neuroradiology 19:119–121
5. Stake G, Borgnes J, Monn E (1979) Urography in children. A double blind study of metrizamide and metrizoate. Ann Radiol (Paris) 22:201–206

# Section G:
# Contrast Media and CT

# Optimal Contrast Media for CT: Ionic or Nonionic, Monomer or Dimer?

P.B. Dean

The continuous development of new contrast agents with lower toxicity gives the radiologist a difficult choice. He must decide whether the reduced toxicity justifies the considerably greater expense of the newer agents. The amount of these expensive agents to be injected becomes another difficult question. The effectiveness of the new agents in CT contrast enhancement is a factor which can help the radiologist decide which to use. This effectiveness appears to be related to osmolarity, ionic nature, molecular size, and hydrophilicity.

I will discuss one of the problems facing a radiologist performing CT examinations once he has decided to give a patient intravenous contrast enhancement: which contrast agent shall he choose? Is any one of them any better or any worse than any of the others? There are a number of factors which can be taken into consideration (Table 1). Are the nonionic agents better than the ionic? The dimers better than the monomers? The hydrophilic better than the lipophilic? The isosmolar better than the hyperosmolar? Is there a use for particles or emulsions? Should the standard, low toxicity urographic agents be replaced by newer agents with still lower toxicity? Can we afford even the expensive standard agents, and can anyone afford any of the newer agents in the large volumes required by CT? Can we use the same agent for both brain and body studies, dynamic and not-so-dynamic studies? Should we give a high dose or an even higher dose? Do we even inject intra-arterially?

I do not promise to answer all these questions, and I intend to show you which of these questions cannot yet be answered. Since some of these questions can be answered from a knowledge of the pharmacokinetics of intravascular contrast media, let me base this discussion on a brief review of contrast media pharmacokinetics.

**Table 1.** Optimal intravenous contrast media for CT

| | | |
|---|---|---|
| Nonionic | vs | Ionic |
| Dimer | vs | Monomer |
| Hydrophilic | vs | Lipophilic |
| Isosmolar | vs | Hyperosmolar |
| Water-soluble | vs | Particles and emulsions |
| Low toxicity | vs | Lower toxicity |
| Expensive | vs | More expensive |
| Brain | vs | Body |
| Dynamic | vs | Less dynamic |
| High dose | vs | Higher dose |
| Intravenous | vs | Intra-arterial |

When a large dose of contrast media is injected into a vein, the contrast is rapidly diluted by blood on its way to the heart. As this contrast media bolus reaches the systemic capillaries, it begins to diffuse through the capillary wall into the interstitial fluid spaces. Diffusion to the immediate perivascular spaces is extremely rapid, but after the contrast media bolus has passed through the capillary, the contrast media diffuses further into the tissue and may already begin to diffuse back again into the capillary. Although the contrast media flux across the capillary wall is initially directed out of the capillary, renal excretion causes the blood contrast concentration to fall to such an extent that the net contrast media flux across the capillary wall soon reaches a momentary equilibrium. At this point in time, the total amount of contrast medium in the tissue under consideration is already falling (as the blood concentration falls faster than the tissue concentration rises at equilibrium flux). We are now beyond the time of interest in CT as the contrast enhancement of the tissue continues to fall [1].

Contrast enhancement will be greatest during or soon after the passage of the contrast medium bolus through the capillaries. The greater the capillary permeability and the smaller the interstitial fluid volume, the sooner the maximum contrast medium concentration will occur.

The brain is a special case. The lack of an available interstitial fluid volume and the relatively low vascular volume give immediate but very low peak contrast enhancement. Blood-brain barrier breakdown usually results in a large interstitial fluid volume and a considerably delayed peak enhancement.

Diffusion into the tissue interstitium depends not only upon the characteristics of the particular tissue in question, but also upon the contrast media concerned. Contrast media which have low protein binding, a low molecular size and a high liposolubility will diffuse more rapidly into the interstitium. However, do we really want such media?

Let us examine the types of intravascular contrast media we presently have available. In the first category we have all the ionic monomeric media in general use today, including metrizoate, iothalamate, diatrizoate, ioxithalamate and iodamide. These media cover a very wide range of hydrophilicity [5]. Although their toxicity is relatively low, with a ratio of only 1.5 iodine atoms per ion in solution, they are extremely hyperosmolar in the concentrated solutions normally injected intravascularly.

In the second category we have a monoacidic dimer, which has a ratio of three iodine atoms per ion in solution, this ratio being twice as advantageous as that of the monoacidic monomers just discussed. The only example of this group presently available is ioxaglate, which is relatively lipophilic [5].

In the third category we have the nonionic monomers, including metrizamide, the first of these low-osmolality agents to be introduced. Metrizamide is even more lipophilic than ioxaglate [5] and also more hyperosmolar at equal iodine concentrations. This group of compounds, which includes iopamidol and iohexol as two other significant examples, also has a ratio of three iodine atoms per ion in solution. These latter two compounds are relatively hydrophilic [5].

The final group under consideration is the nonionic dimers, having a ratio of six iodine atoms per ion in solution. These agents have approximately one-fourth the osmolality of the conventional agents and one-half the osmolality of the agents in the second and third categories. One agent from this group which we have had the opportunity to study, ZK 38 005, is very hydrophilic [5].

The following conclusions are based on studies performed in collaboration with Drs. Kivisaari and Kormano in Turku [4]. In the rat we found the best enhancement from the nonionic agents in the blood, kidneys and brain. The more hydrophilic agents also seem to give the best enhancement to these tissues. We have not been able to determine which of these two factors, ionic nature or hydrophilicity, is more important to this small increase in enhancement at equal total body iodine doses. We have tentatively interpreted this improved enhancement as resulting from the nonionic and hydrophilic agents remaining in higher concentrations intravascularly.

The greater enhancement which the ionic and lipophilic agents produce in the liver and pancreas may be interpreted as a higher interstitial fluid contrast concentration in these organs resulting from more rapid diffusion out of the capillaries [4].

It does not seem to matter very much whether a particular contrast agent is a monomer or a dimer, because this factor had no correlation with the degree of contrast enhancement in our studies in rats [4].

These conclusions appear to be valid in another study performed in Malmö in collaboration with Drs. Ingemann Jensen, Golman, Nyman and Almen [3]. We injected either diatrizoate or iohexol in equal doses of 1 g iodine/kg into pigs and measured the contrast enhancement in the liver and aorta during the first half hour. We also measured the iodine concentration in the arterial blood at the same time. Iohexol, a nonionic, more hydrophilic contrast medium, had a higher concentration in the blood than the ionic monomer diatrizoate. Although the higher blood concentration of iohexol gave it an initially greater liver enhancement, the greater extravascular concentration of diatrizoate caused it to have a higher liver attenuation after 4 min. However, this is really too late to be diagnostically useful, since at 4 min the contrast enhancement has already fallen to less than half of the peak values.

The following conclusions are based on a study performed on rabbits in collaboration with Dr. Violante in Rochester [2]. By increasing the dose of intravenous diatrizoate we obtained a corresponding increase in contrast enhancement in the liver, even though the peak enhancement was very short lived. By increasing the rate of injection of the contrast medium, we produced a greater peak liver enhancement. An additional observation was that there was a linear increase in enhancement with time during the injection, and that the maximum enhancement occurred immediately at the end of the injection. We concluded that in CT of the liver, in order to obtain the greatest increase in hepatic attenuation, the highest dose and fastest infusion rate which can be safely tolerated should be employed [2].

The next question is whether contrast enhancement enables us to detect even smaller tumors. In a study also performed in rabbits with Dr. Violante [7], we could detect all VX2 tumors having a minimum width equal to the scan slice width, 5 mm, before contrast enhancement. With contrast enhancement we could detect tumors down to a size of 2 mm. We still missed some of these smaller tumors at CT, but verified their presence at pathology. The smaller the tumor, the greater the tumor-tissue attenuation difference required for detection. This shows where we need contrast enhancement the most: to demonstrate small lesions which would otherwise remain undetected.

This particular study was done with a particulate, hepatosplenic contrast agent. Both particulate and emulsified contrast agents have considerable diagnostic potential, which is improving with continued improvements in toxicity.

In addition to the detection of lesions, we might also be able to improve our CT differential diagnosis by using the standard urographic agents, the cholangiographic agents and the particulate or emulsified contrast agents.

In a recent study performed in collaboration with Drs. Moss, Axel, Goldberg and Glazer in San Francisco [6], we have followed the passage of a contrast media bolus through the liver with time-enhancement curves. When comparing the maximum difference in attenuation between the liver and different malignant lesions, we sometimes found this maximum difference to occur before contrast enhancement as well as at the time of greatest hepatic enhancement. In between, the malignant lesions were sometimes less well seen, because early arterial enhancement tended to make them isodense with the liver. It is quite clear that contrast enhancement does not always make lesions more detectable: it may obscure them. In conclusion, I think that there can not be a single optimal contrast agent for CT.

The choice of nonionic versus ionic and hydrophilic versus lipophilic will be influenced by the type of organ under consideration. Whether the agent is a monomer or a dimer does not seem to be very important. The question of optimal osmolality has not yet been answered.

Particulate or emulsified agents could play an important role in both detection and differentiation of hepatic and splenic lesions.

The lower the toxicity the better, particularly since much renal toxicity remains unrecognized. Unfortunately we must make compromises as the less toxic agents are currently much too expensive. More than anything we need a hydrophilic nonionic agent with low osmolarity which is as cheap as or cheaper than the current ionic monomers.

And finally, we must have enough humility to realize that we will never image perfectly. Perhaps the worst problem is that so many patients come to us after it is too late for us ever to cure them.

## References


1. Dean PB, Plewes DB (to be published) Contrast media in CT. In: Sovak M (ed) Handbook of experimental pharmacology: contrast media. Springer, Berlin Heidelberg New York
2. Dean PB, Violante MR, Mahoney JA (1980) Hepatic CT contrast enhancement: effect of dose, duration of infusion, and time elapsed following infusion. Invest Radiol 15:158–161
3. Ingemann Jensen L, Golman K, Nyman U, Dean PB, Almen T (1981) Contrast enhancement of the liver after administration of non-ionic and ionic contrast media. In: The 39th Scandinavian congress of radiology, August 12–14, 1981
4. Kivisaari L, Dean PB, Kormano M Contrast enhancement pharmacokinetics of ionic and nonionic contrast agents.
5. Mützel W (1981) Properties of conventional contrast media. In: Felix R, Kazner E, Wegener OH (eds) Contrast media in computed tomography. Excerpta Med Int Congr Ser 561:19–26
6. Moss AA, Goldberg HI, Axel L, Dean PB, Glazer GM (1981) Detection and characterization of hepatic mass lesions by dynamic CT following three modes of contrast delivery: intravenous bolus, intrahepatic arterial bolus and intravenous drip infusion. In: The association of university radiologists 29th annual meeting, April 22–24, 1981
7. Violante MR, Dean PB (1980) Improved detectability of Vx2 carcinoma in the rabbit liver with contrast enhancement in computed tomography. Radiology 134:237–238

# The Value of Nonionic Contrast Media in CT

P. Rossi, S. D'Auria, P. Pavone, S. Minucci, L. Tipaldi, and K. McBride

Angio CT is becoming more and more common as a method for improving the visualization of vascular structures during normal CT examination, and for differentiating shadows belonging to vessels from abnormal tissues (such as lymph nodes). But the intravenous injection of contrast medium is also useful for diagnosing an alteration of a vessel (aneurysm, AV fistula) if a patient is undergoing CT prior to angiography; we have often been able to avoid the more traumatic angiographic examination. However, commonly used urographic water-soluble contrast media have a small molecular size [5], which permits a free passage through the capillary wall and an easy distribution in all the extravascular spaces, decreasing the plasmatic iodine concentration in a few seconds to levels not useful for contrast enhancement [3].

Another problem is that the machine does not allow rapid movements from one slice to another as could be useful for following the full extension of an aneurysm. To prolong the contrast enhancement we must increase the number of bolus injections, increasing at the same time the danger due to the higher amount of contrast medium injected.

Newly synthesized low osmolarity nonionic contrast medium has been proven to give a prolonged plasmatic iodine concentration in experimental animals as well as in man [5]. There is a good correlation between the iodine concentration of a tissue or blood and the contrast enhancement measured in HU (an increase of 1 mg iodine results in an increase of attenuation of 25–30 HU) [2].

We have evaluated the contrast enhancement achieved in vascular and parenchymatous structures after nonionic contrast medium injections and compared it to that obtained after injection of the same iodine amount of ionic contrast media of the type commonly used for urography or angiography. We have been using a new nonionic contrast medium, iopamidol, which is characterized by an osmolarity only two times greater than blood. Clinical trials have already been done with iopamidol, showing its usefulness in other contrastographic examinations.

## Materials and Methods

Sixty patients that were to undergo abdominal CT examination for different reasons not involved with our experiment were divided into two groups of 30 patients. Group A was composed of 15 males and 15 females ranging in age from 6 months to 79 years (mean 42); group B was composed of 16 males and 14 females, aged from 5 to 81 years (mean age 48).

The angio CT was used for clinical reasons, and contrast administered with the multiple bolus injection as described elsewhere. Iopamidol (370 mg I/ml) was used in group A, while in group B different preparations of commercially available contrast media (Uromiro 300, 300 mg I/ml, Bracco, Spa; Pielografin 60, 282 mg I/ml, Schering Corp.; Selectografin 70, 340 mg I/ml, Schering Corp.) were used. Due to the different iodine concentrations, the contrast medium injections were dosed in order to give a final amount of 1 g I/kg body weight.

Four boli were given, starting from time 0 s to 80 s, and scans were taken in between the injections and at 100 s, 120 s, and 180 s respectively.

On the images obtained in this way, we evaluated the contrast enhancement in HU at the level of vascular structures (aorta and IVC) and three parenchymatous organs (liver, spleen, and pancreas). The average of the data of each patients was then measured and a time density analysis was obtained for each organ with both ionic and nonionic contrast media.

## Considerations

For vascular structure the improvement in contrast enhancement is much better with iopamidol. In the aorta peak enhancement is achieved after the third and fourth injection of contrast medium for both ionic and nonionic contrast media, but the contrast enhancement with iopamidol is 74.7 HU more than ionic contrast medium. The decrease in contrast enhancement in the later phase is also slower with iopamidol, with an enhancement still useful at 180 s.

In the IVC iopamidol also reaches peak enhancement values higher than ionic contrast media (28.2 HU difference) and keeps a better enhancement at 180 s (31.3 HU difference).

In the parenchymatous organs iopamidol does not prove better than ionic contrast media, but in the late phase there is a persistent enhancement of liver and spleen as it vanishes with ionic contrast media (difference of 20.8 HU and 35.6 HU at 180 s for liver and spleen respectively).

## Discussion and Considerations

As we should expect, with iopamidol the enhancement of vascular structures is better and more prolonged than with ionic contrast media. In fact, the slower osmolarity avoids the movement of fluids from extravascular spaces to the blood pool. Furthermore, osmolarity is one of the factors responsible for the extravascular diffusion of contrast medium [4], and the persistence of iopamidol in the blood pool allows a prolonged vascular enhancement, useful for the execution of multiple scans.

In the parenchymal organs, iopamidol is not better than ionic, but permits again a prolonged enhancement due to the recirculation of blood still full of contrast medium at the capillary level.

We believe that for these reasons and mainly for the lesser hemodynamics and drug toxicity reactions [1], this nonionic contrast medium will find wide use in angio CT, allowing better images and a higher amount of contrast medium injection without a higher danger of hemodynamic reactions.

Finally, it is not to be forgotten, that the lesser pain sensation with iopamidol permits a good respiratory control for the patient, permitting the execution of scans at the same respiratory level in order to make good comparisons of different slices.

## References


1. Aspelin P (1978) Effects of ionic and non ionic contrast media on whole blood viscosity, plasma viscosity and hematocrit in vitro. Acta Radiol [Diagn] (Stockh) 19:977–989
2. Burgener A (1981) Contrast agents for body computed tomography. In: Fuchs WA (ed) Contrast enhancement in body computerized tomography, 11th international symposium, Thieme-Stratton, New York, pp 5–19
3. Dean PB (1981) Pharmacokinetics of contrast media in body CT. In: Fuchs WA (ed) Contrast enhancement in body computerized tomography, 11th international symposium, Thieme-Stratton, New York, pp 20–27
4. Gardeur D et al. (1980) Pharmacokinetics of contrast media: experimental results in dog and man with CT implications. J Comp Assoc Tomogr 4:178–185
5. Mutzel W (1981) Properties of conventional contrast media. In: Felix R, Kazner E, Wagener OH (eds) Contrast media in computed tomography. Excerpta Medica, Amsterdam Princeton London Geneva New York, pp 19–26

# Comparison of Contrast Enhancement Pharmacokinetics of Contrast Media in Clinical Patients

M. Kormano, R.F. Spataro, S. Soimakallio, and M. Wiljasalo

Experimental evidence suggests that the pharmacokinetic properties of several recently introduced contrast media differ from each other and from the conventionally used ionic monomers, which vary from each other as well. Gardeur et al. [4] observed that tissue distribution volume of ioxithalamate in dogs is higher than that of diatrizoate, ioxaglate, iocarmate, or metrizamide. In rat experiments the nonionic agents had a lower tissue distribution volume than the ionic agents [2]. Blood concentration measurements in man suggest that equal doses of ioxithalamate result in lower blood concentrations than those of ioxaglate and iocarmate [4].

Lower incidence of immediate side effects with nonionic monomers and the monoionic dimer ioxaglate is obvious as compared to conventional media. However, there are no investigations into how the different osmolality and diffusibility of contrast media will influence the resulting contrast enhancement of blood and tissues in clinical CT.

We have compared the contrast enhancement of blood, liver, and spleen in clinical patients after equal intravenous bolus doses of various contrast media.

## Material and Methods

### Nondynamic Studies

Altogether 25 patients undergoing CT scanning of the upper abdomen received a rapid intravenous bolus dose of contrast medium (300 mg I/kg body weight). CT scans were obtained at the end of the injection and 1, 2, 3, 5, and 15 min after the injection using a Siemens Somatom 2, a 5-second scanner (University Central Hospital of Kuopio, Finland). Sodium/meglumine diatrizoate (Urografin 60%, 292 mg I/ml, Leiras-Schering), sodium/meglumine ioxaglate (Hexabrix, 320 mg I/ml, Guerbet), and iopamidol (Iopamidol, 300 mg I/ml, Bracco) was given to seven, ten, and eight patients, respectively. CT numbers were measured in the aorta, liver, and spleen.

### Dynamic Studies

To study the immediate kinetic behavior, another series of 18 patients, using equal doses of the above-mentioned contrast media as well as ioxithalamate (Telebrix, Guerbet), was studied by scanning the patients every 10 s for the first 2 min and thereafter every minute up to 5 min after a 10-s bolus of contrast agent containing 18.5 g iodine and similar measurements were done.

## Results

### Nondynamic Studies

In the first minute after injection both ioxaglate and iopamidol showed a higher blood level of iodine in the aorta (Fig. 1). The contrast enhancement measured in the liver (Fig. 2) and spleen (Fig. 3) were slightly higher within the first minute with the two new contrast media as compared to diatrizoate. After the first minute and after equilibration of contrast media with the extracellular space, no significant difference in contrast enhancement was found in the aorta, spleen, or liver.

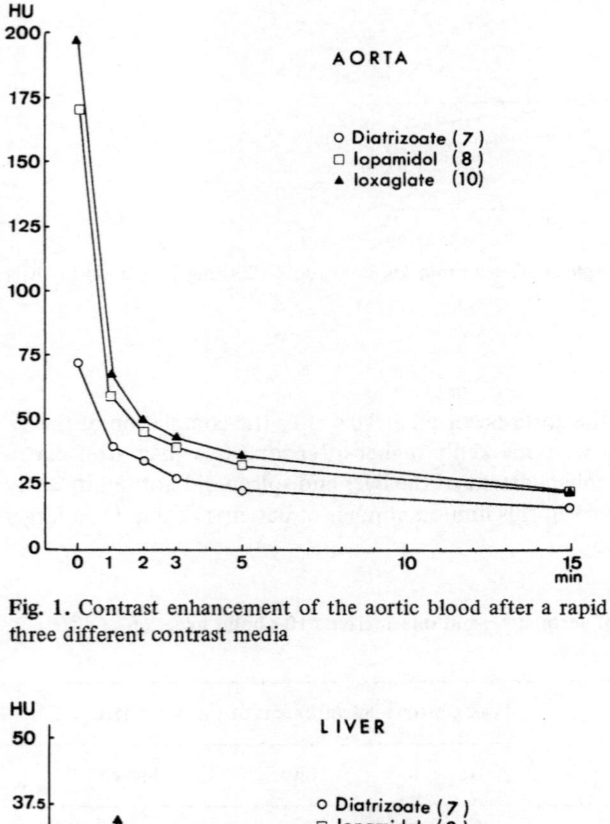


Fig. 1. Contrast enhancement of the aortic blood after a rapid i.v. bolus dose (300 mg I/kg b.w.) of three different contrast media

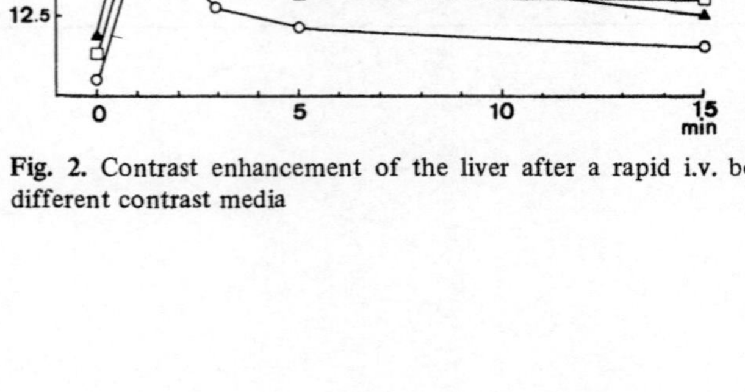


Fig. 2. Contrast enhancement of the liver after a rapid i.v. bolus dose (300 mg I/kg b.w.) of three different contrast media

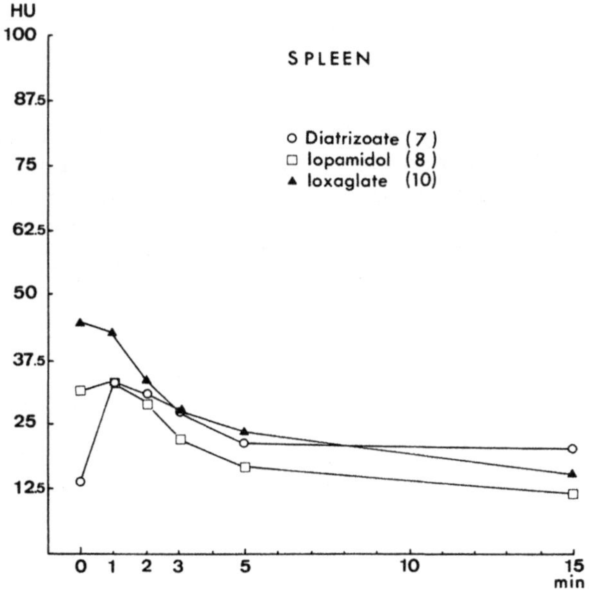


**Fig. 3.** Contrast enhancement of the spleen after a rapid i.v. bolus dose (300 mg I/kg b.w.) of three different contrast media

## Dynamic Studies

Peak concentration of iodine in the aorta occurred at 10 s after the completion of the injection. CT numbers of the aorta were markedly higher after ioxaglate than after diatrizoate or ioxithalamate. Contrast enhancement of the liver and spleen did not significantly differ with different contrast media in this limited number of patients (Table 1). A larger series of experiments is underway.

**Table 1.** Peak contrast enhancement of aorta, liver, and spleen after a 10-s bolus injection of different contrast media (18.5 g iodine in each dose)

| Contrast medium | *n* | Peak contrast enhancement of the organ (HU ± SD) | | |
|---|---|---|---|---|
| | | Aorta | Liver | Spleen |
| Ioxaglate | 5 | 266 ± 57 | 28 ± 5 | 50 ± 13 |
| Iopamidol | 3 | 229 ± 38 | 22 ± 5 | 45 ± 3 |
| Ioxithalamate | 4 | 180 ± 39 | 32 ± 5 | 54 ± 8 |
| Diatrizoate | 6 | 195 ± 12 | 34 ± 4 | 58 ± 17 |

## Discussion

Gardeur et al. [4] consider that the most diffusible contrast media should be used in routine body CT, because they produce a better tissue contrast enhancement, and that higher hydrophilicity will result in higher diffusibility. Our rat experiments [2] do not suggest positive correlation between diffusibility and hydrophilicity. The contrast media used in the nondynamic part of the present study fall into the category of medium hydrophilicity, in the order of diatrizoate, iopamidol and ioxaglate, the latter being most lipophilic [6].

As a matter of fact, the magnitude of contrast enhancement of the liver was in the order of lipophilicity, ioxaglate giving highest readings during the first 5 min. In spleen the pattern after the first minute showed no relationship between hydrophilicity and contrast enhancement. We postulate that the higher contrast enhancement within the first minute, and especially during the first passage of the contrast medium, is due to a slower dilution of the contrast bolus due to lower osmolality of the new contrast media and has no obvious relationship to other pharmacologic properties.

Because of transiently higher blood level of iodine within the first minute after intravenous bolus injection, iopamidol and ioxaglate have advantages over current contrast media in dynamic CT scanning and even more so in digital angiography. After the first minute, however, the contrast enhancement of the organs is not significantly different with different contrast media in the clinical setting during nondynamic CT scanning.

Early scans as a means of detecting small lesions with contrast enhancement is widely recognized [1, 3, 5, 7].

While better visual recognition of lesions in the early phase after bolus injection is obvious in many cases, scanner artifacts pose a problem in quantitative measurements of actual contrast enhancement of the anterior upper abdomen, due to intestinal gas and biological motion. In such circumstances, significant differences in the diffusibility of contrast agents are required to make quantitative measurements significant. Whether normal and abnormal tissues differ in their uptake and washout of different contrast media remains to be explored.

*Acknowledgement:* This investigation was in part supported financially by the Sigrid Jusélius Foundation, Helsinki, Finland.

*Addendum at proof:* An extended series including 71 patients changed the results as follows: Iopamidol produced the highest average peak and 2 minute contrast enhancement, significantly different from the other contrast media [8].

## References

1. Dean P, Kivisaari L, Kormano M (1978) The diagnostic potential of contrast enhancement pharmacokinetics. Invest Radiol 13:533–553
2. Dean P, Kivisaari L, Kormano M (1981) Contrast enhancement pharmacokinetics of five ionic and nonionic contrast agents [Abstr]. XV Int Congr Radiol, 1981, pp 381
3. Galanski M, Cramer BM, Drewes G (1980) Möglichkeiten der Kontrastmittel-Anwendung bei der Computertomographie. ROEFO 132:139–144
4. Gardeur D, Lautrou J, Millard JC, Berger N, Metzger J (1980) Pharmacokinetics of contrast media. Experimental results in dog and man with CT implications. J Comput Assist Tomogr 4:178–185

5. Hübener K-H, Klott KJ (1980) „Statisches“ und dynamisches Kontrastmittelenhancement der Körperstamm-Computertomographie. ROEFO 133:347–354
6. Mützel W (1981) Properties of conventional contrast media. In: Felix R, Kazner E, Wegener OH (eds) Contrast media in computed tomography. Excerpta Med Int Congr Ser 561:19–26
7. Young SW, Turner RJ, Castellino RA (1980) A strategy for the contrast enhancement of malignant tumors using dynamic computed tomography and intravascular pharmacokinetics. Radiology 137: 137–147
8. Kormano M, Partanen K, Soimakallio S, Kivimaki T (1982) Dynamic contrast enhancement of the upper abdomen: Effect of contrast medium and body weight. Submitted for publication in Invest Radiol

# Contrast Materials and the Liver: Application to Scanography X

J.L. Lamarque, J.M. Bruel, J.P. Rouanet, X. Triby, P. Lopez, and F. Jauvion

Despite its great sensitivity in the measurement of attenuation in density, scanography X does not spontaneously and constantly permit adequate imaging at the level of the liver, particularly in small-caliber circumscribed lesions. Based on the hepatic structure (the complex biliary vascular arborization and the various cellular systems), it is possible to enhance the coefficient of attenuation in a relatively selective manner.

Hydrosoluble contrast materials permit the enhancement of the vascular arborization. The quality of the images obtained depends on the route of injection and the timing of hepatic control. Biliary-elimination contrast materials are often inadequate to enhance the density of the hepatic parenchyma significantly and lead for the most part only to opacification of the intra- and extrahepatic biliary canals. Liposoluble contrast materials enable opacification of the parenchyma either by temporary sinusoidal embolization or by fixation of the cells of the reticuloendothelial system.

The diagnostic consequences of these different methods of artificial modification of hepatic coefficients of attenuation have relevance to scanography X. The emphasis is particularly on liposoluble contrast materials administered intravenously, as they alone appear to be capable of improving the detection of small circumscribed lesions, although hydrosoluble contrast materials remain of prime importance in the study of the nature of these lesions.

# Water-soluble Contrast Agents for Computed Tomography of the Liver: Experimental Studies in Dog

W. Mützel, O.H. Wegener, R. Souchon, and H.-J. Weinmann

## Introduction

Despite numerous attempts to develop an X-ray contrast medium (CM) especially for the liver, there is no such CM available today. With the rise of abdominal computed tomography (CT), interest has been revived in an organ-specific CM for the liver.

This interest centers on the diagnosis of smaller lesions in the liver parenchyma. Clinically speaking, there is special desire for the diagnosis of liver metastases of less than 1 cm in diameter. This goal is at best seldom achieved with the degree of image resolution available today in CT, even with the use of additional conventional contrast media.

According to our own evaluations [2], a suitable CM should effect a density gradient of 1.5–2 standard deviations from the mean measured value of the liver parenchyma and the lesion. In the practice of hepatotomography, this corresponds to density contrasts of about 35–40 Houndsfield Units (HU). If a lesion were incapable of absorbing any CM at all, the healthy parenchyma would thus have to be enhanced at least 35–40 HU. With these goals in mind experimental studies in dogs were conducted to find a new contrast media that will improve CT diagnosis.

## Experimental Approaches and Methods

The series of experiments were conducted with water-soluble contrast media for parenteral application of the dimeric hexaiodinated type. The basic type of the 5-unsubstituted dicarboxylic acids, a classic i.v. cholegraphic medium with a well-known ability to flow to the liver, was systematically chemically modified. Variations included representatives of 5,5′-substituted dicarboxylic acids, 5,5′-substituted monocarboxylic acids, and a substance of nonionic type (Fig. 1).

Test animals were predominantly Beagle dogs. The animals were intubated in phenobarbital-Na anesthesia, relaxed with suxamethonium chloride and, except in scanning times, continuously artificially respirated. The examination was conducted with an EMI CT 5005/12 scanner, which works on the rotation-translation principle. Scanning time was 20 s. Before injection of the contrast medium, the density value of the liver without contrast medium was measured with two to three scans on the same slice. Immediately after administration of the CM, and then every 5–90 min thereafter, the same liver slice was scanned. This measured the density values of the parenchyma over the course of time, i.e., it measured the kinetics of the enhancement of the liver.

| Type | Generic Name |
|---|---|
| 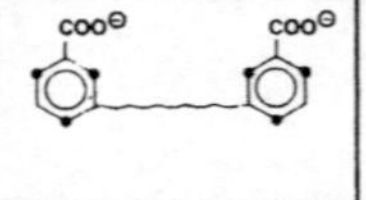 | Iodipamide<br>Iotroxate |
| 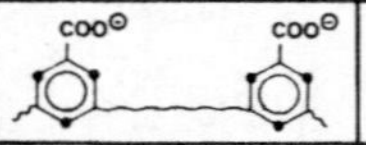 | Iosefamate |
| 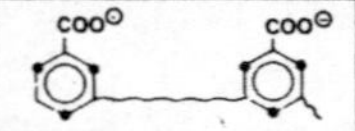 | – |
| 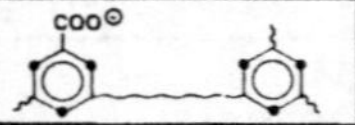 | Ioxaglate |
| 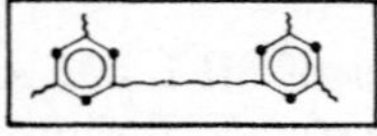 | – |

**Fig. 1.** Water-soluble dimeric hexaiodinated contrast media

## Results

The following are the results in each group of the five structural types tested:
1. Of the classical type of i.v. cholangiographic CM, iotroxate (Biliscopin), was tested, and a structural variant of iodipamide (test substance I). The dosage was 70 mg I/kg of body weight.

Iotroxate's enhancement curve showed that this CM rapidly enhances the liver, resulting in 12 HU 1 min after injection. It evidently flows quickly away by biliary excretion, as is desired in a good cholegraphic contrast medium. Test substance I was transported into the liver more slowly, but this CM also achieved a liver level, even if at a relatively low niveau of about 12 HU over the previous value, for about 60 min.
2. The substitution in a position 5 of the classic i.v. cholegraphic CM type, iotroxate and ioglycamate, led to test substances II, III, and IV. Test substance II acted very similarly to iotroxate itself, but test substances III and IV revealed an enhancement of the liver of 25–50 HU, even with the low dosage of 70 mg I/kg.

With a higher dosage of 360 mg I/kg test substance II did not produce an X-ray density in liver parenchyma that rose proportionally to the dosage increase. This could be traced to increased heterotopic excretion, together with a correspondingly lower maximum transport capacity of the substance in the liver.

Test substance III (Schering Code SH L 433 A) behaved much differently at higher dosage. With increased dosage, an almost directly proportional increase in density values was observed. The question was also examined of whether metabolism of the substance played a role in the specific and especially high enhancement of the liver in dogs after the administration of test substance III. A comparison of the high-pressure liquid chromatogram was made for solutions of the SH L 433 A preparation and aqueous liver extract with identical iodine content. This comparison did not indicate the presence of metabolites in the dogs' livers.

**Table 1.** Maximum difference in enhancement between liver and blood after intravenous injection of a 5-substituted, 5′-unsubstituted dicarboxyl dimer SH L 433 A (360 mg I/kg)

| Species | ΔHU |
|---|---|
| Cat | > 40 |
| Dog | ≈ 70 |
| Guinea pig | < 10 |
| Minipig | < 10 |
| Monkey | ≈ 40 |
| Mouse | ≈ 50 |
| Rat | < 10 |
| Rabbit | < 10 |
| Man | < 10 |

Separate experimental series studied the species-dependent behavior of SH L 433 A in regard to liver enhancement. Table 1 summarizes the results of these studies. It shows that the maximal difference of enhancement between liver and blood varies greatly from species to species after i.v. administration of SH L 433 A at a dosage of 360 mg I/kg. Dogs, mice, monkeys, and cats showed very clear differences, but differences were very small in the other animal species tested, and in humans. Differences on this scale will probably have no great relevance for clinical investigations.

3. The main feature of the third class of substance tests is the substitution of diverse functional groups in position 5 of the benzene rings. A total of seven substances in this group were tested at the lower dosage and, in part, at the higher dosage as well. Chemically, these compounds are derivatives of iodipamide, i.e., compounds with more or less elongated aliphatic chains as links between the triiodinated benzene rings. Some of the compounds are derivatives of ioglycamate or iotroxate.

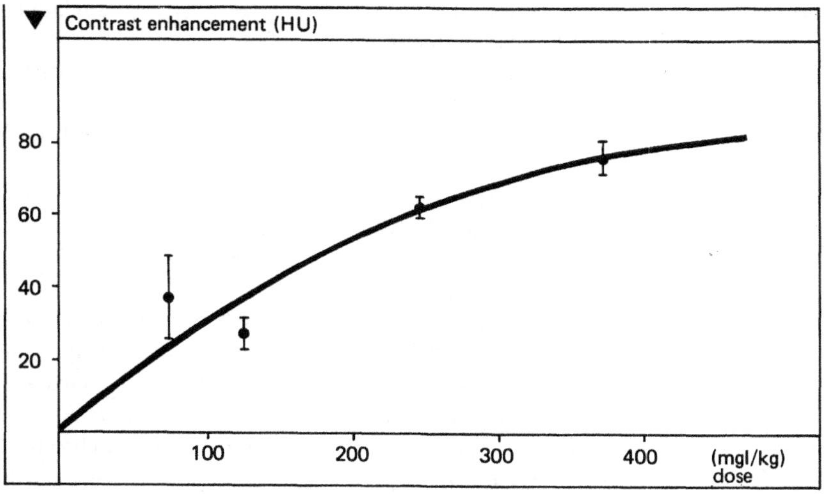


**Fig. 2.** Correlation between dose and maximum enhancement of the liver after intravenous administration of 5-substituted, 5′-unsubstituted dicarboxyl dimer SH L 433 A in dogs

The results of the density measurements can be summarized as follows: With the exception of iosefamate, none of the test substances showed a pronounced, long-lasting concentration in the liver parenchyma. After a single injection of 70 mg I/kg meglumineiosefamate, a longer-lasting enhancement of approximately 30 HU was achieved. With a higher dosage of 360 mg I/kg, the density rose to about 44 HU. Similar results were reported by Koehler et al. [1].
4. As a representative of the 5,5′-substituted dimeric monocarboxcylic acids, ioxaglate was tested, an uroangiographic CM with low osmotic pressure. This compound has relatively high protein-binding and lipophilia for its class of substances. It is therefore excreted to no small extent via the bile and thus, in part, does go into liver cells. Nevertheless, ioxaglate will probably not prove to be specifically suited to CT of the liver.
5. The last hexaiodinated substance tested was a nonionic dimer. Like ioxaglate, it is intended primarily for uroangiography. The extreme hydrophilia and extremely low affinity to proteins and membranes of the nonionic dimer produced a rapid drop in the density value of the liver with a half-life of about 70 min, which lies within the half-life of the substance's renal excretion. Contrast media of this type have a volume of distribution consisting, for all practical purposes, only of the volume of the vessel and extracellular space. They could be used well for checking the degree of vascularization in lesions in dynamic CT, especially when an extremely high dosage is necessary, since the compound is extremely well tolerated.

## Summary and Conclusions

In a homologous series of tests, the following properties were found for dimeric hexaiodinated X-ray contrast media with regard to enhancement of the liver:
1. By means of certain chemical variations of molecules in the classical i.v. cholegraphic contrast media, media result which are better suited than conventional cholegraphic media, and the general tolerance of the compounds can definitely be increased.
2. High density increases of the liver parenchyma, with specific absorption into the liver cell of dogs, are always observable only long after the bolus injection. Non-liver-specific contrast media show their maximal enhancement soon after application.
3. A dosage increase of contrast media with affinity to the liver does not always lead to a proportional density increase (e.g., iosefamic acid). That is, the desired effect cannot always be increased any further.
4. Metabolism of the compounds, and the consequent special concentration of metabolites in the liver, play no apparent role in the types of substances described here.
5. The suitability of hexaiodinated dimeric substances for raising the density of the human liver can be tested less well in dogs, monkeys, and cats than it can, for instance, in rabbits and rats.

## References

1. Koehler RE, Stanley RJ, Evens RG (1981) Iosefamate meglumine: an iodinated contrast agent for hepatic computed tomography scanning. Excerpta Med Int Congr Ser 561:88
2. Wegener OH, Mützel W, Souchon R (1980) Contrast media for computer tomography of the liver. Acta Radiol [Diagn] (Stockh) 21:239

# Contrast Enhancement Pharmacokinetics of Ionic and Nonionic Contrast Agents

L. Kivisaari, P.B. Dean, and M. Kormano

The diagnostic use of computed tomography depends upon differences in tissue attenuation for the demonstration of anatomical and pathological structures. This demonstration can be improved by manipulation of the relative attenuation of adjacent tissues with contrast materials, which can be given intravenously, into the gastrointestinal tract or into body cavities. To improve clinical diagnosis we wish (1) to differentiate the organs from each other as well as possible, (2) to make lesions within an organ detectable and (3) to identify the nature of the lesion. We have previously demonstrated that the tissue concentration of intravenously administered diatrizoate changes remarkably with time and varies considerably among tissues [1]. With the advent of new, low osmolality agents, it is important to know if their contrast enhancement will differ significantly in any organ from that produced by conventional ionic agents with higher osmolality. Knowledge of the speed and intensity of this contrast media accumulation may help us select agents producing optimal contrast media enhancement in a particular organ and help determine the time of maximum enhancement. We have approached the problem by investigating the enhancement produced by six contrast materials in 13 tissues as a function of time.

## Materials and Methods

The following six high-purity $^{125}$I-labeled contrast agents were used:
Ionic monomer: diatrizoate (Schering AG, Berlin)
Nonionic monomers: metrizamide (Nyegaard & Co. A/S, Oslo), iohexol (Nyegaard & Co. A/S, Oslo), iopamidol (Bracco Industria Chimica S.p.A., Milan)
Ionic dimer: ioxaglate (Laboratoire Guerbet, Aulnay-sous-Bois)
Nonionic dimer: iodecol (Schering AG, Berlin)

For each of these contrast agents, 25 rats were sacrificed at five time intervals (0 and 40 s, 2, 5, and 15 min after the end of the contrast media injection). The contrast dose was 612 mg iodine/kg, and contrast concentration was 264–301 mg iodine/ml. Tissue samples were taken from: blood, kidney (a transverse section including cortex and medulla), liver, spleen, stomach, pancreas, duodenum, cecum, heart, lungs, brain, testis, muscle (rectus abdominis).

The $^{125}$I activity was counted in a scintillation counter (LKB, Wallac, Turku) with corrections being made for sample decay and background. Contrast enhancement was calculated assuming 25 Hounsfield units equivalent to an iodine concentration of 1 mg/ml [4].

## Results

The calculated contrast enhancement of all the six contrast materials decreased rapidly in *blood* for the first 2 min and less rapidly after that, in a compound exponential manner. In spite of the equal doses of iodine per unit weight, the contrast enhancement produced in the blood could be divided into three groups (a: iopamidol; b: iohexol and iodeclol; c: diatrizoate, ioxaglate and metrizamide) which differed significantly from each other, iopamidol producing the highest and the last-mentioned group the lowest enhancement in blood.

All the contrast materials produced an initial rise in contrast enhancement in the *kidney*. After 40 s to 2 min the enhancement began to fall slowly. In the kidney the contrast materials could be divided into three groups according to the enhancement (a: iodecol; b: nonionic monomers and ioxaglate; c: diatrizoate) which significantly differed from each other, iodecol producing the highest enhancement.

In the *liver* the contrast enhancement produced by the six agents fell for the first 2 min, after which the enhancement of metrizamide and diatrizoate began to rise and the others continued to fall, iodecol more rapidly than the others. The shape of time-density curves [2] of the six contrast materials in the *pancreas, spleen, lung, brain,* and *heart* followed that of the exponential curves of the blood. In the pancreas, iopamidol gave the highest enhancement during the first 2 min; thereafter metrizamide produced significantly greater enhancement.

The abdominal muscle, opposite to the heart muscle, showed an initial rise in the enhancement from 40 s to 5 min, followed by a slow fall. The nonionic dimer and iopamidol showed a significantly greater enhancement after 2 min.

## Discussion

In spite of a similar iodine dose, the blood enhancement varied with different contrast agents [3]. The higher concentration of nonionic agents in the blood as compared to ionic agents is probably the basis of greater initial enhancement of nonionics in the parenchymal organs: liver, kidney, and pancreas as well as in the brain, heart, and lungs. Of the nonionic agents, the more hydrophilic [6] agents seem to give higher blood enhancement and as a result, higher organ enhancement as well, although in the liver and pancreas there was greater late enhancement with the lipophilic nonionic agent metrizamide. Monomers and dimers seem to give the same enhancement with the same iodine dose. The choice between monomers and dimers appears to be more a question of osmolality than of enhancement, although the nonionic dimer in the kidney showed long-standing, remarkably high enhancement.

In spite of the different biological and chemical properties of the modern contrast agents, the differences in contrast enhancement produced by various contrast agents were, although statistically significant under experimental conditions, not remarkable (except for the nonionic dimer in the kidney). In clinical CT work these differences among the enhancement of different contrast media may be less significant because of other factors; including the type (and speed) of the scanner and the condition of the patient (bowel contents, respiratory movements) with all the associated artifacts [5].

With further development of CT scanners these problems may be minimized and with further development of contrast agents it may be possible to enhance the particular organ or lesion in question at the time which is appropriate for the investigation.

## References


1. Dean PB, Kormano M, Kivisaari L (1978a) The diagnostic potential of contrast enhancement pharmacokinetics. Invest Radiol 13:533–540
2. Dean PB, Kivisaari L, Kormano M (1978b) Contrast enhancement: diagnostic significance from a statistical viewpoint. J Comput Assist Tomogr 2:314–318
3. Gardeur D, Lautou J, Millard JC, Berger N, Metzger J (1980) Pharmacokinetics of contrast media. Experimental results in dog and man with CT implications. J Comput Assist Tomogr 4:178–185
4. Hindmarsh T (1975) Elimination of water-soluble contrast media from the subarachnoid space. In: Lindgren E (ed) Computer tomography of brain lesions. Acta Radiol [Diagn] 346:45–50
5. Kormano M, Spataro RF, Soimakallio S, Wiljasalo M (1982) Comparison of contrast enhancement pharmacokinetics of contrast media in clinical patients. This book page 314–317
6. Mützel W (1981) Properties of conventional contrast media. In: Felix R, Kazner E, Wegener OH (eds) Contrast media in computed tomography. Excerpta Med Int Congr Ser 561:19–26

# Section H:
# New Molecules and New Images

# Futurology of Contrast Media: A Partially Warranted Prophecy

M. Sovak

Mr. Chairman, Ladies and Gentlemen: I was asked to deliver a talk about the future of contrast media. Every talk about future is a private fantasy and my talk can thus hardly be anything else. Worse, my guesses must inevitably be subjective. For those of us who put their hearts and brains into the service of contrast media, out-guessing the future of the field is necessarily an emotional game in which we mix rationality with instincts. But, for the same reason, we can often not only perceive the yet ill-defined clues to the future but sometimes also influence future's formation. Thank you for allowing me to play a prophet.

Is there a future for contrast media? If so, it is predetermined by the evolution of radiology. After decades of steady evolvement, the discipline is in the process of making a major quantitative leap forward. There is plenty of evidence that from an essentially morphologically descriptive field, diagnostic radiology is becoming a conglomerate of dynamic methods of which imaging may, in the future, be only a part. Noninvasive procedures based on ultrasound, CT, and NMR will dominate the field. Studies of dynamics of the physiologic compartments will have increasing diagnostic importance. Minimal invasiveness will be in great demand. It is probable that in the near future a by-product of NMR imaging will also emerge: analysis of the magnetic resonance signal characteristically identifying specific pathologic tissue states.

So far, noninvasive techniques have been based on advanced electronic registration of the classical physiological parameters. Novel physiological information of diagnostic importance will be supplied by CT, ultrasound, and NMR.

In the near future, the need for a blood-pool contrast agent will be generally recognized. I venture to make this statement because I believe that it will become generally obvious that to improve quantitatively morphological and dynamic information of ultrasound, CT, and possibly NMR, a reliable, stable blood-pool contrast medium (BPCM) will be indispensable. A CM confined to the vascular compartment for a reasonable period of time would allow development of new imaging techniques. A CM which does not leak from the capillary bed into the overlying tissues, thus degrading the image contrast, would make chasing time by rapid injection of large doses of CM unnecessary. Consequently, problems of systemic toxicity and anaphylactoid reactions caused by CM should be ameliorated. It is conceivable that a combination of BPCM and conventional CM in conjunction with subtraction techniques would provide new diagnostic information.

So far, polymers developed as BPCM have not been successful and I do not think them likely to succeed in the future. A BPCM must be deliverable and large polymers with molecular weight over 40 000 are too viscous. Polymers of various conventional triiodinated benzene derivatives with molecular weight varying from 10 000 to 40 000 proved also to be very toxic. Polymeric BPCM must be rapidly biodegradable which is practically impossible to achieve in a truly predictable manner.

I think it is safe to predict that the future of BPCM belongs not to the polymers, but to the concept of particulate contrast media. So far, toxicity of particulate iopamide esters coated with albumin [10], as well as the various inorganic colloids including the rare earth oxides [8], is not acceptable. These particulate CM are immediately recognized by the organism and thus engulfed by the RES. This feature limits their usefulness to potential employment only as hepatographic agents. Nevertheless, it is possible that organic compounds will be developed which will lead to useful hepatographic agents of low toxicity. For vascular imaging, other ways will be pursued. New biodegradable polymers will be developed; substances more stable and more inert in vitro and in vivo than proteins. This concept will be applied to stable encapsulation of gases to give a useful contrast medium for ultrasound vascular imaging and derivation of hemodynamic parameters. For CT scanning, a reliable BPCM will also be found.

Liposomes encapsulating conventional contrast media were themselves enveloped in great expectations which, nevertheless, failed to materialize. I am afraid that liposomes as we know them today, because of their inherently high thermodynamic instability, will not be able to reach the stage of pharmaceutical preparation. Yet, with the help of polymerization, the liposome concept should prove viable.

What will the future CT scanning be like? I venture to predict that in view of the economic realities, optimistic predictions about availability of high resolution scanners will have to be revised. Although the total number of CT units will increase, the latest generation of high resolution scanners will not be generally available soon. This will have some impact on the choice of alternative procedures, especially in intrathecal and vascular imaging whose share of the radiologist's armamentarium will not decrease markedly. We will see substantial improvement in CT cardiac imaging when new ultra-fast scanners based on completely new concepts, now operational in certain physics laboratories, will emerge. They will make the gating technology obsolete and hopefully decrease the cost.

In neuroradiology, barring the limitation imposed by availability of high resolution scanners, intrathecal contrast media will be used to a lesser degree. In the future, discopathies will be diagnosed almost exclusively by CT, although the neurosurgical preoperative evaluation will require a standard contrast media-assisted myelogram. Such was the opinion of five leading neuroradiologists and five neurosurgeons asked. It is also likely that radiopaque media will continue to be used in the cranial space but high resolution CT will rediscover the air and CT visualization of extremely small structures will thus become possible.

It is very likely that angiography is going to stay with us for many years to come. It may be partially improved by the digital procedures but neither CT, ultrasound nor NMR scanners will be able to replace the quintessential information supplied by angiography and standard radiography. There is little doubt that better contrast media are needed and will be needed, but economic realities will, for a long time, prevent a large-scale switch from the current ionic CM to new generation CM. Yet, as evidence of lower patient discomfort and lower toxicity of new CM accumulates, there will be a more vocal demand for improved CM in the future. Realistically, toxicity of current ionic contrast media is not unacceptable and the idiosyncratic toxicity will be minimized by detecting the potential reactors, thus eliminating the anaphylactoid catastrophies [7]. Evidence will accumulate that the likelihood of an anaphylactic reaction in a known or a diagnosed potential patient-reactor could be significantly diminished if new generation contrast media is used. Yet, it is unlikely that either United States or European health systems would accept the new expensive CM for general use. Therefore, compromises will appear. Variants on the current molecules will be made, and cost containment will dictate revival of older design concepts like those of radiopaque cations or usage of cheap substituents for the triiiodinated aromatic ring. If the latter succeeds, nonionic monomers may become cheaper and contrast materials for large dose application, such as angio, urography, and CT enhancement will become available.

Widespread use of lymphography has always been limited by the technique of selective cannulation. With the advent of CT, lymphography's use decreased even further. It can be expected that the method will be revived when the new two-phase contrast media appear [9]. Even though the new contrast medium may prove to opacify lymph nodes following subcutaneous limb injection, CT and possibly NMR will become diagnostically more important in this area.

We can expect that oral cholecystopaque will stay with us, based on the unsuccessful record of some 200 attempts to qualitatively improve the now ancient Iopodate and Iopanoate molecules [1].

There will be new efforts to make an agent for CT hepatography which could be administered orally or, more likely, intravenously. Therefore, it is probable that the future will bring, as a by-product, new CM for IV cholecystography.

Greatest advances will be made in nuclear magnetic resonance (NMR). The likelihood of truly revolutionary events occurring in this area is so high that I should like to digress for awhile and dwell on the present rather than on the future which in fact, for NMR, may almost be the same. Confusing modesty with uncertainty, a number of investigators have voiced their skepticism about NMR developing into a universal clinically applicable diagnostic tool, based on the long scanning times and high cost. I am certain that such skepticism will not stop development and that NMR scanning other diagnostic applicability will make this new modality an extremely important part of modern medicine. NMR will evolve not as an outright competitor to CT, but as an entirely new diagnostic tool which will also involve imaging. NMR will have a number of obvious advantages: no ionizing radiation, no known biological hazards and most importantly, a capability to obtain in a noninvasive manner biophysical signals from any part of the organism. The radiologist will have to reorient his mind in order to interpret his findings not only in terms of the gray scale contrast differences, but in terms of biophysical characteristics of normal and abnormal tissue states. He will no longer be looking at a map of electron densities such as the X-ray, but at a record of proton density in combination with a record of proton behavior in the magnetic field.

An inevitable question is sensed in this room: will NMR need contrast media and will there be any? Aye to both, in future's name. Here is why I think this way: for the moment, NMR is basically a challenge to physics. Remarkable improvements were made in a short time. This is obvious when one compares the first NMR images with those produced by the latest NMR technology utilizing superconducting magnets [4]. While most laboratories (and there are six of them of significance) expend all their efforts on grappling with the formidable technological challenges of achieving a homogenous magnetic field and other scale-up problems, researchers at University of California in San Francisco also study the basics of physiologic interpretation of NMR, working with a 6-cm NMR camera [2, 5]. In addition to other findings, these studies indicated that, with the possible exception of the CNS structures in the head, NMR imaging would be greatly enhanced if a suitable contrast material could be found. Specifically, the heart and the great vessels cannot be imaged satisfactorily with the up-to-date NMR scanning technology (Fig. 1a). It can be gleaned from Fig. 1 that the muscles, the spinal cord and the fat are imaged well while bones are not. The latter is attributed to the relative absence of hydrogens in bone tissue.

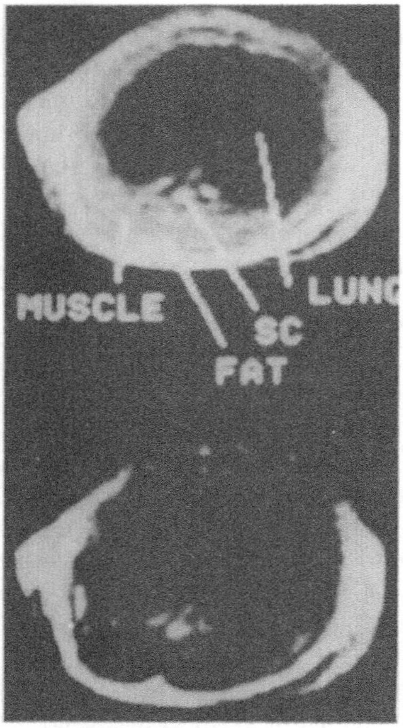

a

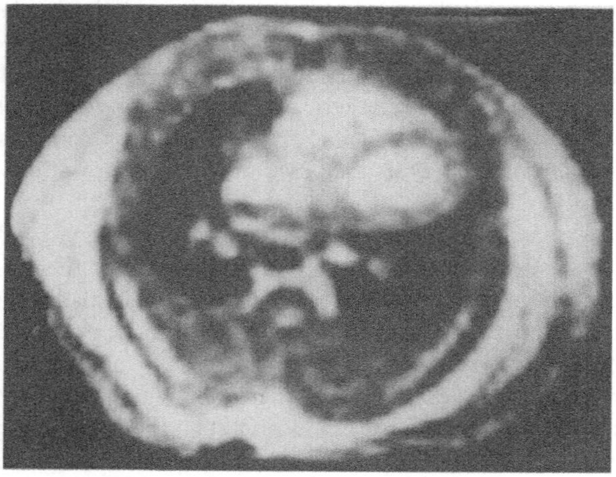
b

**Fig. 1a, b.** NMR scan of a rat's mid-thorax before (a) and after (b) intravenous experimental contrast media

Why the heart and the great vessels containing blood fail to produce an image remains to be explained, since these structures certainly contain plenty of hydrogen. The only explanation at this time is that the behavior of protons in those structures is apparently such that it prevents generation of a useful signal.

A question could be asked: why not increase the magnetic energy akin to the increase of energy in X-ray technology? Unfortunately for NMR, nature plays against this concept: more potent magnets would require higher radiofrequencies which in turn would weaken the biological NMR signal even more [6]. Thus, it is obvious that contrast must be enhanced by other means: either by introducing another atom with a magnetizable nucleus other than the proton, or by introducing substances which would affect the behavior of the body protons. The former concept has not been adequately explored, but most experimental NMR systems are based on imaging hydrogen. In a pilot experiment, using the 6-cm NMR camera at University of California at San Francisco and working with Drs. Kaufman and Crooks, one of the experimental substances which we developed as a potential NMR-CM was injected into a rat. This resulted in imaging of the heart's structures and of the great vessels (Fig. 1b). It should be noted that the rat was living and that the reasonably sharp cardiac image can possibly be explained by a minimal motion of the rat's heart in the transversal plane. Another medium was later seen on a pelvic scan as a "fluid" level within the opacified urinary bladder (Fig. 2), suggesting potential usefulness of injectable para- and ferromagnetic substances.

Protons produce the relatively strongest NMR signal and even the next strongest signal generator, fluorine, produces a signal which, for imaging purposes, is about 20 times weaker than that of hydrogen. Neither does injection of heavy metals seem to be promising due to their extreme toxicity. Oxygen, which was reported previously, is a nontoxic paramagnetic substance but it has not proved useful in imaging [3]. In the future, NMR contrast media will have to develop as a completely new class of substances designed along the familiar theme of biological inertness, rapid excretion, etc. In addition, such compounds may also have to be generating a strong NMR signal or affect the protons in

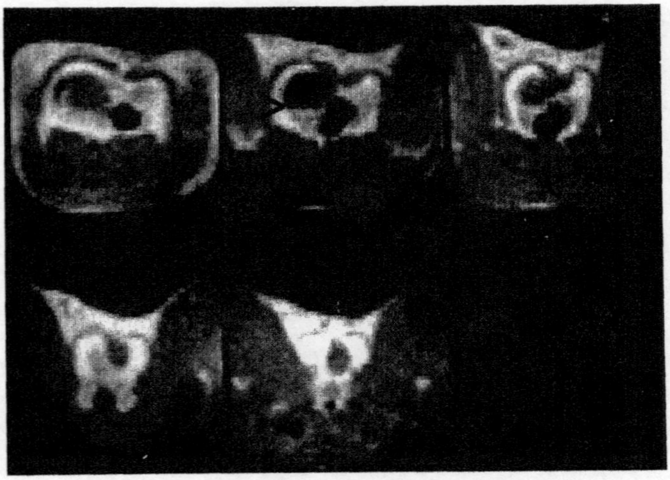

**Fig. 2.** NMR transversal cut through a rat's pelvis and the bent lower limbs: a urinary bladder containing a level of CM within the urine can be appreciated

the body in a specific way, possibly in specific compartments and/or organs. I strongly believe that it will happen. Contrast media in general will undergo a metamorphosis from adjuncts of morphological elucidation to dynamic diagnostic aids reflecting pathophysiology. We will have to reread the textbook on histochemistry and create new ones on histo- and organophysics, and it will all be great fun! I hope that you share my conclusion that contrast media's future is bright.

*Acknowledgement:* Supported in part by NIH grant CA 32852-06.

## References

1. Barnhart JL (1982) Biliary contrast materials and methods in hepatobiliary physiology. In: Sovak M (ed) Handbook of experimental pharmacology, contrast media agents volume. Springer, Berlin Heidelberg New York
2. Crooks LE, Herfkens R, Davis PL (1981) Nuclear magnetic resonance imaging at the Univ of Calif San Francisco. SPIE 273:11 Application of optical instrumentation in medicine IX
3. Gore JC, Doyle FH, Pennock JM (1981) Nuclear magnetic resonance (NMR) imaging at Hammersmith hospital. SPIE Vol. 273, Application of Optical Instrumentation in Medicine IX, 1981
4. Hawkes RC, Holland GN, Moore WS, Worthington BS (1980) Nuclear magnetic resonance imaging: an overview. Radiography 46:253
5. Herfkens R, Davis P, Crooks L, Kaufman L et al. (to be published) NMR imaging of the abnormal live rat and correlation with tissue characteristics. Radiology
6. Hoult J (1980) In: Marks JL (ed) NMR opens a new window into the body. Science 210:302
7. Lasser EC, Lang JH, Lyon SG, Hamblin AE, Howard MM (1981) Prekallikrein-Kallikrein conversion rate as a predictor of contrast material catastrophies. Radiology 140:11–15
8. Seltzer SE, Adams DF, Davis MA et al. (1979) Development of new hepatic contrast agents for CT scanning: high atomic number particulate materials. Invest Radiol 14:292–298
9. Siefert HM, Mutzel W, Schobel C, Weinmann H-J, Wenzel-Hora BI, Speck U (1980) Iotasul, a water soluble contrast agent for direct and indirect lymphography. Results of preclinical investigations. Lymphology 13:150–157
10. Violante MR, Mare KO, Owunwanne A, Fischer HW (to be published) Particulate contrast agents: characterization of albumin binding to iodipamide ethyl ester and its effect on efficacy and toxicity. [Abstr] 29th annual AUR meeting, April 1981. Invest Radiol

# Two New Classes of Low-Osmotic Contrast Agents: Triiodinated Cations and Nonionic Dimers

U. Speck and W. Mützel

In 1969 Almen proposed in a paper published in the *Journal of Theoretical Biology* several approaches to decrease the osmotic activity of currently used urographic and angiographic contrast media by reduction of the number of particles dissolved in a solution containing the usual iodine concentration. The principals proposed by Almen were: polymerization, synthesis of nonionic agents and the use of triiodinated cations instead of meglumine or sodium. With the introduction of Amipaque it became abvious that nonionic low-osmotic contrast agents are superior to the hypertonic ionic media at least in myelography and certain angiographic examinations. Thus, in the meantime the chemists have synthesized a large number of low-osmotic contrast agents according to the abovementioned principals.

Four types of low-osmotic contrast agents derived from the diatrizoate-type agents in the middle are shown in Fig. 1. On the right side the ionic compounds are shown, on the left side the nonionic agents, at the top the monomers, and at the bottom the dimers. Two compounds have already been introduced into clinical practice: metrizamide as nonionic monomer and in some countries ioxaglate, a monocarboxydimer. The comparison of these agents with new compounds of both the other types was performed in our laboratories on the basis of physicochemistry and animal experiments.

The chemical structure of one of the nonionic dimers and a group of triiodinated cations is shown in Figs. 2 and 3. Both are extremely hydrophilic due to a number of hydroxy groups. In the case of the cations the electrical charge of the amino- or methylamino-group increases the hydrophilicity and makes the molecule suitable for the formation of salts with triiodoacids like diatrizoate, iothalamate, or others. (First triiodoca-

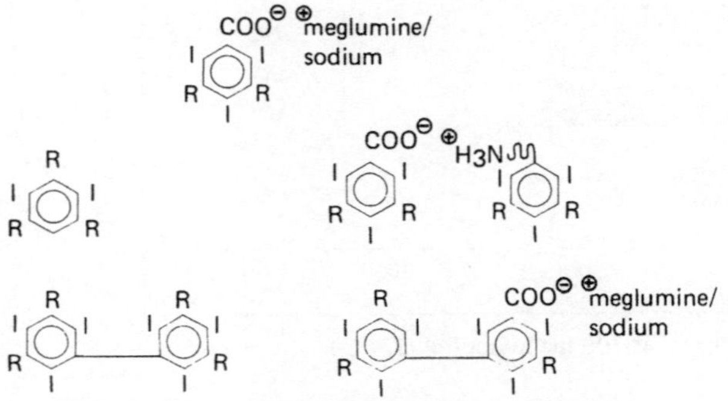


**Fig. 1.** Design of contrast agents with reduced osmotic pressure

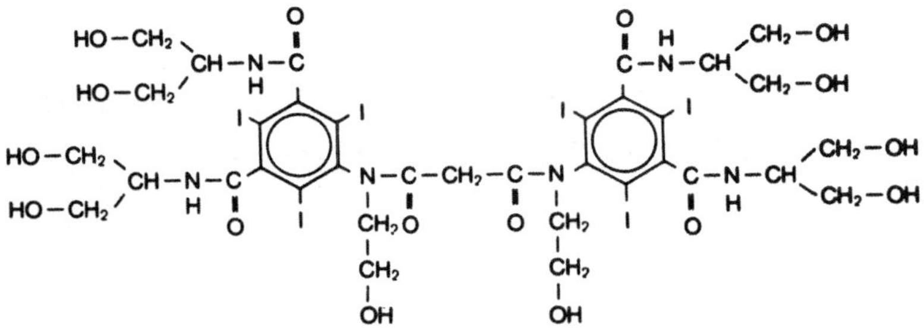

**Fig. 2.** Nonionic dimer for angiography: iodecol

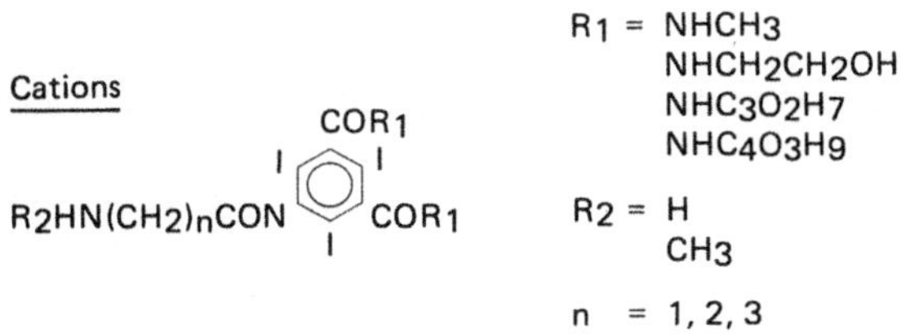


**Fig. 3.** Triiodinated cations

tions were described by M. Sovak, F.L. Weitl, J.H. Lang, and C.B. Higgins; Eur. J. Med. Chem. 14:257–260, 1979. The compounds proved to be rather toxic.)

The main reason why these new contrast agents were synthesized was to lower the osmotic pressure. Figure 4 compares the osmolality of blood and various agents at concentrations of 300 mg iodine/ml. Whereas diatrizoate is strongly hypertonic, ioxaglate and salts of triiodinated cations (and iopromide as an example of a nonionic agent) range between twice and 1.5 times the osmotic pressure of blood. From the theoretical point of

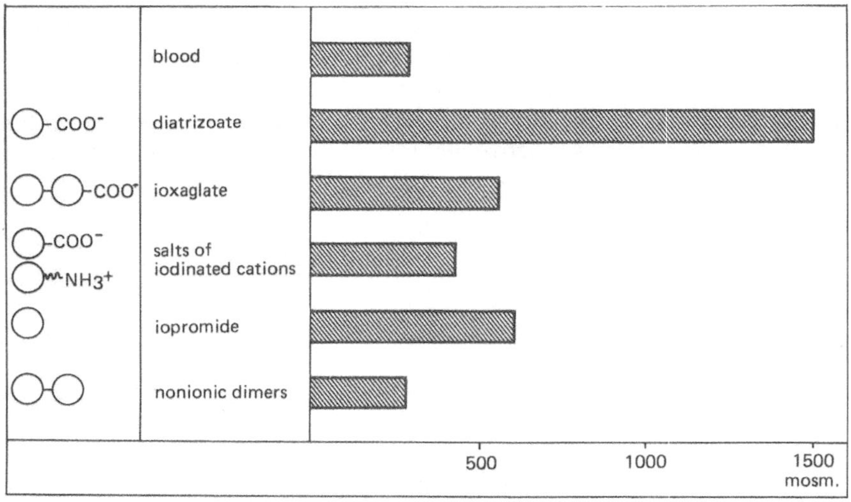


**Fig. 4.** Osmolality of various contrast agents at 300 mg iodine/ml, 37 °C

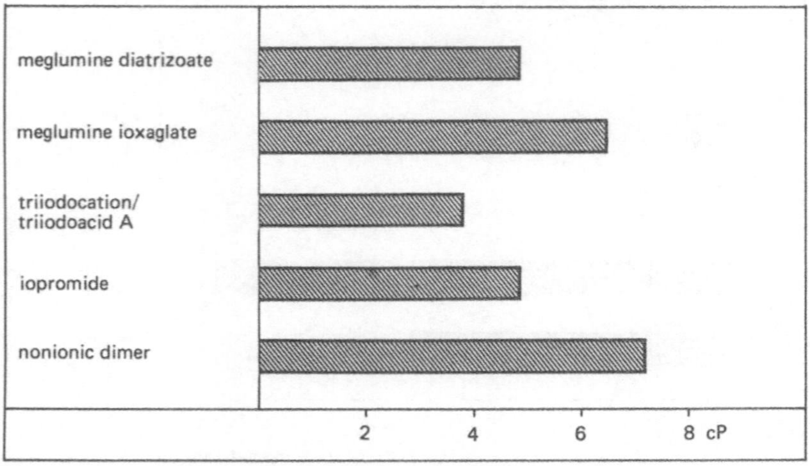


**Fig. 5.** Viscosity of various contrast agents at 300 mg iodine/ml, 37 °C

view each of these three types of contrast agents should have the same osmotic pressure. The differences observed are caused by an association of molecules and ions in the solution, which is especially marked in the case of triiodinated cations.

Viscosity of contrast medium solutions should stay within certain limits to allow rapid injection or infusion. A clear difference can be observed between the monomers of different types on the one hand and the ionic and nonionic dimers on the other hand (Fig. 5). Whereas the dimers are at the upper limit with regard to viscosity, viscosity of salts of triiodinated cations is low.

A very important property of a contrast medium is its electrical charge and the occurrence of ions. The ions move independently according to their special pharmacokinetic properties, for example, through biological membranes. This may result in an unequal distribution of electrical charge at membranes of nerve cells, thus disturbing their normal function and excludes ionic CM from the use in myelography.

On the other hand the electrical charge contributes to an extremely high degree to the solubility and hydrophilicity of ionic contrast agents. The crucial question regarding the potential use of triiodinated cations is whether there is any principal disadvantage of ionic molecules compared to nonionic compounds in intravascular application as in the subarachnoic space. The results of the following experiments may answer part of the question.

As can be predicted, ionic agents are far less tolerated by the nervous system than nonionic contrast media. A comparison of the results obtained after subarachnoidal injection in rats according to the method described by Siefert et al. 1980 demonstrates that none of the ionic agents achieved an $LD_{50}$ value similar to metrizamide (Fig. 6).

In contrast to the neurotoxicity, tolerance after i.v. injection is not influenced by the electrical charge of ions in such a striking way (Fig. 7). The $LD_{50}$ of contrast agents after intravenous injection in rats was found to be about 7 g iodine/kg in the case of a conventional ionic agent and ioxaglate. High osmotic pressure may contribute to the toxicity of the first-mentioned compound, and lipophilicity may cause the toxicity of ioxaglate. Salts of triiodocations and nonionic monomers such as iopromide, iopamidol, and metrizamide

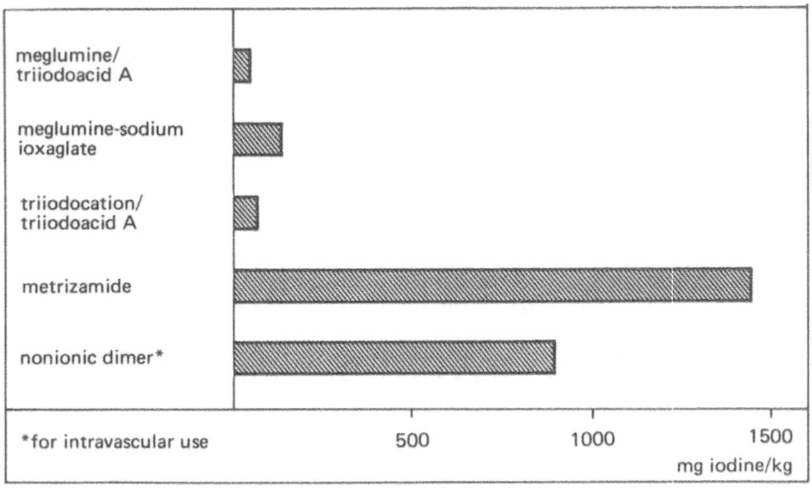


**Fig. 6.** Neural tolerance of various contrast agents after pericerebral injection in rats; $LD_{50}$ (mg iodine/kg)

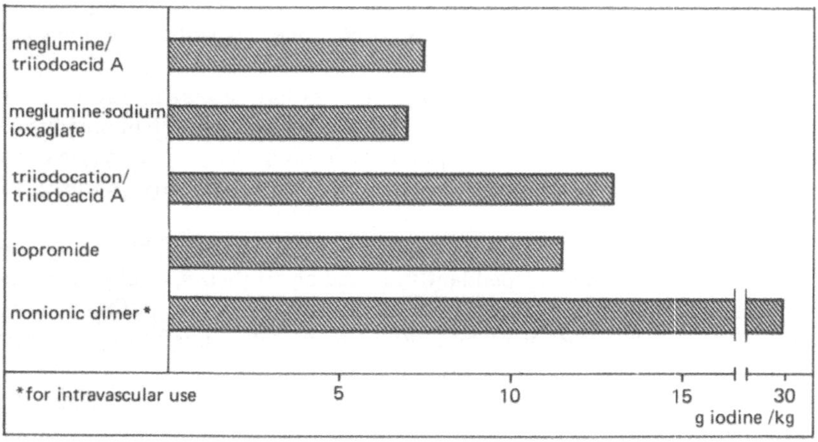


**Fig. 7.** $LD_{50}$ of various contrast agents after intravenous injection in rats, 300 mg iodine/ml, 2 ml/min

are tolerated at higher dosages since osmotic pressure and lipophilicity are lower. Optimization of the chemical structure of nonionic dimers in the recent past has led to extremely untoxic compounds. One of these dimers especially designed for angiographic use was tested in direct comparison to metrizamide. The $LD_{50}$ of this dimer was at least twice that of nonionic monomers.

None of the CM with reduced osmotic pressure causes pain in peripheral arteriography. This was concluded from experiments performed in conscious mobile rats by injecting the contrast media into the femoral artery (Speck et al. 1980). No difference could be observed between ionic and nonionic agents in this regard.

An angiographic examination in which a number of pharmacological properties of the contrast agent are decisive for the overall tolerance is cerebral angiography. Injection

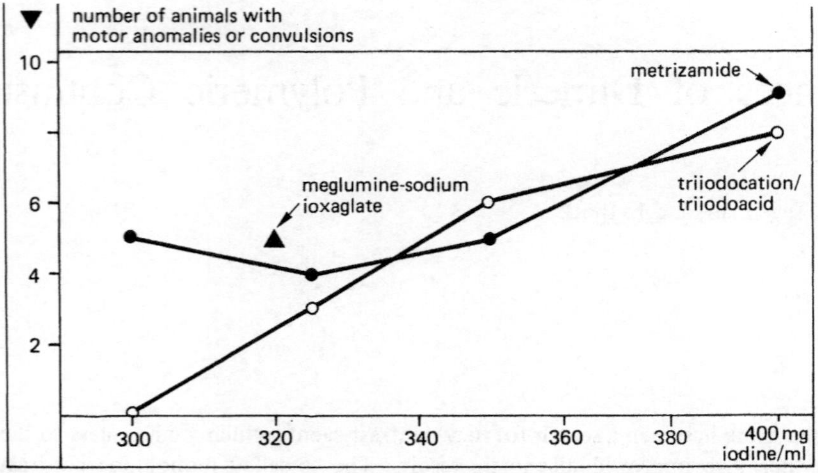


**Fig. 8.** Neurotoxicity of various contrast agents after intracarotid injection in rats; 1.0 ml/animal, 300–400 mg iodine/ml, $n = 10$ per concentration

of contrast material was performed in the carotid artery of rats (Siefert et al. 1980). The number of animals with unequivocally neurotoxic reactions to various iodine concentrations of the contrast solution was registered. In this experiment the salt of a triiodocation proves to be at least as well tolerated as metrizamide and ioxaglate, the last two being used in this indication in clinical practice (Fig. 8).

The following conclusions may be drawn from the physicochemical data and pharmacological studies:

Nonionic monomers and salts of triiodocations should be most suitable for angiography, urography and CT enhancement due to their low viscosity and low local and systemic toxicity. Dimers will only be useful if the tolerance is far superior to monomers, thus compensating for the higher viscosity.

Some pharmacological experiments do point to such advantages in the case of nonionic dimers.

For myelography ionic contrast agents should definitely be discarded. Nonionic dimers look most promising because higher viscosity is an advantage in myelography, and the pharmacological properties of these compounds should be superior to all other contrast agents (Sovak et al., 1982).

## References

1. Almen T (1969) Contrast agent design. Some aspects on the synthesis of water soluble contrast agents of low osmolality. J Theor Biol 24:216
2. Siefert H-M, Press W-R, Speck U (1980) Tolerance to iohexol after intracisternal, intracerebral and intraarterial injection in the rat. Acta Radiol [Suppl] (Stockh) 362:77
3. Sovak M, Ranganathan R, Speck U (1982) Nonionic dimer: Development and initial testing of an intrathecal contrast agent. Radiology 142:115
4. Speck U, Mützel W, Mannesmann G, Siefert H-M (1980) Pharmacology of nonionic dimers. Invest Radiol [Suppl] 15:317

# Experiences of Dimeric and Polymeric Contrast Agents

U. Erikson, B. Ingelman, and L. Björk

For a long time there has been a search for new contrast agents which are harmless to the patient and which give improved diagnostic results. The so-called monomeric contrast agents very often cause the patients discomfort in the form of a sensation of heat and intense pain, and frequently also have effects upon the blood pressure and blood flow. Apart from the unpleasantness for the patients, this discomfort may give rise to involuntary movements and thus disturb the angiographic investigation.

Since the early 1960s, a team in Uppsala including the three present authors has conducted research on dimeric and polymeric contrast agents. This communication will briefly present some of the results.

## Dimeric Contrast Agents

Within the group of dimeric compounds which were synthesized, a compound which was given the code number PhDZ 59A was chosen for further studies. This compound was later named iozomic acid. Its chemical structure is given in Fig. 1. A solution containing 235 mg I/ml of its methylglucamine salt (PhDZ 59B) was used for clinical investigations. We have previously reported our experiences with this contrast agent in angiocardiography, thoracic angiography, peripheral, coronary, carotid, and renal arteriography, hysterosalpingography, and arthrography [1, 2, 4].

The results were quite favorable. In double-blind studies we have now tested the new contrast agent in 123 patients. For comparison, monomeric contrast agent solutions with the same iodine content were used, such as diatrizoate, metrizoate, and iothalamate preparations. As seen in Table 1, this dimeric contrast agent caused much less discomfort to the patients than the compared monomeric contrast agents. Ninety-three patients reported that the dimer caused least discomfort. Only six patients stated that the dimer caused most discomfort, but in these cases the degree of discomfort was very low. Studies have

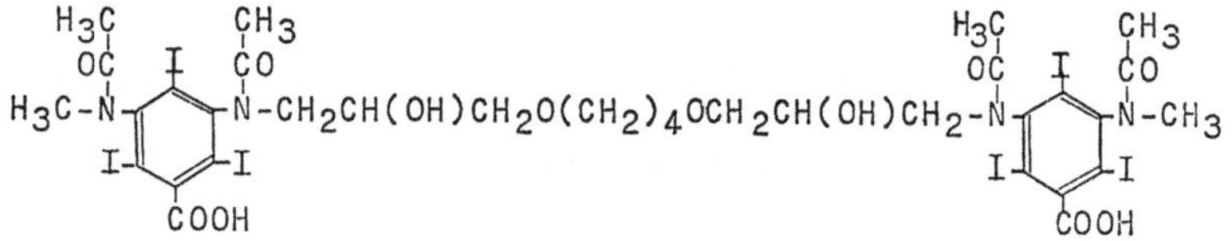


**Fig. 1.** Chemical structure of the new contrast agent (iozomic acid) in its acid form. The methylglucamine salt of this acid was used in the clinical investigations

**Table 1.** Summary of double-blind studies of adverse subjective effects after angiography in 123 patients in whom the methylglucamine salt of iozomic acid was compared with diatrizoate, metrizoate, and iothalamate preparations (monomeric compounds)

| | Contrast agent | |
|---|---|---|
| | PhDZ 59B | Other contrast agent |
| Least discomfort | 93 | 6 |
| Most discomfort | 6 | 93 |
| No difference | 24 | 24 |

also shown that this dimeric contrast agent has a favorably low effect upon the blood pressure and blood flow. It is therefore an improvement in several respects over the generally used ionic monomeric contrast agents. The reduced degree of pain after injection is a particular advantage, a finding which confirmed our initial theory of the value of dimeric contrast agents for intravascular use. This contrast agent has now been submitted for registration in Holland under the name of Neoangiobrine.

In recent years, favorable results have also been reported from tests with other dimeric contrast agents, for example, ioxaglate, which is marketed as Hexabrix [7].

The desire to introduce agents which cause as little trouble as possible for both the patient and the investigator has meant an increased interest in dimeric as well as in nonionic contrast agents.

## Water-soluble Polymeric Contrast Agents

Different water-soluble polymeric contrast agents of varying average molecular weights were synthesized, both for gastrointestinal and vascular use, and tested in animal investigations [3, 5]. As the polymers for gastrointestinal use were also soluble in the acid gastric juice, and had other favorable properties, they are interesting alternatives in some situations to the contrast agents generally used for this purpose. Polymeric contrast agents with molecular weights of 4000–40 000 were also employed for angiography in rabbits and dogs. Good filling of both arteries and veins was obtained, although the agents were rapidly excreted in the urine. The research in this area is still at an early stage and there is much to be done before the best molecular sizes and structures of the polymer molecules are ascertained for various uses. This ought to prove a rewarding field for future research. It may be mentioned that we initially started our studies with an interesting research model with a colloidal thorium dioxide preparation called Thorotrast, in animal experiments [6].

## Suspensions of Water-insoluble Polymeric Gel Particles

Complete new types of insoluble polymeric contrast agents, for example, for use in the gastrointestinal tract, have been synthesized by Dr. Ingelman. These agents consist of very small polymeric particles. The polymers have a three-dimensional network structure held together by covalent bonds. The structure also includes covalent bound, iodine-substituted aromatic groups as well as hydrophilic groups. The particles are insoluble, but swell in water to small soft gel particles. If the particles are sufficiently small it is possible to prepare stable suspensions. The specific gravity of the water-swollen particles is very low, compared with that of barium sulphate. Particles which do not grow or aggregate in the suspensions can also be prepared. Therefore, small particles of these agents will show less sedimentation and flocculation than barium sulphate. The contrast-giving, small, swollen, soft, inert gel particles in the suspension have very little effect on gastrointestinal function. These new types of contrast agents are described in the British patent 1400985 and the French patent 2200018.

## Method, Material, and Results

Six dogs weighing 15–20 kg were given suspensions of such small contrast-giving gel particles orally, to allow visualization of the gastrointestinal tract. The radiographs were of good quality and the passage time was normal. No adverse effects were noted. An example of this is shown in Figs. 2–4.

In Figs. 2–4 the dog was given 100 ml of such a suspension of very small gel particles. The suspension had an iodine content of about 5%. Good contrast filling was obtained in the stomach, intestine, and colon.

These interesting new types of contrast agents should be explored further for different applications.

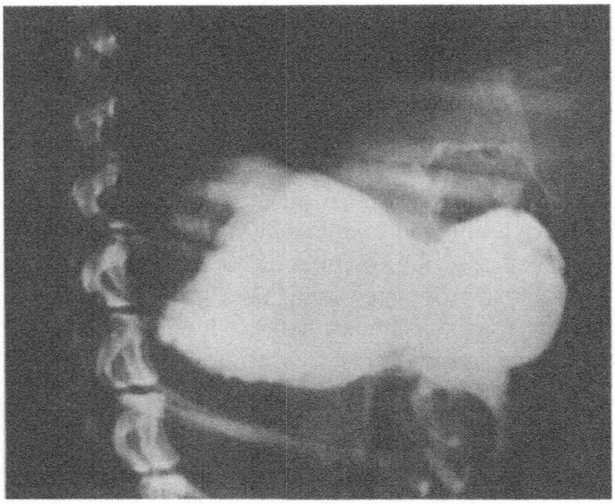

Fig. 2

**Figs. 2–4.** A dog weighing 15 kg was given 100 ml of a suspension of small, contrast-giving, soft, polymeric gel particles. Good contrast filling of the stomach, intestine, and colon was obtained. There were no adverse effects

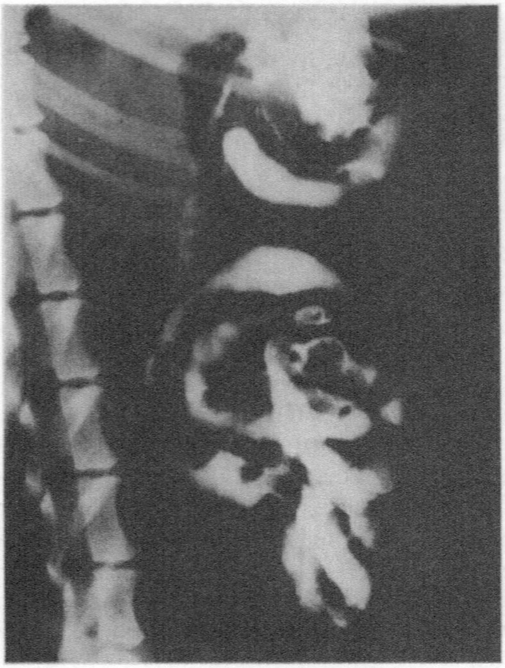

Fig. 3

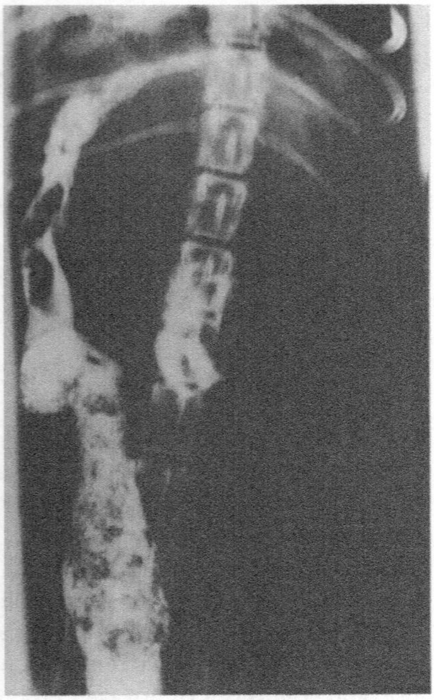

Fig. 4

## References


1. Björk L, Erikson U, Ingelman B (1969) Clinical experiences with a new type of contrast medium in peripheral arteriography. Amer J Roentgenol 106:418–424
2. Björk L, Erikson U, Ingelman B (1972) A new type of contrast medium in selective coronary arteriography. Ups J Med Sci 77:19–21
3. Björk L, Erikson U, Ingelman B, Zaar B (1974) Improved polymeric contrast agents for roentgenologic examination of the gastrointestinal tract. I. Preliminary report on the chemistry of the polymers. Ups J Med Sci 79:103–105
4. Björk L, Ekholm J, Erikson U, Ingelman B, Lindblad G (1975) Effects of carotid artery injections of some roentgen contrast agents on the EEG in the unanaesthetized dog. Ups J Med Sci 80:83–87
5. Björk L, Erikson U, Ingelman B (1976) Preliminary report on angiography with polymeric contrast agents in rabbits and dogs. Ups J Med Sci 81:183–187
6. Ekholm J, Erikson U, Skoglund S (1964) An improved method for experimental angiography. Brit J Radiol 37:839–842
7. Erikson U, Hemmingsson A (1981) Experiences with ioxaglate (Hexabrix) in cardioangiography and peripheral angiography. Acta Radiol Diagn. In press.

# Corporeal Distribution of Iodinated Lipid Emulsions in Terms of Particle Size

M. Laval-Jeantet and A.M. Laval-Jeantet

New contrast media with cellular fixation have been investigated since 1971 [3]. High doses are necessary in classical radiology. Low doses are sufficient with CT scanner, and with these doses the toxicity is low. These facts explain the renewed interest in the iodinated lipid emulsions [1, 7]. However, the emulsion is still experimental. The optimal size of the particles is a condition for the stability of the emulsion, but also an important factor of its biodistribution and metabolism.

The purpose of this work is to report the results of investigations of the tissue distribution of the particulate agent in the rat as a function of the size of particles, of the dose, and conditions of intravenous injection.

## Materials and Methods

We have described the contrast material AG 52315 and AG 6099 in previous publications [3, 4].

AG 52315 is a coarse emulsion (mean size 7 μm, SD4 μm), the AG 6099 a stable emulsion of iodized fatty acid esters of poppy seed oil containing 0.20 gI/ml. The particles have an average diameter of 1.3 microns (S.D 1 μm). The very fine emulsion was prepared immediately before use by mechanical dispersion of AG 52315 in glucose solution followed by filtration (mean diameter 0.7 μm).

The 5 groups of 4 animals were sacrificed at 15 min, 1, 3 and 24 h and 15 days post injection. Iodine content dosage and histologic examinations were performed. Complementary experiments with coarse and fine emulsions using radioactive iodine (131 I) were done in three groups of two rats studied by classical scintigraphy and quantitative measurements with scintillation counter.

## Results

At 15 min post-injection, we had detected the following amounts of the iodinated lipid in selected tissues of the rat, expressed in percentage of injected dose:
coarse emulsion: liver 50%, lung 44%, spleen 2.4%
fine emulsion: liver 66%, lung 16%, spleen 6%
ultra-fine emulsion: liver 6%, lung 0.5%, spleen 4.6%

At 24 h the dose in the liver remains high for the coarse emulsion (45%), and is only 22% for fine and 4% for ultra-fine.

At 15 days the clearance of fine and ultra-fine emulsions is almost complete. The coarse emulsion remains in the liver (23%) and in the lung (2%).

The best concentration in the liver is between 1 and 3 h post injection, with the fine emulsion. The decline of contrast concentration is slow with coarse emulsion, and faster with fine. Lung fixation for coarse emulsion is very similar to that observed for the liver: high concentration and slow decrease; in the case of fine emulsion a short peak is achieved at 1 h followed by a fast decrease.

These great differences appears on scintigrams: At 12 h post injection radionuclide uptake appears in both lungs and liver for coarse emulsion, and only in liver for fine (60 99), emulsion (Fig. 1).

*Histologic studies* show that the coarse emulsion accumulates within the lumina of the liver sinusoïds immediately after the injection. Thirty minutes later, fine droplets of sudanophilic material are phagocytized by the Kupffer cells. Fine and ultra-fine emulsions are not present in the vessels and sinusoïds at 15 minutes, but are rapidly taken up by both the hepatocytes and Kupffer's cells. Three hours after the injection the phagocytized lipidic amount decrease in the Kupffer's cells and more sudanophilic material appears in the hepatocytes (Fig. 2).

The lipidic exogenous substances decrease rapidly, and by the 15th day after injection of AG 60 99 the hepatocytes are free of sudanophilic lipids. Late examinations (3 months) of rats injected with radioactive emulsions show a normal structure of liver tissue and cells.

In the lungs a certain quantity of sudanophilic material is present with coarse emulsion in the macrophages of the alveolar septa. Pulmonary edema was observed only with

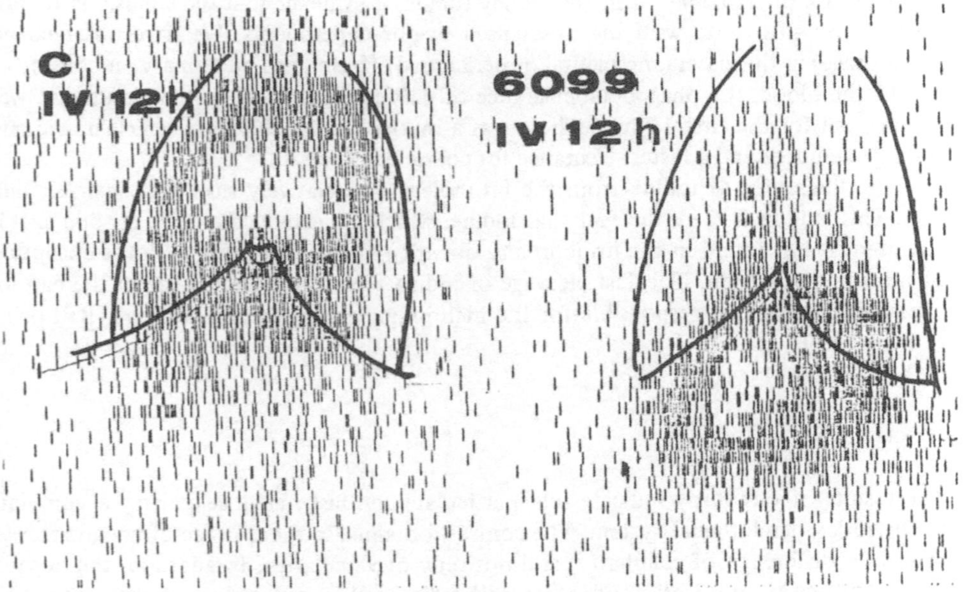


**Fig. 1.** Comparison between fixation at 12 h of radioactive (131 I) for coarse and fine emulsions. Note the high persistent pulmonary uptake of coarse emulsion

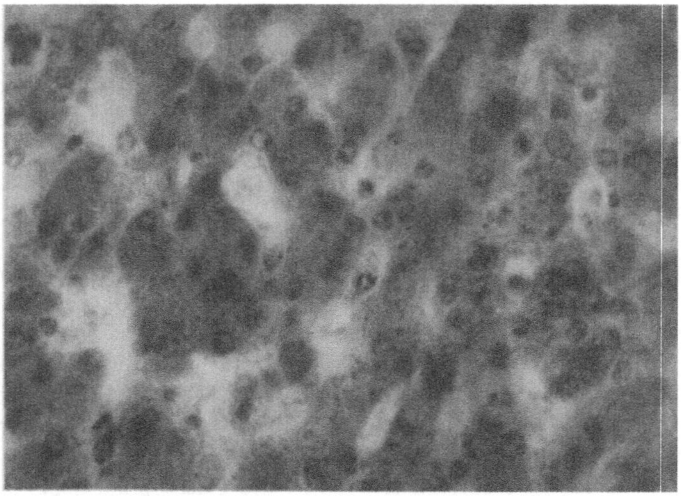

**Fig. 2.** Histologic examination of the liver 3 h after injection of fine emulsion. Sudanophilic material is present in Kupffer's cells and hepatocytes

intravenous injections of coarse emulsion. With fine and ultra-fine emulsions, the cells lining alveoli are practically devoid of such particles after 24th hour.

In the spleen, the sudanophilic material is concentrated in the marginal zone of the spleen red pulp (reticulo endothelial cells and reticular cells of the ellipsoïds).

The lack of stainable fat in the kidney tubules is evidence that the emulsions are not excreted by this route with the doses used in our experiments. We have observed no hemorrhages in the viscera, no pleural or pericardial effusion, no pulmonary embolism.

In the blood, the phagocytic clearance of particulate lipid from the circulation was exponential for the first 10 min. There was a inverse relationship between clearance rate and injected dose and a fastest clearance for coarse emulsion.

The liberation of iodine from the fat molecule is relatively slow with coarse emulsion. This is indicated by the fact that iodine, which appears in the urine as soon as it is liberated, is not found in the urine in any quantity in the first hour, with the exception of ultra-fine emulsion. The fast cleavage of iodine from the fat molecule in the case of ultra-fine emulsions is responsible for the high iodine concentration in blood (RBI rising to 4 mg/liter).

## Discussion

The results of our study indicate that particulate contrast media selectively accumulate in the reticuloendothelial system. The contrast obtained in the CT scan of hepatic masses reflects a difference of cellularity, and not only of vascularity. In addition, the hepatogram resulting from injection of iodinated lipidic emulsions is of long duration, with no density variations between the successive CT scans obtained from a liver. This retention eliminates the need to perform rapid examinations.

Ultra-fine emulsions, with size similar to liposomes [2] are phagocitized by reticulo-endothelial cells, with a preferential relative uptake in the spleen.

The important pulmonary fixation of some of the emulsions experimented could, therefore, limit their clinical application, and respiratory disturbances have been described after intravenous hepatography in man [4]; the knowledge of relative liver/lung fixation and histologic studies for different sizes of the particles are essential: our experiments show that very fine emulsion has the higher ratio between liver and lung fixation.

But, however, the absolute uptake of contrast media by the liver remains low with these very fine emulsions, blood concentration is high, and very fast degradation could rise serum iodine up to toxic levels.

From our data it is not possible to determine the rate of metabolism of the iodinated or deiodinated fat. Comparison of data on concentration of iodine in different tissues are interesting with respect to this question: fine emulsions are fixed in the reticuloendothelial system, but the coarse emulsions are fixed in lung capillaries and liver sinusoïds by embolization. In the latter case deiodination and resorption of fat deposits is slow. If the emulsion is fine the liver loses it much more rapidly, the reticuloendothelial cell having a well-known catabolism function [6].

The most effective and less dangerous opacification of the liver is obtained by intravenous injection of low doses (0.2 ml/kg) of a fine emulsion (1–2 μm). Coarse emulsions had an important lung fixation; very fine emulsions did not give a good hepatography and had too a fast disappearance.

## References


1. Alfidi RJ, Laval-Jeantet M (1976) AG 60 99: A promising contrast agent for computed tomography of the liver and spleen. Radiology 121:491
2. Havron A, Seltzer SE, Davis MA, Shulkin P (1981) Radiopaque liposomes: A promising contrast material for computed tomography of the spleen. Radiology 140:507–511
3. Laval-Jeantet M, Tristant H, Guerbet M et al. (1972) Une nouvelle méthode d'hépatographie lipiodolée par voie intra-artérielle. J Radiol Electrol 53:29–34
4. Laval-Jeantet M, Lamarque JL, Dreux P, Laval-Jeantet AM, Launay J (1976) Hepatosplenography by intravenous injection of a new iodized oily emulsion. Acta Radiol 17:19–60
5. Pellerin F (1970) Dosage de l'iode dans les composés organiques iodés. Ann Pharm Fr 28:685–696
6. Thompson SW (1974) The pathology of parenteral nutrition with lipids. C Thomas Springfield IL
7. Vermess M, Chatterji DC, Doppman JL, Grimes G, Adamson RH (1979) Development and experimental evaluation of a contrast medium for computed tomographic examination of the liver and spleen. J Comput Assist Tomogr 3:25–31

# Contrast Media for Long-term (Blood Pool) Opacification of the Vascular System

L. Björk

The ideas behind this paper go back to 1964 when Eriksson and Björk published the first proposal for a new type of contrast medium that would remain in the circulating blood for a considerable time and would allow imaging of the vascular system for extended periods of time, 30 min to several hours.

The advantages of such a contrast agent are several and obvious to everyone interested in radiology of the cardiovascular system. The approach that was tried followed two lines.

*One consisted* of adding *iodine to dextran molecules.* The dextran molecules were attractive because their pharmacology was well known and well studied and their elimination from the body was also well known and complete within a relatively short time. Also dextran could be used as very large molecules approaching the size of particles. Dextran has an extremely low toxicity.

At that time with the imaging system available, an iodine concentration of approximately 40 mg iodine per ml blood was necessary for identification of the heart chambers and the larger vessels. It turned out difficult or impossible to add enough iodine to dextran molecules to achieve this goal without using excessive volumes of dextran solution.

The *other approach* tried was *polymers of known conventional triiodated contrast agents.* Such polymers could be made into very large molecules. These molecules would eventually be phagocytized and would remain in the body for a long time. This could be overcome by introducing in certain parts of the polymer chain bonds that would be attacked by enzymes in the body, leading to breakdown of the chain and consequently relatively rapid and controlled elimination of the contrast agent. The problems with the production of such breakable bonds and the problems of control of the molecule size, etc. turned out to be considerable.

The projects were abandoned for two reasons. First the difficulty in achieving high iodine concentration and secondly because of the difficulty in guaranteeing and proving total complete elimination of the compound from the body within a short time.

In the last few years several things have changed. First of all we have imaging modalities such as CT and digital electronic angiography. These will reduce the need for iodine concentration in the blood for imaging of the vessels from a previous 40 mg iodine per ml to 1 or 5 mg per ml.

Secondly the demand from authorities and others for complete elimination of the diagnostic compound from the body within 24 h may have been modified and an elimination of the diagnostic compound over several days or even weeks might be acceptable.

The problems with these compounds can be listed as follows:

1. Synthesis
2. A narrow average molecular weight distribution
3. How to find suitable breakdown points in the molecules
4. Control of the elimination
5. Balance between time of opacification of the blood vessels and phagocytosis
6. A suitable molecular weight. If too small osmotic effect. If too high, rapid phagocytosis with granolomas and possibly fibrosis as results.
7. Cost effectiveness
8. Approval of authorities like FDA

These compounds certainly are well worth studying again in the light of the developments that now appear. They are quite promising and research along this line should be instituted again.

In the meantime I have tried some other methods for achieving the same goal, i.e., using *suspensions of small particles.* These are true particles with a size less than 1 μm. We have tried two types of such particle suspensions. One is emulsions of particles of perfluorocarbonhexylbromide. This is the same compound that has been used by Dr. Long in California. We have tried this compound mainly using CT imaging modality. When these emulsions are injected in the dog and the attenuation in the aorta is measured over time the following results are obtained.

After the initial peak an increased level of opacification remains relatively constant and falls off slowly during the 4 h the experiment continues.

The emulsions are somewhat difficult to prepare. They are relatively unstable even when kept frozen. This means that the emulsions have to be zonicated and controlled immediately before injection. If this is not done, there is a risk of clumping together of the particles, which will produce pulmonary embolism and other side effects. Also relatively large volumes have to be used because of the low attenuation of bromide, which can only be added in an amount a relatively few percent of the total weight of perfluorocarbon. Perfluorocarbon per se is, as you may know, completely harmless and can be used as a blood substitute. The obvious improvement would be to use perfluorocarbon with iodine added instead of bromide. Such compounds are known. However, they seem to be less stable than bromide compounds and in animal experiments they can, too, produce unpredictable side effects.

The main problem is, however, the slow elimination of these particles. They are phagocytized and although they seem to be eventually eliminated from the body this takes several months.

The other approach is to use *liposomes with contrast material included in the vesicles.* Liposomes are little vesicles composed of lipides. By special technology they can be made to any size and also by special technique different compounds can be included in them. These little vesicles are then carried through the blood stream and eventually phagocytized in different organs in the body. The technique has been used as a transport vehicle for drugs to different organs.

Such vesicles can be made with inclusion of contrast agents. We have tried the well-known contrast Renografin for inclusion in the vesicles. With this technique with vesicles of a size of 0.1 μm results similar to those with perfluorocarbon bromides were obtained. Again we have a high peak immediately after injection followed by a slow drop to a plateau which remains constant for at least 2 h. The problem is the low concentration of

Urografin in the vesicles. This requires that large volumes are injected. The elimination of the Renografin part is complete usually in 24–48 h. The elimination of the liposome capsule as such is not completely known but on theoretical grounds it should be complete and harmless, since it contains only naturally occurring compounds. With the liposomes the elimination problem seems to be under control. The problem of achieving a high enough iodine concentration in the blood without using excessive volumes remains. This problem will remain as long as water-soluble contrast agents are used for inclusion in the vesicles. If other contrast-giving compounds that are not water soluble could be included, a higher concentration of iodine in the vesicles could be achieved and maintained but, on the other hand, these non-water-soluble compounds would be phagocytized and the control of their elimination would probably be much more difficult.

# Summary of the Round Table

M. Sovak

This Round Table addressed two aspects of possible contrast media improvement: development of larger molecules and use of new emulsions of the iodinated oils.

Usefulness of the novel emulsions in hepatography has been by now, I think, firmly established. The work which we have just heard makes it evident that the toxicity and pharmacokinetics of these new preparations is not only a function of dose but also of the particle size. The conclusion, it seems, is that a balance must be found in a pharmaceutical preparation to reconcile two opposites: on one hand, use of small size particles which do not interfere with the circulation but increase the contact area between the hydrophobic surface of the oils and the body milieu; on the other hand, use of large size particles which may become trapped in the microcirculation but whose contact surface, for the dose injected, is smaller.

Development of molecules larger than the current monomeric water-soluble contrast media is motivated by the desire to decrease osmolality of CM solutions without reducing their iodine content. Hyperosmolality has been firmly established as an important toxicological factor responsible for pain in limb angiography, untoward hemodynamic effects, endothelial injury, and a number of sequelae related to the electrolytic disbalance. To decrease the osmolality two ways have been proposed: in current ionic CM to replace the sodium or meglumine cation with an iodine-containing cation or, to make nonionic or ionic oligomers and/or polymers.

The first opaque cations were synthesized in our laboratory in 1975, but these compounds had unacceptable neurotoxicity. The concept, however, was correct as witnessed by the development at Schering reported here today. It appears that although the radiopaque cation-based salts would probably be ill suited for neuroradiological application, due to their low cost they may well become the new media for improved urography and angiography. For these applications, therefore, I think that they are more promising than the nonionic oligomers. A number of nonionic oligomers based on triiodinated benzene moieties have been synthesized at Bracco, Nyegaard and at Schering AG. They have not been further developed, probably mainly because of slow renal excretion caused by the extremely low osmolality and possible tubular recirculation of these compounds.

Ionic oligomers are easily excretable, but compared to the new generation of nonionic monomers, they seem to be less well tolerated and less economical. The polymers, as we have just heard, have so far shown a disappointing record: when too large, the molecules tend to be water insoluble; when smaller and soluble, they prove rather toxic. Therefore, a useful blood-pool contrast medium does not yet exist.

In the development of nontoxic uro- and angiography contrast media of low osmolality, the most promising and feasible concepts seem to be the opaque cations, the nonionic monomers, monovalent dimers, and possibly nonionic dimers biotransformable to ionic species.

# Subject Index

Adverse reactions, general 3
–, prevention 1
–, survey 7, 14
Albumin, binding 251
Anaphylaxy 3, 16
Angiography, cerebral 269
–, intravenous 227
–, limbs 257, 274, 279
–, reactions 265, 276
Antibody-antigen 3, 16
Arthrography 241

Blood volume 233
Brain, toxicity on 113, 115, 141

Cardiac effects 58
Cardiac function see left ventricular function
Cells 44, 49, 52
Cholecystography 295, 299
Coagulation 3, 31
Complement 3, 20, 31
Coronary, artery or angiography 57, 76, 79, 94, 98, 108
–, flow 91
CT, contrast media and 305, 311

Dimeric contrast agent 335, 340

EEG, studies by 123, 134, 141
Embolisation 237
Endothelium of vessels 223
Enzymes and Isoenzymes 3, 28

Futurology 329, 344, 348

Heart 57
–, electrolythe shifts 80
–, electrophysiological effects 60, 80
–, hemodynamic effects 63
–, infants and pediatric 101, 104
Hemodynamic effects 285, 288
Hepatobiliary see liver 292
Histamine 3

Idiosyncrary 3
Intrathecal space 123, 129, 134–159
Ischemic state of heart 57, 64, 84

Kidney 189

Left ventricular function 57, 64, 70, 94, 108
Limbs, angiography of 257, 279
Lipidic, contrast media 344
Liver 292–320

Myelography 123, 129, 134, 170, 175, 179, 182
Myocardial effects 57, 59, 68, 70

NMR 329
Nephrotoxicity 195, 211, 215
Nervous system, effects on 113
Neurotoxicity 113
–, animal studies 123, 129, 134, 141, 148, 154, 159, 164
–, human studies 170, 174, 175, 179, 269

Pharmacokinetics, of contrast media 314, 324
Phlebography, side effects 231
Platelets 40
Polymeric, contrast agent 340, 348

Side effects see adverse reactions
Subarachnoid spaces 123, 129, 134, 148, 170

Thyroid, side effects 245, 251
Toxicity, cardiac 57
–, general 1
–, nephrologic 189
–, neurologic 113
–, systemic 3
–, vessels 257

Urinary concentration, radio-contrast drugs of 201, 207

Vessels, side effects 223, 257

GPSR Compliance

*The European Union's (EU) General Product Safety Regulation (GPSR) is a set of rules that requires consumer products to be safe and our obligations to ensure this.*

*If you have any concerns about our products, you can contact us on ProductSafety@springernature.com*

In case Publisher is established outside the EU, the EU authorized representative is:

Springer Nature Customer Service Center GmbH
Europaplatz 3
69115 Heidelberg, Germany

**Batch number: 10723355**

Printed by Printforce, the Netherlands